Hallucinations

Hallucinations
A guide to treatment and management

Edited by

Frank Larøi

André Aleman

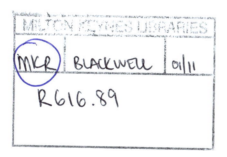
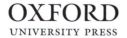

OXFORD
UNIVERSITY PRESS

OXFORD
UNIVERSITY PRESS

Great Clarendon Street, Oxford ox2 6DP

Oxford University Press is a department of the University of Oxford.
It furthers the University's objective of excellence in research, scholarship,
and education by publishing worldwide in

Oxford New York

Auckland Cape Town Dar es Salaam Hong Kong Karachi
Kuala Lumpur Madrid Melbourne Mexico City Nairobi
New Delhi Shanghai Taipei Toronto

With offices in

Argentina Austria Brazil Chile Czech Republic France Greece
Guatemala Hungary Italy Japan Poland Portugal Singapore
South Korea Switzerland Thailand Turkey Ukraine Vietnam

Oxford is a registered trade mark of Oxford University Press
in the UK and in certain other countries

Published in the United States
by Oxford University Press Inc., New York

British Library Cataloguing in Publication Data
Data available

Library of Congress Cataloging-in-Publication Data
Data available

Typeset in Minion by Glyph International, Bangalore, India
Printed in Great Britain
on acid-free paper by
CPI Antony Rowe Chippenham, Wiltshire

ISBN 978–0–19–954859–0

10 9 8 7 6 5 4 3 2 1

Contents

Contributors

Eduardo J Aguilar
Psychiatric Unit
Clinic Hospital
Valencia
Cibersam
Spain

André Aleman
BCN Research School and University
Medical Center
Groningen
The Netherlands

Francesc Artigas
Department of Neurochemistry
and Neuropharmacology
Institut d'Investigacions Biomediques
de Barcelona
Barcelona
Spain

Vaughan Bell
Institute of Psychiatry
London
United Kingdom

Paul Bebbington
Research Department of
Mental Health Sciences
University College London
London
United Kingdom

Max Birchwood
Department of Psychology University of
Birmingham
YouthSpace Youth Mental Health
Programme
Birmingham
United Kingdom

Daniel Collerton
Northumberland, Tyne &
Wear NHS Trust
Clinical Psychology Department
University of Newcastle upon Tyne
Gateshead
United Kingdom

Frank Eperjesi
Optometry
School of Life and Health Sciences
Aston University
Birmingham
United Kingdom

Sandra Escher
Drees 11B
Gravenvoeren
Belgium

John Farhall
School of Psychological Science
La Trobe University
Melbourne
Australia

Gilles Fénelon
Service de Neurologie
Hôpital Henri Mondor
Créteil
France

David Fowler
School of Medicine, Health Policy
and Practice
The University of East Anglia
Norwich
United Kingdom

Daniel Freeman
Department of Psychology
Institute of Psychiatry
King's College London
London
United Kingdom

Philippa Garety
Department of Psychology
Institute of Psychiatry
King's College London
London
United Kingdom

Michael Garrett
Department of Clinical Psychiatry
State University of New York Downstate
Medical Center
New York, NY
United States

Jean-Louis Goëb
Service de Psychiatrie de l'Enfant et de
l'Adolescent
Centre Hospitalier Universitaire
Lille
France

Ralph Hoffman
Department of Psychiatry
Yale School of Medicine
New Haven, CT
United States

Renaud Jardri
Service de Psychiatrie de l'Enfant et de
l'Adolescent, Center Hospitalier
Universitaire
Lille
France

Jack A. Jenner
University Medical Center Groningen
Section F, Groningen the Netherlands &
Jenner Consultants
Haren
The Netherlands

Louise Johns
PICuP Clinic
South London and Maudsley NHS
Foundation Trust
Denmark Hill
London
United Kingdom

Kees Korrelboom
Parnassia Bavo Psychiatric Institute
The Hague
The Netherlands

Elizabeth Kuipers
Psychology Department
King's College London
Institute of Psychiatry
London
United Kingdom

Frank Larøi
Cognitive Psychopathology Unit
Department of Cognitive Sciences
University of Liège
Liège
Belgium; Intercommunale de Soins
Spécialisés de Liège
Mental Health Sector
Liège
Belgium

Eleanor Longden
Bradford Early Intervention Service
Bradford & Airedale Teaching Primary
Care Trust
Bradford
United Kingdom

Rufus May
Bradford Assertive Outreach Team,
Bradford District Care Trust
West Yorkshire
United Kingdom

Alan Meaden
Birmingham and Solihull Mental
Health Trust
Birmingham
United Kingdom

Eric Morris
Lambeth Early Onset Services
South London & Maudsley Trust
London
United Kingdom

Urs Peter Mosimann
Department of Psychiatry
University of Bern
Bern
Switzerland

Brendan O'Sullivan
C/o Dr.Ben Smith
Research Department of Mental Health
Sciences
University College London
London
United Kingdom

Juliana Onwumere
King's College London
Institute of Psychiatry
London
United Kingdom

Andrea Raballo
Danish National Research Foundation:
Centre for Subjectivity Research
University of Copenhagen
Denmark

Marius Romme
Psychiatric Unit
Faculty of Medicine
Valencia University
Cibersam
Spain

Julio Sanjuan
Unidad Psiquiatría
Facultad de Medicina
Avda
Spain

Ben Smith
Research Department of Mental Health
Sciences
University College London
London
United Kingdom

Peter Trower
School of Psychology
University of Birmingham
Birmingham
United Kingdom

Lucia R. Valmaggia
Department of Psychological Medicine
Institute of Psychiatry
London
United Kingdom

Mark van der Gaag
Van der Boechorststraat 1
Free University
Amsterdam
The Netherlands

Philip Watson
Division of Community Health Sciences
University of Edinburgh
Edinburgh
United Kingdom

Til Wykes
Institute of Psychiatry
King's College London
London
United Kingdom

Chapter 1

Introduction

Frank Larøi and André Aleman

Hallucinations are complex experiences that can be highly distressing and burdening for a number of individuals. Research has come a long way the past few decades in attempting to better understand these multifaceted experiences. Admittedly, this is only the beginning and much still remains poorly understood. Nevertheless, thanks to this resurgence of research, a number of intervention strategies for hallucinations do exist and novel approaches are being developed. We hope that this book provides evidence of this and furthermore that the various contributions will render these strategies as accessible as possible to readers.

The purpose of this book is to bring together the current knowledge of the various intervention strategies for hallucinations and to provide practical and extensive presentations of these strategies. This book will interest a wide range of professionals (clinical psychologists, psychotherapists, counsellors, psychiatrists, neurologists, child psychiatrists, old-age psychiatrists, nurses, and social workers) who work with persons presenting hallucinations, whether in a clinical or a research context. In this context, we hope that this book will not only extend the 'toolkits' of clinicians, but also provide a better understanding of the experiences themselves. In addition, we hope that certain contributions will also provide interesting and noteworthy reading for those who experience hallucinations and also for those who are in contact with these individuals, such as family and friends, on a more personal level.

Leading experts in the area of the treatment of hallucinations contribute with their expertise in their specific area. Although essentially a practical guide, chapters also contain overviews (empirical and/or theoretical) of the pertinent areas of research. Each contribution contains concrete methods of evaluation and specific techniques of the treatment strategy itself, oftentimes with clinical vignettes and/or case studies so that the intervention strategy is illustrated as clearly as possible. Finally, chapters end with discussions concerning various issues such as future directions, possible limitations of the intervention strategy presented in the chapter, or any overlaps with other treatment strategies. Where applicable, treatments are evidence-based, and any claims regarding efficacy are backed up with references to empirical evidence. However, since some strategies presented in the book are also relatively novel and recent in the literature, and therefore no studies have tested its efficacy, these are also mentioned, although with a cautionary note regarding the need of empirical support.

It is beyond the scope of this book to give exhaustive and detailed overviews of the research that has been carried out in the past decades on hallucinations. For the reader who wishes more detail concerning general, historical, or philosophical accounts of hallucinations, a number of excellent books are available such as Leudar and Thomas (2000), Watkins (1998), Fish (2009), Smith (2007), and Blom (2010). For the reader interested in overviews of recent empirical findings, they may consult Aleman and Larøi (2008) and Spence and David (2004). It is important to emphasize that many of the intervention strategies are based on models of hallucinations. We believe this to be an essential constituent: research increases knowledge, which produces theoretical paradigms and which ultimately provides inventive and helpful treatment strategies. The ultimate goal is thus unmistakable—to provide ways of improving the lives of the many people who are distraught and burdened by these experiences.

A wide variety of issues, strategies, populations, and types of hallucinations are addressed in this book. Strategies vary from those on the individual to those on the group level. Some are well-known and established strategies, whilst others represent more recent arrivals in the literature. Certain chapters deal with hallucinations in general; others focus on specific types or modalities of hallucinations. Contributions also touch upon how we view these experiences, at the level of individual patients, but also on a wider, societal level. Target populations involve the full developmental range from children, adolescents, adults, and elderly persons. There is a myriad of types of intervention strategies—extending from primarily biological to primarily psychological.

In their chapter entitled 'Pharmacological treatment of hallucinations', Sanjuan and colleagues begin with a summary of the neurochemical basis of hallucinations (drugs that induce hallucinatory experiences, drugs that eliminate or reduce hallucinations, and the neurochemistry of hallucinations). They then provide practical guidelines for the pharmacological treatment of hallucinations (including a section on special populations such as children and adolescents, organic hallucinations, and non-psychotic subjects), in addition to a section on psychological treatments in combination with anti-psychotics. This is followed by a detailed presentation of two case examples, and the chapter ends with suggestions for future directions in the field.

Aleman and Hoffman provide a chapter concerning the use of Transcranial Magnetic Stimulation in the context of auditory hallucinations. A summary of the technique is provided, followed by a review of the efficacy of Transcranial Magnetic Stimulation for hallucinations. This is followed by a section regarding various issues concerning Transcranial Magnetic Stimulation in the context of auditory hallucinations, including location of stimulation, number of stimuli and sessions, cognitive changes after TMS treatment, side effects and safety, measurement of hallucinations in Transcranial Magnetic Stimulation studies, and blinding.

Concerning Cognitive-Behavioural Therapy, separate chapters are consecrated for individual and group Cognitive-Behavioural Therapy, respectively. Smith *et al.*, consider individual Cognitive-Behavioural Therapy for auditory–verbal hallucinations. In this chapter, the theoretical and empirical literature is reviewed, and the treatment strategies used are outlined. This is followed by a clinical case of individual Cognitive-Behavioural Therapy for Auditory–Verbal Hallucinations. Interestingly, they describe the change processes from the perspective of both client and therapist. In particular, the authors consider the role of illness perceptions in the maintenance and psychological treatment of hallucinations. Finally, they provide reflections on future directions and limitations of the Cognitive-Behavioural Therapy strategies described in the chapter.

Group Cognitive-Behavioural Therapy is addressed in Johns and Wykes' chapter. The chapter begins with an extensive and up-to-date review of the evidence of the beneficial effects of group Cognitive-Behavioural Therapy for psychotic patients with auditory hallucinations, followed by detailed descriptions of the group Cognitive-Behavioural Therapy manuals developed for treatment trials, in addition to the various adaptations that have been made to these manuals. Finally, the authors consider various issues such as the advantages and disadvantages of group Cognitive-Behavioural Therapy, discussing factors that influence outcome and pointing to feasibility of group Cognitive-Behavioural Therapy.

In their chapter entitled 'Appraisals: Voices' power and purpose', Trower and colleagues argue that interventions should target the client's reactions (e.g., the distress and associated behaviour) to auditory hallucinations. Furthermore, these reactions will vary to a large degree between individuals, which are largely a consequence of each individual's appraisal of their voice. Beliefs can be identified, which specifically give rise to these reactions. The origins and development of the cognitive model of voices that this approach is based on is described. Then, the authors show how a formulation based on the cognitive model can be used as a guide to the assessment of these beliefs and their intervention, and their role in perpetuating the problem when they give rise to safety behaviours. These various steps are illustrated with the help of a clinical case.

A particular type of auditory–verbal hallucination, command hallucinations, is addressed in the chapter by Meaden *et al.* The key feature that distinguishes command hallucinations from 'ordinary' auditory–verbal hallucinations is that the voice is experienced or interpreted as commanding, rather than commenting. Such hallucinations can be even more distressing and disruptive than commenting 'voices'. The authors base their intervention on the cognitive model described in the chapter by Trower and colleagues, albeit adapted for cognitive therapy for command hallucinations. Like all cognitive therapies for psychosis, cognitive processes are conceptualized as central to understanding psychotic experiences and thus working with them are crucial in the therapeutic process. The intervention described in the chapter also clarifies the psychological processes that underlie many of the risk behaviours tenuously linked to command hallucinations and offers a set of therapeutic principles for reducing such risk. Throughout the chapter, several key case examples are detailed, in addition to other brief vignettes, to further illustrate key points. Finally, evidence for this form of cognitive therapy for command hallucinations is presented, which is then terminated by a section on the limitations and future directions in cognitive therapy for command hallucinations.

Valmaggia and Morris provide examples of the utility of two types of interventions in the context of distressing auditory hallucinations: Attention Training Technique and

Acceptance and Commitment Therapy. Briefly, attention training technique aims to alleviate psychological problems through both cognitive and metacognitive modification, and Acceptance and Commitment Therapy may be described as a form of behaviour therapy that incorporates mindfulness and acceptance processes in order to help clients with unwanted private experiences. Evidence for the efficacy of both techniques is provided, and each technique is illustrated with detailed accounts of a case example for each type of intervention: 'Peter' for attentional training technique and 'Amanda' for Acceptance and Commitment Therapy.

Competitive Memory Training is a relatively novel intervention form that is based on the idea that, since psychopathology often involves dysfunctional meanings that are triggered too often in the wrong circumstances, therapy should influence the retrieval competition such that the chances of functional meanings to be retrieved are increased. This is achieved via a number of different techniques, all of which attempt to make the positive and incompatible meanings emotionally more salient. In their chapter, van der Gaag and Korrelboom describe the competitive memory training protocol for auditory hallucinations in detail, in addition to illustrations of the protocol via numerous case examples. A section devoted to presenting the evidence for the effectiveness of competitive memory training is also included.

Hallucinations-focused Integrative Therapy, a multi-faceted form of psycho-social intervention specifically tailored for auditory hallucinations, is described in Jenner's chapter. The main goals of Hallucinations-focused Integrative Therapy include optimizing compliance, reducing the burden of the disorder and related symptoms, and improving control, quality of life, and social functioning. In this chapter, the format (e.g., therapeutic alliance, the diagnostic protocol), content (including descriptions of the various hallucinations-focused integrative therapy treatment modules), and long-term effects and cost effectiveness of Hallucinations-focused Integrative Therapy are described. Finally, a description of indications and contraindications for hallucinations-focused integrative therapy concludes the chapter.

'Normalizing' within the continuum model emphasizes the similarities between psychotic symptoms, such as hallucinations, and everyday experience. In his chapter on how this has implications for intervention strategies, Garrett shows how an appreciation of the continuum between psychosis and ordinary mental life becomes a practical clinical tool in the form of 'normalizing' interventions in the psychotherapy of psychosis. He provides specific examples of 'experiential exercises' that can be used to normalize psychosis. Furthermore, the uses of these techniques are illustrated with the help of various case examples.

A great majority of individuals who experience hallucinations try to do something about reducing the negative impact these have on their lives, that is, they use one or several coping strategies. Farhall begins his chapter with a literature review on the efficacy of various coping strategies and provides a discussion of the implications these findings have for clinical practice. Then, the author turns to programmes and therapies that have utilized a coping approach and considers the approaches taken and their effectiveness.

A coping model (stress-appraisal-coping model of voices) specifically developed for the experience of hearing voices is then presented. This is followed by a comprehensive and highly illustrative (with numerous case illustrations) section on assessment and treatment for coping enhancement. Finally, a section addressing various issues (limits of the coping strategies literature, the aim of the treatment of voices, effectiveness of strategies, and styles of adaptation) and an account of ideas for future directions bring the chapter to an end.

Romme and Escher's approach is based on the observation that many mental problems, including hearing voices, are reactive patterns to socio-emotional problems in daily life and/or problems in the person's past and upbringing. In that voices are considered meaningful personal phenomena, their approach consists of making sense of the voices, which involves exploring the relationship between the voices and a person's life experiences. In their chapter 'Personal history and hearing voices', Romme and Escher discuss the theoretical background behind their approach, they describe how they gather information about the experience itself, how this information is used in a psychological formulation of the person's problems, what voice hearers themselves reveal about their recovery, and how all this information can be used in a therapy plan. The specific steps involved in the interview and therapeutic process are described in detail throughout the chapter, with numerous cases examples to help illustrate.

Self-help in the context of hearing voices refers to approaches to healing and recovery on either a group or individual level. It is based on the idea of learning to respect and support the experience of hearing voices rather than on the traditional medical approach of attempting to 'cure' it. Self-help in the context of hearing voices is based on the groundbreaking work of Marius Romme and Sandra Escher in the 1980s, which later on provided the basis for the hearing voices movement, which now represents a world-wide movement (represented across Europe, Australia, Japan, and elsewhere) in the form of research, forums, conferences, publications, and self-help groups. In their chapter 'Self-help approaches to hearing voices', May and Longden trace the roots of this movement up to the present day. They then depict the nature and goals of these self-help groups, in addition to providing a list of helpful self-help organizations. Several examples of individuals who have participated in self-help groups, and the benefits for these individuals, are also provided.

Hallucinations are not only present in adult populations, but both epidemiological and clinical studies clearly show that a substantial number of children and adolescents may also experience hallucinations. Goëb and Jardri provide the reader with a review of the epidemiological studies concerning hallucinatory experiences during childhood. A detailed account of issues associated with the assessment of hallucinations in this population is provided, followed by an account of the psychiatric causes of hallucinations in children and adolescents. Finally, treatment strategies are presented, which include psychotherapeutic interventions and psychoeducative programmes in addition to an examination of the role of other intervention strategies (anti-psychotics, transcranial magnetic stimulation) in non-adult populations. A detailed clinical observation (and follow-up) of a child experiencing hallucinations is also provided in the chapter.

Charles Bonnet syndrome refers to a condition where visual hallucinations result from visual impairment due to ocular disease. This syndrome remains a largely under-recognized and unfamiliar condition to both health care practitioners and the general public. Eperjesi provides a review of the diagnostic criteria, prevalence, clinical characteristics, pathogenesis, and management of visual hallucinations in Charles Bonnet syndrome. Treatment is addressed in detail, which includes treatment of the underlying cause of visual impairment, and psycho-social-based and pharmacologically based interventions. Finally, a section on future therapies is included.

Hallucinations in the context of dementing illnesses are depicted by Mosimann and Collerton. In this comprehensive chapter, the authors review the current epidemiological, clinical, and biological evidence on the relationships between hallucinations and dementing illnesses. They then compare dementia specific models for their genesis with models derived in other disorders. Lastly, the authors evaluate assessment, treatment, and support options and look to unresolved issues and the potential for further developments. Clinical vignettes are presented throughout the chapter, providing concrete and illustrative examples of the various issues developed in the chapter.

The second most common neurodegenerative disease, Parkinson's disease, where hallucinations are also common, is dealt with in the chapter by Fénelon. Although previously considered as coincidental, end-stage non-specific phenomena or a mere side effect of anti-parkinsonian (dopaminergic) treatment—hallucinations in this condition—are now considered as the product of complex interactions between treatment- and disease-related factors. The author provides an overview of hallucinations in Parkinson's disease (including definitional issues and diagnostic criteria, phenomenology, prevalence, clinical course, and prognosis), followed by a presentation of associated (pharmacological, disease-related, and genetic) factors. A review of the pathophysiology of hallucinations in Parkinson's disease is also provided. This is followed by a large section on assessment issues (evaluating the impact of hallucinations, contributory factors, an account of useful coping strategies, and the importance of providing reassurance to caregivers), followed by a presentation of first-line (pharmacological and non-pharmacological) and second-line (anti-psychotics) treatment options. Other therapeutic considerations are also provided (primary prevention, electroconvulsive therapy, and deep brain stimulation), and the chapter concludes with a section on therapeutic perspectives. A detailed clinical vignette 'Seeing fish on the bed' is also included in the chapter.

Finally, Bell, Raballo, and Larøi (Assessment of hallucinations) provide information concerning important issues to take into account when assessing hallucinations. They emphasize that it is not only important to assess the hallucinations themselves in detail (including perceptual, cognitive, and emotional aspects), but that other facets should also be evaluated, such as the contexts in which they appear, the consequences for the person and their entourage, and the assessment of medical and psychiatric problems and adverse life events. Assessment of hallucinations furthermore represents a crucial element in the therapeutic process: it is an important step towards tailored treatment, provides an understanding of the maintaining factors and the strengthening of basic coping strategies, and continued assessment will help guide treatment over time. The essential elements that constitute an assessment instrument (e.g., possessing adequate psychometric properties, allowing a comprehensive and detailed evaluation) are outlined by the authors, and specific hallucination assessment instruments are detailed in this respect. In particular, various issues related to the assessment of auditory–verbal hallucinations are presented in detail (e.g., the emergence of auditory–verbal hallucinations, perceptual properties, emotional and social aspects, and appraisals of hallucinations), as are hallucinations in other modalities, such as visual and somatic hallucinations.

We would like to take this opportunity to thank our colleagues for having accepted our invitation to contribute to this book and for their highly captivating, innovative, scholarly, and accessible chapters. Your contributions will no doubt help provide ways of improving the lives of the many people who are troubled and burdened by these experiences.

References

Aleman, A., & Larøi, F. (2008). *Hallucinations: The science of idiosyncratic perception.* Washington D.C.: American Psychological Association.

Blom, J.D. (2010). *A dictionary of hallucinations.* New York: Springer.

Fish, W. (2009). *Perception, Hallucination, and Illusion.* Oxford: Oxford University Press.

Leudar, I., & Thomas, P. (2000). *Voices of reason, voices of insanity: Studies of verbal hallucinations.* London: Routledge.

Smith, D.B. (2007). *Muses, madmen, and prophets: Rethinking the history, science, and meaning of auditory hallucination.* New York: Penguin Press.

Spence, S.A., & David, A.S. (2004). *Voices in the Brain: The cognitive neuropsychiatry of auditory verbal hallucinations.* Hove: Psychology Press.

Watkins, J. (1998). *Hearing voices: A common human experience.* Melbourne: Hill of Content.

Chapter 2

Pharmacological treatment of hallucinations

Julio Sanjuan, Eduardo J. Aguilar, and Francesc Artigas

A significant number of studies exist that consider the pharmacological treatment of schizophrenia as a global disorder. However, to date, very few researchers have considered the use of drugs specifically to treat hallucinations. On the other hand, with the exception of Transcranial Magnetic Stimulation (TMS; see Aleman & Hoffman, this volume), most clinical trials that involve patients with persistent hallucinations are psychologically oriented and are not based on biology. There are two main reasons for this lack of interest in the pharmacology of hallucinations:

1. Psychiatrists use a categorical diagnostic system instead of a symptom-oriented approach (for more information concerning the symptom-oriented approach, see Aleman & Larøi, 2008). Most research uses instruments such as the Positive and Negative Syndrome Scale (PANSS; Kay *et al.*, 1987) and consequently reports on positive symptoms as a cluster, and not separately on hallucinations.

2. Recent research into new anti-psychotics has focused more on cognitive symptoms and relatively less on psychotic symptoms such as hallucinations (Snyder & Murphy, 2008).

In this chapter, we will first summarize the neurochemical basis of hallucinations. Second, we will provide practical guidelines for the pharmacological treatment of hallucinations. Finally, we will suggest future directions in this field.

The neurochemical basis of hallucinations

To understand the pharmacological treatment of hallucinations, first, it is important to summarize the neurochemistry of the hallucinatory experience. The neurochemistry of hallucinations is based on three kinds of data: (a) drugs that can induce hallucinatory experiences, (b) drugs that eliminate or reduce the hallucinations, and (c) neuroimaging studies.

Drugs that can induce hallucinatory experiences

The use of some natural substances to voluntarily provoke perceptual abnormalities has been commonplace across many cultures. The best known of these are angel's trumpet

(*Brugmansia*), henbaene (*Hyoscyamus niger*), magic mushrooms (*Psilocybine*), ayahuasca (*Beniteropsis caapi*), marijuana (*Cannabis*), peyote (*Lephora Willamsi*), fly agaric (*amanita muscaria*), and others (Cunningham, 2008). Nevertheless, the discovery of highly potent synthetic hallucinogenic drugs, in particular the hallucinogenic capacity of lysergic acid diethylamide (LSD) by Albert Hofmann in 1943, was probably the most relevant historical issue in neurochemical studies concerning hallucinations (Dyck, 2005). Nowadays, there are many synthetic hallucinogenic drugs. The hallucinogenic potency and the subjective effect of these synthetic drugs vary considerably. Taking LSD as a prototype, the effects vary among individuals, but the drug usually produces perceptual abnormalities, mainly involving the visual modality. Paradoxically, 'hallucinogenic' drugs rarely induce 'true psychopathological hallucinations.' As a pharmacological group, hallucinogens include a wide range of drugs with many different mechanism of action. These span from cannabinoid agonists (*Cannabis*) to *N*-methyl-D-aspartate (NMDA) antagonists (*Phencyclidine*), muscarinic receptor antagonists (*Scopolamine*), opioid agonists (*Salvinorin*), monoamine release agents (*Methilanphetamine*), and others. Although these drugs act via different neurotransmitter systems, particular attention has been paid to drugs that display agonistic effects at 5-HT$_{2A}$ receptors, and this has been suggested as a common target to induce perceptual abnormalities (Nichols, 2004; Fantegrossi *et al.*, 2008). Different synthetic compounds such as LSD or 1-2,5-dimethoxy-4-iodophenyl-2-aminopropane (DOI) and chemically related compounds as well as natural compounds such as dimethyltryptamine (DMT) or 5-methoxydimethyltryptamine (5-MeO-DMT) that contain the indoleamine ring (present in the serotonin molecule) display potent hallucinogenic properties by activating 5-HT$_{2A}$ receptors. Some of these products (DMT, 5-MeO-DMT) confer the hallucinogenic properties of some ethnic beverages, such as ayahuasca, a potent psychotropic drug that has been used for centuries for magico-religious purpose in the Amazon and Orinoco river basins (Dobkin de Rios, 1972; Riba & Barbanoj, 2005). The reasons why these exogenous 5-HT$_{2A}$ agonists (but not serotonin itself, the physiological 5-HT$_{2A}$ agonist) display hallucinogenic properties are unclear. Different explanations have been suggested, including differences in the ability to modify neuronal properties (Aghajnaian & Marek, 1999), the activation of different intracellular transduction mechanisms (González-Maeso *et al.*, 2007), or the modification of cerebral network properties (Celada *et al.*, 2008). The administration of exogenous 5-HT$_{2A}$ agonists, such as DOI, evokes a marked increase in the activity or projection neurons in the frontal lobe (Puig *et al.*, 2003), decreasing at the same time the cortical synchrony at low frequencies (Celada *et al.*, 2008). These effects can possibly mediate the perceptual abnormalities induced by agents acting at 5-HT$_{2A}$ receptors and are strikingly similar to those produced by the non-competitive NMDA receptor antagonist phencyclidine (Kargieman *et al.*, 2007), which also displays psychotomimetic properties. Thus, a disruption of the activity of certain areas of the prefrontal cortex may underlie hallucinogenic properties. Given the role of the prefrontal cortex to integrate and process external (e.g., sensory) and internal (e.g., propioceptive, memories, etc.) stimuli, the hallucinogen-induced alteration of frontocortical processing may result in an abnormal perception (i.e., hallucination) despite the signals reaching primary sensory areas remain unaltered (Celada *et al.*, 2008).

However, it is worth noting that, apart from the so-called 'hallucinogenic' drugs, many other drugs that affect the brain can induce perceptual abnormalities and hallucinations in vulnerable individuals. Table 2.1 lists the most common drugs that have been associated with hallucinations. Although Hofmann's discovery provoked an enormous research interest, this curiosity disappeared in subsequent years, probably because the study of these drugs was associated with esoteric and mystical ideas and poor research methodologies. Nevertheless, recently we have observed a resurgence of interest in hallucinogenic research (Nichols, 2004; Fantegrossi *et al.*, 2008).

Table 2.1 Drugs associated with hallucinations

Group	Drug
Hallucinogens	LSD
	Dimethyltryptamine
	Psilocibina
	Psilocin
	Harmine
	Mescaline
	Tetrahydrocannabinol
	Phencyclidine
	Ketamine
	Nitrous oxide
	DOI
Antidepressants	Imipramine
	Maproptiline
Anti-parkinsonian	Anti-cholinergic
	Amantadine
	Levodopa
	Bromocriptine
Hormonal agents	Steroids
	Thyroxin
Antibiotics	Sulfonamides
	Penicilin
	Tetracycline

(Continued)

Table 2.1 (continued) Drugs associated with hallucinations

Group	Drug
Drugs associated with withdrawal syndromes	Alcohol
	Barbiturates
	Benzodiazepines
	Chloral hydrale
	Paraldehyde
	Meprobamate
	Methaqualone
	Opiates
	Cocaine
Miscellaneous	Bromide
	Digoxine
	Sympathomines
	Cimetidine
	Propanolol
	Phenacetin
	Disulfiram
	Narcotics
	Anti-malarials
	Heavy metals
	Metrizamide

Drugs that can eliminate or reduce hallucinations

The introduction, by serendipity, of chlorpromazine in the 1950s was the beginning of the 'psycho-pharmacological revolution' in psychiatry, together with the discovery of new kinds of drugs, first called neuroleptics and now known as anti-psychotics. Since the discovery of chlorpromazine, dozens of drugs with anti-psychotic properties have been developed. In clinical terms, 'anti-psychotics' are substances that are potentially anti-delusional or anti-hallucinatory. Apart from anti-psychotics, other drugs with anti-hallucinatory properties have been reported (see Table 2.2). The main questions are

◆ Is there a common mechanism of action for all these anti-hallucinogenic drugs?

◆ How, in clinical and psychological terms, can a drug reduce hallucinations?

◆ Why do some patients suffer from persistent hallucinations in spite of anti-psychotic treatment?

Soon after the discovery of anti-psychotics, it was proposed that these pharmaceutical agents acted to block the dopamine system. Later on, this proposal was apparently

Table 2.2 Drugs used in the treatment of hallucinations

Group	Drug	Recommended dosage range (mg/day)
First-generation anti-psychotics	Chlorpromazine	300–1000
	Haloperidol	5–20
	Thioridazine	300–800
	Perphenezine	16–64
	Trifuoperazine	10–50
	Thiothixene	15–50
	Fluphenazine	5–20
	Pimozide	2–8
	Molindone	30–100
Second-generation anti-psychotics	Clozapine	150–600
	Risperidone	2–9
	Olanzapine	7,5–30
	Quetiapine	300–750
	Ziprasidone	40–200
	Aripiprazole	15–30
	Paliperidone	3–15
	Zotepine	75–300
	Asenapine	5–10
	Lloperidone	14–24
	Sertindole	12–24
Antidepressant	Velafaxine	75–300
Cholinesterase inhibitors	Fluoxetine	20
	Donepezil	5–10
	Rivastigmine	1,5–6
Anticonvulsant	Carbamazepine	600–1200
	Lamotrigine	50–200
	Valproate	400–1500
	Diazepan	5–30
	Loracepan	3–6

confirmed, and researchers suggested that the neurochemistry of schizophrenia (and particularly its positive symptoms: delusions and hallucinations) was related to an excess of dopaminergic activity. In the last 20 years, the role of dopamine was confirmed through neuroimaging techniques. Such techniques, particularly Positron Emission Tomography (PET), taught us that the anti-hallucinogenic power of these drugs was specifically related to their capacity to block dopamine D_2 receptors in the limbic system. All typical anti-psychotics require 60–70% blockade of dopamine D_2 receptors in order to achieve anti-hallucinogenic effects (Kapur & Mamo, 2003). The discovery in the 1980s of a new drug, clozapine, with a lower (e.g., 40–50%) D_2 receptor occupancy was an important development with respect to the dopaminergic hypothesis. Paradoxically, clozapine is until now the most powerful anti-psychotic (for both positive and negative symptoms) and the only drug with evidence based for treatment-resistant schizophrenia (Kane *et al.*, 1988, Chakos *et al.*, 2001; Tandon *et al.*, 2008). This deviation from the classical rule led researchers to discover a new group of anti-hallucinogenic drugs: the so-called atypical or second-generation anti-psychotic. These atypical anti-psychotics, apart from blocking D_2 receptors, exhibit a preferential anti-serotonergic activity, blocking 5-HT_{2A} and 5-HT_{2C} receptors, while acting as partial agonists at 5-HT_{1A} receptors. Overall, these second-generation anti-psychotics are not as effective as clozapine in positive symptoms (Chakos *et al.*, 2001) but have less side effects (particularly in extrapiramidal symptoms) than first-generation anti-psychotics (Bishara & Taylor, 2008; Leucht *et al.*, 2009). It has been suggested that D_2 receptor blockade remains critical to their anti-hallucinogenic action, and their efficacy is associated with their faster receptor dissociation rate from D_2 receptors (Kapur & Seeman, 2001). Recently, researchers have proposed an anti-hallucinogenic drug that involves no anti-dopamine blocking action (Patil *et al.*, 2007). Nevertheless, such hypotheses remain controversial (Weinberger, 2007).

How may a drug reduce hallucinations? To date, the most comprehensive attempt to explain the mechanism of action of anti-psychotics was the hypothesis put forward by S. Kapur (Kapur, 2003). He proposed that the positive symptoms of schizophrenia (particularly delusions, but also hallucinations) could be explained as an 'aberrant salience' mediated by a dysfunction in the dopamine system (Kapur, 2003; Kapur *et al.*, 2005). Kapur's hypothesis is based on two sets of data:

1. From many experiments using animal models, there is a general agreement on the central role of dopamine in reward and reinforcement.

2. Dopamine blockade is critical for anti-psychotic response.

The central issue of Kapur's model is to conceptualize schizophrenia as an aberrant assignment of salience to external objects and internal representations due to dopamine overactivity. In this context, hallucinations arise as a direct result of this abnormal salience in the context of internal representations of perceptions and memories. In this hypothesis, the anti-psychotic effect is not directly related to the symptoms (delusions or hallucinations) but is only indirectly linked. In one patient's words, the most common acute effect of anti-psychotics in hallucinations is 'I still hear voices, but they don't bother me as much anymore.' In half of all patients, these voices disappear after several weeks,

25% of the patients hear voices only occasionally, and in the remaining 25%, the anti-psychotics have no effect (Gonzalez *et al.*, 2006).

Neurochemistry of hallucinations based on neuroimaging

Another important source of data about the neurochemistry of hallucinations came from neuroimaging studies on drug-naïve patients. Several studies on untreated patients with schizophrenia found an increased occupancy of D_2 receptors and 5-HT_{2A} receptors in the striatal system and caudate nucleus, respectively, when compared to the healthy controls (Abi-Dargham *et al.*, 2002; Schmitt *et al.*, 2006; Erritzoe *et al.*, 2008; Hurlemann *et al.*, 2008). Moreover, one study found a significant correlation between frontal D(2/3) receptor binding values and positive symptoms in male patients with schizophrenia (Glenthoj *et al.*, 2006). Although some studies did not confirm these results (Corson *et al.*, 2002, Lomeña *et al.*, 2004) overall, these findings provide some evidence of a relationship between changes in dopamine/serotonin activity in the limbic system and hallucinatory experience in patients with schizophrenia.

Furthermore, in a Magnetic Resonance Spectroscopy (MRS) study on a metabolic ratio differences between schizophrenic patients with and without auditory hallucinations and control subjects, we found that choline and *N*-acetyl-aspartate ratio abnormalities in the thalamus may be related to the pathogenesis of auditory hallucinations (Martinez-Granados *et al.*, 2008).

In summary, many drugs with different mechanisms of action can induce or reduce the hallucinatory experience. Several neurotransmitters have been associated with hallucinations: dopamine, acetylcholine, serotonin, and glutamate. However, the most common mechanisms to reduce hallucinations are 5-HT_{2A} and D_2 receptor antagonism.

Pharmacotherapy of hallucinations

There is no specific pharmacotherapy for hallucinations in any sensory modality. Anti-psychotics are the mainstay of most treatment programmes, but they are also active against other types of symptoms such as delusions and depressive or cognitive symptoms. Auditory Hallucinations (AH) are considered to be most responsive to treatment compared with other symptoms in patients with schizophrenia and related psychotic disorders (Gunduz-Bruce *et al.*, 2005). However, the symptoms persist in spite of treatment in 32% of chronic patients (Curson *et al.*, 1988) and 56% of acutely ill patients (Miller, 1996). In the last decade, a great amount of interest has been devoted to alternative treatments for persistent AH, such as Cognitive-Behavioural Therapy (CBT) and TMS. To date, no strategy has been shown to be the pharmacological treatment of choice for persistent hallucinations. As specificity is still a goal, treatment should be individualistic and several therapeutic strategies should be used simultaneously (Aleman & Larøi, 2008).

There is tremendous individual variability in anti-psychotic response. Clinical and pathogenic heterogeneity adds more difficulty when constructing treatment guidelines. Moreover, no follow-up study has evaluated the efficacy of anti-psychotics on AH in the long term. It is therefore not surprising that we lack clear guidelines for the pharmacological treatment of AH. Many clinicians use a high-affinity receptor model when choosing an anti-psychotic drug for treating AH, but research has repeatedly shown that no anti-psychotic is best for treating these symptoms. Only clozapine has been consistently shown to be effective, and this also applies to treatment-refractory schizophrenia (Tandon *et al.*, 2008). Clozapine is also the drug of choice in the context of comorbid substance abuse (Green, 2006). Olanzapine and risperidone may be good alternatives before clozapine is considered. In fact, these drugs have shown similar efficacy in treating hallucinations in first-episode patients (Robinson *et al.*, 2006).

In spite of the traditional view of delayed-onset action of anti-psychotics, recent studies suggested an early-onset action within the first day (for review, see Agid *et al.*, 2006). Nevertheless, definitions of clinical 'response' and 'non-response' greatly differ from one study to another (for review, see Kane & Leucht, 2008). Current guidelines for the treatment of schizophrenia suggest a period of 2–8 weeks, using at least one conventional and one atypical anti-psychotic in doses equivalent to 600 mg of chlorpromazine, before considering non-response (Lehman *et al.*, 2004, Falkai *et al.*, 2005). Similar trial durations (4–6 weeks) have been applied in TMS studies when considering medication-resistant AH (Hoffman *et al.*, 2003; Horacek *et al.*, 2007). However, certain data suggest that an anti-psychotic trial lasting 2 weeks may be sufficient to determine non-response and evaluate an alternative therapeutic approach in the treatment of patients with schizophrenia (Kinon *et al.*, 2008; Leucht *et al.*, 2008). A change will be required if no response or intolerable side effects appear. First, however, dosing should be increased. An individualized gradual switching strategy is advisable. Finally, efficacy and safety drug profiles, symptomatology, comorbidity, and side effects will be taken into consideration for the second treatment attempt (Buckley & Correll, 2008).

Ziprasidone has recently been receiving support for its use in treatment-refractory schizophrenia (Loebel *et al.*, 2007), and quetiapine might also be an option for treatment-resistant AH (Mosolov & Kabanov, 2005). Sertindole should not be dismissed when treating AH, particularly in treatment-resistant patients, because of its efficacy (Azorin *et al.*, 2008). Anti-psychotic co-treatment should also be considered in certain situations (Correll *et al.*, in press). Amisulpride (Shiloh *et al.*, 1997), because of its D_2 specificity, as well as risperidone (Josiassen *et al.*, 2005), seem to be good options for clozapine augmentation. Estradiol may be a future possibility as an adjunct therapy for treating positive symptoms in women with schizophrenia (Kulkarni *et al.*, 2008). Finally, long-acting injectable anti-psychotic medications are an option when compliance is not guaranteed.

Several special situations should be considered when treating hallucinations pharmacologically (Fig. 2.1):

1. *Children and adolescents* (see Goëb & Jardri, this volume): A substantial number of children and adolescents report hallucinations both in clinical and non-clinical populations. Although they may increase the likelihood of psychiatric symptoms both in childhood and later in life, they do not have a clear predictive value for the appearance of psychoses in adult life (Larøi *et al.*, 2006). In fact, they are in many cases

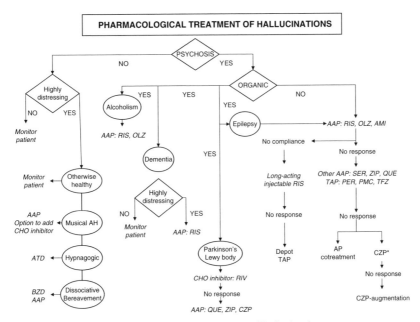

Fig. 2.1 Decision tree in the pharmacological treatment of hallucinations.

*Except for epileptic hallucinations.

AAP, atypical anti-psychotic; TAP, typical anti-psychotic; RIS, risperidone; OLZ, olanzapine; AMI, amisulpride; SER, sertindole; ZIP, ziprasidone; PER, perphenazine; PMC, pimozide; TFZ, trifluorperazine; CZP, clozapine; CHO inhibitor, cholinesterase inhibitor; RIV, rivastigmine; QUE, quetiapine; ATD, antidepressant; BZD, benzodiacepine.

of a transient nature and no medication is required. In such cases, they are often related to negative life events such as childhood abuse. Thus, non-pharmacological interventions including both children and their families (education, normalization, coping strategies, and treatment of co-morbidity) are the best options in many cases (Larøi *et al.*, 2006). Therefore, hallucinations should be carefully evaluated to decide whether they are psychotic or non-psychotic, and treatment should be congruent with this clinical decision (Edelsohn, 2006). Olanzapine (at higher than usual doses if required) and risperidone are better accepted than first-generation anti-psychotics in adolescents with psychosis. Clozapine is known to be superior to haloperidol and olanzapine in refractory schizophrenia, but data are not always specific for AH, and this drug is not easy to use in children and adolescents because of its side effects. There is now an emerging consensus that aripiprazole and risperidone are effective drugs for the first-line treatment of an acute psychotic episode in this setting. Both drugs may soon have a formal FDA indication for this population (Kumra *et al.*, 2008).

2. *Organic hallucinations*: An organic aetiology should be investigated in the presence of substance abuse, accompanying atypical symptoms, late age of onset, no response to conventional treatment, predominating visual sensory modality, fever, or in the case of a systemic disease that potentially damages the brain.

a. *Dementia* (see Mosimann & Collerton, this volume): Psychotic symptoms are relatively frequent in patients with Alzheimer's disease and vascular dementias. As happens in other neurological disorders, visual hallucinations are more frequent than auditory in this setting (Lautenschlager & Forstl, 2001). Although second-generation anti-psychotics are now frequently used for the treatment of psychotic symptoms in Alzheimer's disease, their use is controversial, particularly because of their adverse effects profile (Schneider *et al.*, 2006). Another dementia, Lewy body disease, is likely to present with psychosis, especially visual hallucinations (Lautenschlager & Forstl, 2001). These patients are usually treated with second-generation anti-psychotics such as quetiapine or ziprasidone but can also be treated with cholinesterase inhibitors as some studies have suggested (McKeith *et al.*, 2005). The decision of treating hallucinations in patients with dementia should be individualized, since the hallucinations may often not be distressing for these individuals and their caregivers, they may not cause practical management problems, or they may resolve without treatment. The introduction of anti-psychotic drugs should be done with great caution in these patients, since (1) they are usually polymedicated and a new drug will increase the risk of potential drug interactions and side effects, (2) elderly persons are more sensitive to side effects than non-elderly persons, (3) compliance may be non-adequate if they do not have enough external support, and (4) psychiatric patients differ in many ways from patients with dementia and generalizations from the former patients may imply risks for the latter ones. Patients may be monitored for a period up to 3 months and, if needed, treated with low doses of a second-generation anti-psychotic (Aleman & Larøi, 2008).

b. *Parkinson's disease* (see Fénelon, this volume): Complex visual hallucinations, minor phenomena such as passage hallucinations and visual illusions, and, less frequently, auditory hallucinations (approximately 25–40% of patients) usually appear together (Fénelon, 2008). All these phenomena should probably be treated when discovered (Goetz *et al.*, 2008) with second-generation anti-psychotics (i.e., quetiapine or clozapine) and/or cholinesterase inhibitors (i.e., rivastigmine), if reduction of dopamine agonist drugs is not possible because of worsening motor symptoms (Zahodne *et al.*, 2008).

c. *Epilepsy* (in adults, frequently related to stroke, brain tumours, trauma, degenerative disorders, and alcoholism): Hallucinations may occur during seizures, particularly when the focus is in the left temporal lobe, but also in the context of schizophrenia-like psychotic episodes post- and inter-ictally (Kanner, 2004). Psychoses in patients with epilepsy are usually treated with a combination of anticonvulsants and anti-psychotics. Although anti-psychotics lower the seizure threshold, a careful use of second-generation anti-psychotics, particularly risperidone, is adequate except for clozapine, which has the highest risk (Koch-Stoecker, 2002).

d. *Charles Bonnet Syndrome* (see Eperjesi, this volume): The course of hallucinations may or may not be related to the course of the visual impairment. No established treatment has been stated in the literature; anticonvulsant drugs, second-generation anti-psychotics, 5-HT3 antagonists, and SSRI have been proven to be effective. Their pharmacological treatment is controversial (Rovner, 2006; Lang *et al.*, 2007).

  e. *Alcoholism*: Hallucinosis, usually auditory and with conserved insight, is commonly treated with anti-psychotics, but a randomized controlled trial recently suggested the use of valproate (Aliyev & Aliyev, 2008).

  f. *Delirium*: Second-generation anti-psychotics are widely used, although well-designed studies are not available. For now, data support the use of risperidone, olanzapine, and quetiapine in the treatment of delirium (Boettger *et al.*, 2005).

3. *Non-psychotic subjects*: Hallucinations can be present under a wide range of circumstances, including sensory deprivation, dissociative disorders, bereavement, and other high-emotion situations. It is now widely accepted that they may also occur in non-psychotic patients, even in otherwise healthy individuals (Johns & van Os, 2001; Johns *et al.*, 2002; Choong *et al.*, 2007). In particular, sensory impairment hallucinations may not respond to anti-psychotics. A particular type, musical hallucinations, which typically occur among elderly individuals and are associated with hearing impairment, has been shown to improve with other drugs such as donepezil (in combination with anti-psychotics), a cholinesterase inhibitor (Ukai *et al.*, 2007). Finally, tricyclic antidepressants, selective serotonin reuptake inhibitors (SSRIs), and venlafaxine may be effective treatments for hypnagogic hallucinations (Morgenthaler *et al.*, 2007). Hallucinations appearing in bereavement, dissociative disorders, and other high-emotion situations may better benefit from benzodiacepines or non-pharmacological approaches and are not usually treated with anti-psychotic drugs unless they are associated with intense distress.

Psychological treatments in combination with anti-psychotics

In psychotic patients with hallucinations, psychological treatments are given in addition to, and not instead of, anti-psychotic medication. The hallucinatory experience may be so overwhelming for the patient that it is impossible to manage without medication. In contrast, many studies have reported compliance as a major problem in the treatment of schizophrenia. A large non-commercial clinical trial in the United States has shown that 74% of patients with chronic schizophrenia discontinued their randomized treatment over 18 months (Lieberman *et al.*, 2005). In considering how to improve compliance, it is worth remembering that Sarwer-Former long ago considered the psychotherapeutic use of anti-psychotics as crucial to the overall therapeutic process (Sarwer-Foner, 1963).

    To integrate psychological and pharmacological treatments in a patient with hallucinations, the therapist should consider at least two relevant issues: (a) the emotional impact of the hallucinations in each individual patient and (b) the subjective experience induced by anti-psychotics.

Emotion may play an important role in the hallucinatory experience, particularly in psychotic patients. Some studies have pointed out that the main effect of both anti-psychotics and CBT would be to reduce the anxiety induced by voices rather than the voices (Kapur, 2003; Sanjuan *et al.*, 2007; Costafreda *et al.*, 2008; Murray *et al.*, 2008). Under a strict medical model, hearing voices is always considered a pathological phenomenon and must therefore always be treated. However, hallucinations, even in psychotic patients, are not always related to anxiety or distressing experiences. In a study of fifty hallucinating acute in-patients, many of them reported some positive effects of hallucinations (Miller *et al.*, 1993). Moreover, in 106 psychotic outpatients with AH, 28 had pleasant experiences with the voices and in 10 cases, this positive experience was very frequent (Sanjuan *et al.*, 2004b). Therefore, the rational approach would be to analyze the emotional impact of the voices and assess their adaptive functions before deciding on the most appropriate pharmacological or psychological treatment.

On the other hand, the introduction of an anti-psychotic leads to the subjective interpretation by the patient of the physiological changes that accompany therapy, which, in turn, influences the behavioural response to treatment and ultimately the clinical outcome (Awad, 1989). Traditionally, the notion of the dysphoric response to neuroleptics was considered a disorder of subjective tolerability associated with the interaction of pharmacodynamic features of these agents with individual neurobiological features. However, the subjective experience is also related to personality and the social context of the patient (Hellewell, 2002; Vorugati & Awad, 2004). The patient's ultimate view of the effectiveness of a drug may in fact be very different from that of the clinician. For example, the calming and relaxing effect might be much more valued than anti-psychotic (anti-hallucinatory) activity (Angermeyer *et al.*, 2001, Fitzgerald *et al.*, 2003).

Case presentation 1

Mr AD is 27 years old. He was diagnosed with paranoid schizophrenia 9 years ago. He has continuously been on anti-psychotic treatment during all these years, and he seems to be compliant with treatment. Almost all second-generation anti-psychotics (except for aripiprazole) and several first-generation anti-psychotics (haloperidol, pimozide, trifluorperazine, and levomepromacine) have been tried, with mild responses that have usually lasted for no longer than 1–2 months. After that period, he has usually suffered highly distressing AH and persecutory delusions with negative consequences both socially and in the workplace. Two years after the onset of his illness, he was considered as suffering from treatment-resistant auditory hallucinations and delusions, and six courses of electroconvulsive therapy were tried with only mild improvement. Clozapine was also attempted but had to be interrupted because of intolerable side effects. More recently, a second trial of electroconvulsive therapy (nine courses) was administered with no response. He is now being treated with a combination of quetiapine (900 mg/day) and sertindole (20 mg/day) that has proved to be the most successful therapeutic approach. He was put on individual CBT 6 months ago. His therapist has focused on his AH. He has not been very cooperative with his psychologist and his AH are still present.

However, they are less distressing, and he has been able to improve his ability to cope with these chronic symptoms.

This case presentation illustrates the refractoriness of some AH in spite of a comprehensive pharmacological approach. Alternative options such as CBT are necessary in these cases and may also be a good choice as a concomitant treatment in less severe cases.

Case presentation 2

Mrs MJ is 39 years old. She is married, has two children, and is employed. She was diagnosed with paranoid schizophrenia 10 years ago. She has been maintained for several years on low doses of anti-psychotic medication, namely, trifluorperazine (5 mg/day) and quetiapine (100 mg/day). Recently, she consulted because of a relapse consisting of persecutory delusions and auditory hallucinations that provoked marital troubles and job loss. She was reluctant to modify her quetiapine dosage since previous trials had caused increasing appetite and weight gain. She accepted to take up to 15 mg/day of trifluorperazine, but this was partially ineffective and extrapyramidal symptoms made biperiden (4 mg/day) necessary. On subsequent appointments, she finally recognized cocaine abuse in the beginning of the psychotic episode, although she had lately interrupted it. A lack of response and potential irregular compliance with treatment made depot medication advisable. A combination of zuclophentixol decanoate and acetate was started while maintaining trifluorperazine (10 mg/day). Extrapyramidal symptoms remitted after biperiden was introduced. Her psychotic symptomatology fully disappeared after one month and there was considerable improvement in her social performance, although she is still not working. At this moment, she is under zuclophentixol (400 mg/2 weeks), biperiden (2 mg/day), and trifluorperazine (5 mg/day). Therapeutical efforts are now centered on treatment compliance, substance abuse prevention, and family counselling.

Two issues come across in the context of this case presentation. Substance abuse and non-compliance are frequently responsible for sub-optimal treatment response. Depot medication may be a good option in these cases. Long-acting risperidone might have been a good option, but its delayed action and the antecedents of optimal response with a typical anti-psychotic made the clinician think of this psychopharmacological approach. Psychoeducation and counselling may make oral posology possible after stabilization phase is reached.

Future directions

Almost all recent research models for biological treatments in schizophrenia have been focused on cognitive and negative symptoms. The rationale for this is the assumption that anti-psychotics are usually efficacious in treating hallucinations, whereas cognitive and negative symptoms are more relevant in outcome measures. But these arguments are not applicable to persistently or acutely hallucinating patients. Nevertheless, certain animal models for hallucinations have recently been developed, which examine overall cortical activity (Celada *et al.*, 2008). The neurophysiological changes induced by a hallucinogenic drug, a partial 5-HT2A agonist (DOI, dimethoxi-4-iodophenyl-2amino-propane), were reversed by typical (haloperidol) and atypical (clozapine) anti-psychotic treatment. This model has also been used to examine the effects of other psychotomimetic substances, such as phencyclidine, whose effects are also reversed by haloperidol and clozapine (Kargieman *et al.*, 2007). These observations indicate that the cortical alterations induced by psychoactive agents with different pharmacological mechanisms (5-HT$_{2A}$ receptor agonism, NMDA receptor antagonism) can be reversed by drugs acting also through different mechanisms (preferential D$_2$ receptor or 5-HT$_{2A}$ receptor antagonism). This offers new perspectives to examine the ability of drugs as potentially useful in the treatment of hallucinations.

On the other hand, one of the most controversial issues in schizophrenia treatment nowadays is how to measure clinical response. In most clinical trials, it is defined by a percentage (20–30%) improvement over baseline on a global clinical scale (Lasser *et al.*, 2007). However, this concept is neurobiologically unspecific and highly dependent on baseline severity (Kane & Leucht, 2008). An important methodological problem in anti-psychotic drug trials is the lack of quality of data about the efficacy of a drug to treat a specific symptom such as hallucinations (Leucht *et al.*, 2008). The strategy of a 'core symptom approach' historically proposed by cognitive-behavioural therapists (Aleman & Larøi, 2008) may solve this problem. To select the best anti-hallucinogenic drug, we need qualitative information about how powerful a specific drug is in reducing hallucinations.

With the aim of personalizing the treatment for each patient, many studies on the pharmacogenetics of anti-psychotics have been published. A large number of associations have been discovered with generally small effect size. However, a useful test for clinical practice is still missing (Arranz & Kapur, 2008; Foster *et al.*, 2007). One possible explanation is that most pharmacogenetic research has been conducted blind to environmental influences. Another possible reason is the poor neurobiological validity associated with treatment response. Certain genetic studies have been conducted in order to analyze susceptibility to hallucinations in psychotic patients (Sanjuan *et al.*, 2004a, 2006a,b, 2007; Toirac, 2007; Aguilar *et al.*, 2008). These studies may open the field to a pharmacogenetic approach in hallucination treatments, in order to predict differences in individual response to anti-psychotic drugs.

As mentioned previously, old and new anti-hallucinogenic drugs should ideally be used in an integrated approach together with other treatment schemes such as CBT and psychoeducation, to name but a few (see contributions in this volume for other examples). To date, only a small number of attempts have been made to integrate psychological and biological treatments in psychotic patients with persistent hallucinations (Jenner *et al.*, 2004; see Jenner, this volume). Nevertheless, in medical settings, when psychological interventions are possible, integrated approaches are the rule, since most patients who are undergoing psychological treatment for persistent hallucinations also receive anti-psychotic treatment. Kapur's model, which focuses on the emotional basis of hallucinations (salience due to excessive dopamine activity), is, in our opinion, an excellent starting point to integrate psychological and pharmacological treatments (Kapur, 2003; Mizrahi *et al.*, 2007; Menon *et al.*, 2008), yet probably requiring the involvement of other neurotransmitter systems or brain networks. Accordingly, we need studies with 'complex' interventions including psycho-social and pharmacological treatments.

In summary, a new interest in the neurobiology of hallucinations, including animal models, has recently experienced a slight resurgence (Celada *et al.*, 2008, Fantegrossi *et al.*, 2008). This new interest is encouraging in the search for new anti-hallucinations drugs. Future anti-psychotic clinical trials should include qualitative information at a symptom level using specific and multidimensional scales for hallucinations (Mizrahi *et al.*, 2006). The pharmacogenetics of hallucination treatments should be further elucidated in the future. Finally, additional studies with integrated pharmacological and psychosocial interventions in patients with hallucinations are needed to improve the clinical outcomes of these patients.

References

Abi-Dargham, A., Rodenhiser, J., Printz, D., *et al.* (2002). Increased baseline occupancy of D2 receptors by dopamine in schizophrenia. *Proc Natl Acad Sci USA*, **97**, 8104–9.

Aghajnaian, G.K., & Marek, G.J. (1999). Serotonin and hallucinations. *Neuropsychopharmacology*, **21** (suppl 2), 16S.

Agid, O., Seeman, P., & Kapur, S. (2006). The 'delayed onset' of antipsychotic action—an idea whose time has come and gone. *J Psychiatry Neurosci*, **31**, 93–100.

Aguilar, E.J., Sanjuán, J., García-Martí, G., Lull, J.J., & Robles, M. (2008). MR and genetics in schizophrenia: focus on auditory hallucinations. *Eur J Radiol*, **67**, 434–9.

Aleman, A., & Larøi, F. (2008). *Hallucinations: the science of idiosyncratic perception*. Washington, DC: American Psychological Association.

Aliyev, Z.N., & Aliyev, N.A. (2008). Valproate treatment of acute alcohol hallucinosis: a double-blind, placebo-controlled study. *Alcohol*, **43**, 456–9.

Angermeyer, M.C., Loffler, W., Muller, P., Schulze, B., & Priebe, S. (2001). Patients' and relatives' assessment of clozapine treatment. *Psychol Med*, **31**, 509–17.

Arranz, M.J., & Kapur, S.(2008). Pharmacogenetics in psychiatry: are we ready for widespread clinical use?. *Schizophr Bull*, **34**, 1130–44.

Awad, A.G. (1989). Drug therapy in schizophrenia: variability of outcome and prediction of response. *Can J Psychiatry*, **34**, 711–20.

Azorin, J.M., Murteira, S., Hansen, K., & Toumi, M. (2008). Evaluation of patients on sertindole treatment after failure of other antipsychotics: a retrospective analysis. *BMC Psychiatry*, **8**, 16.

Bishara, D., & Taylor, D. (2008). Upcoming agents for the treatment of schizophrenia: mechanism of action, efficacy and tolerability. *Drugs*, **68**, 2269–92.

Boettger, S., & Breitbart, W. (2005). Atypical antipsychotics in the management of delirium: a review of the empirical literature. *Palliat Support Care*, **3**, 227–37.

Buckley, P.F., & Correll, C.U. (2008). Strategies for dosing and switching antipsychotics for optimal clinical management. *J Clin Psychiatry*, **69** (suppl 1), 4–17.

Celada, P., Puig, M.V., Díaz-Mataix, L., & Artigas, F. (2008). The hallucinogen DOI reduces low-frequency oscillations in rat prefrontal cortex: reversal by antipsychotic drugs. *Biol Psychiatry*, **64**, 392–400.

Chakos, M., Lieberman, J., Hoffman, E., Bradford, D., & Sheitman, B. (2001). Effectiveness of second-generation antipsychotics in patients with treatment-resistant schizophrenia: a review and meta-analysis of randomized trials. *Am J Psychiatry*, **158**, 518–26.

Choong, C., Hunter, M.D., & Woodruff, P.W. (2007). Auditory hallucinations in those populations that do not suffer from schizophrenia. *Curr Psychiatry Rep*, **9**, 206–12.

Correll, C.U., Rummel-Kluge, C., Corves, C., Kane, J.M., & Leucht, S. (2009). Antipsychotic combinations vs. monotherapy in schizophrenia: A meta-analysis of randomized controlled trials. *Schizophr Bull*, **35** (2), 443–57.

Corson, P.W., O'Leary, D.S., Miller, D.D., & Andreasen, N.C. (2002). The effects of neuroleptic medications on basal ganglia blood flow in schizophreniform disorders: a comparison between the neuroleptic-naïve and medicated states. *Biol Psychiatry*, **52**, 855–62.

Costafreda, S.G., Brébion, G., Allen, P., McGuire, P.K., & Fu, C.H. (2008). Affective modulation of external misattribution bias in source monitoring in schizophrenia. *Psychol Med*, **38**, 821–4.

Cunningham, N. (2008). Hallucinogenic plants of abuse. *Emerg Med Australas*, **20**, 167–74.

Curson, D.A., Patel, M., Liddle, P.F., & Barnes, T.R. (1988). Psychiatric morbidity of a long stay hospital population with chronic schizophrenia and implications for future community care. *BMJ*, **297**, 819–22.

Dobkin de Rios, M. (1972). *Visionary vine: hallucinogenic healing in the Peruvian Amazon.* San Francisco: Chandler Publishing.

Dyck, E. (2005). Flashback: psychiatric experimentation with LSD in historical perspective. *Can J Psychiatry*, **50**, 381–8.

Edelsohn, G.A. (2006). Hallucinations in children and adolescents: considerations in the emergency setting. *Am J Psychiatry*, **163**, 781–5.

Erritzoe, D., Rasmussen, H., Kristiansen, K.T., *et al.* (2008). Cortical and subcortical 5-HT2A receptor binding in neuroleptic-naïve first-episode schizophrenic patients. *Neuropsychopharmacology*, **33**, 2435–41.

Falkai, P., Wobrock, T., Lieberman, J., Glenthoj, B., Gattaz, W.F., & Moller, H.J. (2005). World Federation of Societies of Biological Psychiatry (WFSBP) guidelines for biological treatment of schizophrenia, Part 1: acute treatment of schizophrenia. *World J Biol Psychiatry*, **6**, 132–91.

Fantegrossi, W.E., Murnane, K.S., & Reissig, C.J. (2008). The behavioral pharmacology of hallucinogens. *Biochem Pharmacol*, **75**, 17–33.

Fénelon, G. (2008). Psychosis in Parkinson's disease: phenomenology, frequency, risk factors, and current understanding of pathophysiologic mechanisms. *CNS Spectrums*, **13** (suppl 4), 18–25.

Fitzgerald, P.B., de Castella, A.R., Filia, K., *et al.* (2003). A longitudinal study of patient- and observer-rated quality of life in schizophrenia. *Psychiatry Res*, **119**, 55–62.

Foster, A., Miller, del D., & Buckley, P.F. (2007). Pharmacogenetics and schizophrenia. *Psychiatr Clin North Am*, **30**, 417–35.

Glenthoj, B.Y., Mackeprang, T., Svarer, C., *et al.* (2006). Frontal dopamine D(2/3) receptor binding in drug-naive first-episode schizophrenic patients correlates with positive psychotic symptoms and gender. *Biol Psychiatry*, **60**, 621–9.

Goetz, C.G., Fan, W., & Leurgans, S. (2008). Antipsychotic medication treatment for mild hallucinations in Parkinson's disease: positive impact on long-term worsening. *Move Disord*, **23**, 1541–5.

González, J.C., Aguilar, E.J., Berenguer, V., Leal, C., & Sanjuán, J. (2006). Persistent auditory hallucinations. *Psychopathology*, **39**, 120–5.

González-Maeso, J., Weisstaub, N.V., Zhou, M., *et al.* (2007). Hallucinogens recruit specific cortical 5-HT(2A) receptor-mediated signalling pathways to affect behavior. *Neuron*, **53**, 439–52.

Green, A.I. (2006). Treatment of schizophrenia and comorbid substance abuse: pharmacologic approaches. *J Clin Psychiatry*, **67** (suppl 7), 31–5.

Gunduz-Bruce, H., McMeniman, M., Robinson, D.G., *et al.* (2005). Duration of untreated psychosis and time to treatment response for delusions and hallucinations. *Am J Psychiatry*, **162**, 1966–9.

Hellewell, J.S. (2002). Patients' subjective experiences of antipsychotics: clinical relevance. *CNS Drugs*, **16**, 457–71.

Hoffman, R.E., Hawkins, K.A., Gueorguieva, R., *et al.* (2003). Transcranial magnetic stimulation of left temporoparietal cortex and medication-resistant auditory hallucinations. *Arch Gen Psychiatry*, **60**, 49–56.

Horacek, J., Brunovsky, M., Novak, T., *et al.* (2007). Effect of low-frequency rTMS on electromagnetic tomography (LORETA) and regional brain metabolism (PET) in schizophrenia patients with auditory hallucinations. *Neuropsychobiology*, **55**, 132–42.

Hurlemann, R., Matusch, A., Kuhn, K.U., *et al.* (2008). 5-HT2A receptor density is decreased in the at-risk mental state. *Psychopharmacology*, **195**, 579–90.

Jenner, J.A., Nienhuis, F.J., Wiersma, D., & van de Willige, G. (2004). Hallucination-focused integrative treatment: a randomized controlled trial. *Schizophr Bull*, **30**, 133–45.

Johns, L.C. & van Os, J. (2001). The continuity of psychotic experiences in the general population. *Clin Psychol Rev*, **21**, 1125–41.

Johns, L.C., Nazroo, J.Y., Bebbington, P., & Kuipers, E. (2002). Occurrence of hallucinatory experiences in a community sample and ethnic variations. *Br J Psychiatry*, **180**, 174–8.

Josiassen, R.C., Joseph, A., Kohegyi, E., *et al.* (2005). Clozapine augmented with risperidone in the treatment of schizophrenia: a randomized, double-blind, placebo-controlled trial. *Am J Psychiatry*, **162**, 130–6.

Kane, J., Honigfeld, G., Singer, J., & Meltzer, H. (1988). Clozapine for the treatment-resistant schizophrenic. A double-blind comparison with chlorpromazine. *Arch Gen Psychiatry*, **45**, 789–96.

Kane, J.M. & Leucht, S. (2008). Unanswered questions in schizophrenia clinical trials. *Schizophr Bull*, **34**, 302–9.

Kanner, A.M. (2004). Recognition of the various expressions of anxiety, psychosis, and aggression in epilepsy. *Epilepsia*, **45**(suppl 2), 22–7.

Kapur, S. & Seeman, P. (2001). Does fast dissociation from the dopamine d(2) receptor explain the action of atypical antipsychotics?: A new hypothesis. *Am J Psychiatry*, **158**, 360–9.

Kapur, S. (2003). Psychosis as a state of aberrant salience: a framework linking biology, phenomenology, and pharmacology in schizophrenia. *Am J Psychiatry*, **160**, 13–23.

Kapur, S. & Mamo, D. (2003). Half a century of antipsychotics and still a central role for dopamine D2 receptors. *Prog Neuropsychopharmacol Biol Psychiatry*, **27**, 1081–90.

Kapur, S., Mizrahi, R., & Li, M. (2005). From dopamine to salience to psychosis—linking biology, pharmacology and phenomenology of psychosis. *Schizophr Res*, **79**, 59–68.

Kargieman, L., Santana, N., Mengod, G., Celada, P., & Artigas, F. (2007). Antipsychotic drugs reverse the disruption in prefrontal cortex function produced by NMDA receptor blockade with phencyclidine. *Proc Natl Acad Sci U S A*, **104**, 14843–8.

Kay, S.R., Fiszbein, A., & Opler, L.A. (1987). The positive and negative syndrome scale (PANSS) for schizophrenia. *Schizophr Bull*, **13**, 261–76.

Kinon, B.J., Chen, L., Ascher-Svanum, H., *et al.* (2008). Predicting response to atypical antipsychotics based on early response in the treatment of schizophrenia. *Schizophr Res*, **102**, 230–40.

Koch-Stoecker, S. (2002). Antipsychotic drugs and epilepsy: indications and treatment guidelines. *Epilepsia*, **43** (suppl 2), 19–24.

Kulkarni, J., de Castella, A., Fitzgerald, P.B., *et al.* (2008). Estrogen in severe mental illness: a potential new treatment approach. *Arch Gen Psychiatry*, **65**, 955–60.

Kumra, S., Oberstar, J.V., Sikich, L., *et al.* (2008). Efficacy and tolerability of second-generation antipsychotics in children and adolescents with schizophrenia. *Schizophr Bull*, **34**, 60–71.

Lang, U.E., Stogowski, D., Schulze, D., *et al.* (2007). Charles Bonnet Syndrome: successful treatment of visual hallucinations due to vision loss with selective serotonin reuptake inhibitors. *J Psychopharmacol*, **21**, 553–5.

Larøi, F., Van der Linden, M., & Goëb, J.L. (2006). Hallucinations and delusions in children and adolescents. *Current Psychiatry Reviews*, **2**, 473–85.

Lasser, R.A., Nasrallah, H., & Helldin, L. (2007). Remission in schizophrenia: applying recent consensus criteria to refine the concept. *Schizophr Res*, **96**, 223–31.

Lautenschlager, N.T., & Forstl, H. (2001). Organic psychosis. *Curr Psychiatry Rep*, **3**, 319–25.

Lehman, A.F., Lieberman, J.A., Dixon, L.B., *et al.* (2004). Practice guideline for the treatment of patients with schizophrenia, second edition. *Am J Psychiatry*, **161**, 1–56.

Leucht, S., Shamsi, S.A., Busch, R., Kissling, W., & Kane, J.M. (2008). Predicting antipsychotic drug response—replication and extension to six weeks in an international olanzapine study. *Schizophr Res*, **101**, 312–9.

Leucht, S., Corves, C., Arbter, D., Engel, R.R., Li, C., & Davis, J.M. (2009). Second-generation versus first-generation antipsychotic drugs for schizophrenia: a meta-analysis. *Lancet*, **373**, 31–41.

Lieberman, J.A., Stroup, T.S., McEvoy, J.P., *et al.* (2005). Clinical Antipsychotic Trials of Intervention Effectiveness (CATIE) Investigators. Effectiveness of antipsychotic drugs in patients with chronic schizophrenia. *N Engl J Med*, **353**, 1209–23.

Loebel, A.D., Khanna, S., Rajadhyaksha, S., Siu, C.O., Giller, E., & Potkin, S.G. (2007). Ziprasidone in treatment-resistant schizophrenia: a 52-week, open-label continuation study. *J Clin Psychiatry*, **68**, 1333–8.

Lomeña, F., Catafau, A.M., Parellada, E., *et al.* (2004). Striatal dopamine D2 receptor density in neuroleptic-naive and inneuroleptic-free schizophrenic patients: an 123I-IBZM-SPECT study. *Psychopharmacology*, **172**, 165–9.

Martínez-Granados, B., Brotons, O., Martínez-Bisbal, M.C., *et al.* (2008). Spectroscopic metabolomic abnormalities in the thalamus related to auditory hallucinations in patients with schizophrenia. *Schizophr Res*, **104**, 13–22.

McKeith, I.G., Dickson, D.W., Lowe, J., *et al.* (2005). Diagnosis and management of dementia with Lewy bodies: third report of the DLB Consortium. *Neurology*, **65**, 1863–72.

Menon, M., Mizrahi, R., & Kapur, S. (2008). 'Jumping to conclusions' and delusions in psychosis: relationship and response to treatment. *Schizophr Res*, **98**, 225–31.

Miller, L.J., O'Connor, E., & Di Pasquale, T. (1993). Patients' attitudes toward hallucinations. *Am J Psychiatry*, **150**, 584–8.

Miller, L.J. (1996). Qualitative changes in hallucinations. *Am J Psychiatry*, **153**, 265–7.

Mizrahi, R., Korostil, M., Starkstein, S.E., Zipursky, R.B., & Kapur, S. (2007). The effect of antipsychotic treatment on Theory of Mind. *Psychol Med*, **37**, 595–601.

Morgenthaler, T.I., Kapur, V.K., Brown, T., *et al.* (2007). Standards of Practice Committee of the American Academy of Sleep Medicine. Practice parameters for the treatment of narcolepsy and other hypersomnias of central origin. *Sleep*, **30**, 1705–11.

Mosolov, S.N. & Kabanov, S. (2005). Quetiapine in the treatment of patients with resistant auditory hallucinations: two case reports with long-term cognitive assessment. *Eur Psychiatry*, **20**, 430.

Murray, R.M., Lappin, J., & Di Forti, M. (2008). Schizophrenia: from developmental deviance to dopamine dysregulation. *Eur Neuropsychopharmacol.* **18** (suppl 3), S129–34.

Nichols, D.E. (2004). Hallucinogens. *Pharmacol Ther*, **101**, 131.

Patil, S.T., Zhang, L., Martenyi, F., *et al.* (2007). Activation of mGlu2/3 receptors as a new approach to treat schizophrenia: a randomized Phase 2 clinical trial. *Nat Med*, **13**, 1102–7.

Puig, M.V., Celada, P., Díaz-Mataix, L., & Artigas, F. (2003). In vivo modulation of the activity of pyramidal neurons in the rat medial prefrontal cortex by 5-HT$_{2A}$ receptors. Relationship to thalamocortical afferents. *Cereb Cortex*, **13**, 870.

Riba, J. & Barbanoj, M.J. (2005). Bringing ayahuasca to the clinical research laboratory. *J Psychoactive Drugs.* **37**, 219–30.

Robinson, D.G., Woerner, M.G., Napolitano, B., *et al.* (2006). Randomized comparison of olanzapine versus risperidone for the treatment of first-episode schizophrenia: 4-month outcomes. *Am J Psychiatry*, **163**, 2096–102.

Rovner, B.W. (2006). The Charles Bonnet syndrome: a review of recent research. *Curr Opin Ophthalmol*, **17**, 275–7.

Sanjuan, J., Toirac, I., González, J.C., *et al.* (2004a). Possible association between the CCK-AR gene and persistent auditory hallucinations in schizophrenia. *Eur Psychiatry*, **19**, 349–53.

Sanjuan, J., Gonzalez, J.C., Aguilar, E.J., Leal, C., & van Os, J. (2004b). Pleasurable auditory hallucinations. *Acta Psychiatr Scand*, **110**, 273–8.

Sanjuan, J., Tolosa, A., González, J.C., *et al.* (2006a). Association between FOXP2 polymorphisms and schizophrenia with auditory hallucinations. *Psychiatr Genet*, **16**, 67–72.

Sanjuan, J., Rivero, O., Aguilar, E.J., *et al.* (2006b). Serotonin transporter gene polymorphism (5-HTTLPR) and emotional response to auditory hallucinations in schizophrenia. *Int J Neuropsychopharmacol*, **9**, 131–3.

Sanjuan, J., Lull, J.J., Aguilar, E.J., *et al.* (2007). Emotional words induce enhanced brain activity in schizophrenic patients with auditory hallucinations. *Psychiatry Res*, **154**, 21–9.

Sarwer-Foner, G.J. (1963). On the mechanisms of action of neuroleptic drugs: a theoretical psycho-dynamic explanation. *Recent Adv Biol Psychiatry*, **6**, 217–32.

Schmitt, G.J., Meisenzahl, E.M., Frodl, T., *et al.* (2006). The striatal dopamine transporter in first-episode, drug-naive schizophrenicpatients: evaluation by the new SPECT-ligand[99mTc] TRODAT-1. *J Psychopharmacol*, **19**, 488–93.

Schneider, L.S., Tariot, P.N., Dagerman, K.S., *et al.* (2006). Effectiveness of atypical antipsychotic drugs in patients with Alzheimer's disease. *New Eng J Med*, **355**, 1525–38.

Shiloh, R., Zemishlany, Z., & Aizenberg, D. (1997). Sulpiride augmentation in people with schizophrenia partially responsive to clozapine. A double-blind, placebo-controlled study. *Brit J Psychiatry*, **171**, 569–73.

Snyder, S.H. (2008). A complex in psychosis. *Nature*, **45**, 38–9.

Snyder, E.M. & Murphy, M.R. (2008). Schizophrenia therapy: beyond atypical antipsychotics. *Nature Reviews*, **7**, 471–2.

Tandon, R., Belmaker, R.H., Gattaz, W.F., *et al.* (2008). World Psychiatric Association Pharmacopsychiatry Section statement on comparative effectiveness of antipsychotics in the treatment of schizophrenia. *Schizophr Res*, **100**, 20–38.

Toirac, I., Sanjuán, J., Aguilar, E.J., *et al.* (2007). Association between CCK-AR gene and schizophrenia with auditory hallucinations. *Psychiatr Genet*, **17**, 47–53.

Ukai, S., Yamamoto, M., Tanaka, M., Shinosaki, K., & Takeda, M. (2007). Donepezil in the treatment of musical hallucinations. *Psychiat Clin Neuros*, **61**, 190–2.

Voruganti, L., & Awad, A.G. (2004). Neuroleptic dysphoria: towards a new síntesis. *Psychopharmacology*, **171**, 121–32.

Weinberger, D.R. (2007). Schizophrenia drug says goodbye to dopamine. *Nat Med*, **13**,1018–19.

Zahodne, L.B., & Fernandez, H.H. (2008). Course, prognosis, and management of psychosis in Parkinson's disease: are current treatments really effective? *CNS Spectrums*, **13** (suppl 4), 26–33.

Chapter 3

Transcranial Magnetic Stimulation

André Aleman and Ralph Hoffman

Introduction

Transcranial Magnetic Stimulation (TMS) is emerging as a novel treatment modality in neurology and psychiatry (Wasserman; Epstein & Ziemann, 2008). TMS aims to modify neural excitability in defined cortical regions. This method of brain stimulation was introduced in 1985 (Barker *et al.*, 1985) and takes advantage of Faraday's law of induction for time-varying currents. Thus, a rapidly changing external magnetic field induces electric current intracranially, i.e., in brain tissue. The time-varying magnetic field is generated by a current pulse through a stimulator coil placed over a certain scalp position. The rapid rise and fall of the magnetic field induces a flow of current in the underlying brain tissue (diameter of approx. 2–3 cm) resulting in membrane depolarization and neural activation (Hallet, 2000). In particular, 1 Hz (or slow) repetitive TMS (rTMS) is usually used in the context of hallucination treatment because it reduces brain excitability (for review, see Hoffman & Cavus, 2002). In contrast, fast rTMS (>5 Hz) is generally used in depression treatment studies, as it has been shown to enhance neuronal excitability.

Intensity of stimulation is usually set at a certain percentage of the individual motor threshold. Motor threshold refers to the strength of the stimulus provided, which is the percentage of the total machine output that is required to produce movement of thumb or fingers. This is relevant, as intensities that are considerably higher than the motor threshold of a participant are associated with a higher risk of inducing an epileptic seizure (at least for rTMS at frequencies > 1 Hz). We should emphasize, however, that when precautions listed in internationally agreed guidelines (Wasserman, 1998) are taken into account, rTMS appears to be very well tolerated. Contraindications for TMS are pace maker, aneurysm clip, heart/vascular clip, prosthetic valve, intracranial metal prosthesis, personal or familial history of epilepsy, medications that reduce the threshold for seizure, and high alcohol or drug consumption. Pregnant women and young children are also excluded from research studies, although they might be subject to TMS for clinical or therapeutic purposes. Since the introduction of the international safety guidelines occurrence of seizures has been very rare. There has, however, been one report of a seizure during 1-Hz temporoparietal rTMS in a patient with tinnitus (Nowak *et al.*, 2006).

In psychiatry, most studies until now concerned the treatment of depression, with recent meta-analyses indicating a significant improvement after TMS as compared with placebo (Gross *et al.*, 2007; Schutter, 2009). A recent meta-analysis has also found beneficial effects of rTMS in reducing negative symptoms in schizophrenia, using high frequency stimulation over the frontal cortex, although this concerned only six studies (De Lange *et al.*, 2010). In studies targeting depression, typical rTMS sessions are conducted daily for 2–3 weeks. rTMS is delivered at a high frequency, in most cases 10 Hz. The location of stimulation is usually the left dorsolateral prefrontal cortex. Location and frequency are based on the hypothesis that the left DLPFC is underactivated in depression. Indeed, there is neuroimaging evidence that supports that hypothesis (Fitzgerald *et al.*, 2008). Positron Emission Tomography (PET) studies confirm the putative activating effect of rTMS on frontal areas (Baeken *et al.*, 2009; Cho & Strafella, 2009). Most studies determined the location of stimulation, left DLPFC, by localizing the motor cortex and moving 5 cm in the anterior plane. It has been shown, however, that this might be a poor localization of DLPFC. Recent studies that targeted the DLPFC in depression using MRI-guided neuronavigation observed stronger improvement of symptoms as compared to the classic method of localization, i.e., 5 cm anterior to the motor strip (Fitzgerald *et al.*, 2009; Herbsman *et al.*, 2009). MRI-guided neuronavigation involves making an MRI scan of the subject's brain, which can then be used during the TMS session to navigate to the spot on the scalp that corresponds to the targeted brain region. The neuronavigator itself consists of special hardware and software to enable the matching of the space of the subject's head to the MRI space. There are three types of neuronavigators: based on magnetic fields (e.g., Neggers *et al.*, 2004), based on infrared (Fernandez *et al.*, 2002), and based on ultrasound (Sack *et al.*, 2006). For the infrared method, trackers are monitored or 'seen' by an infrared optical position sensor. For the ultrasound method, stereotaxic data for the localization of the TMS stimulation site are recorded using an ultrasound-based co-registration system. This system consists of several miniature ultrasound senders, which are attached to the participant's head as well as to the TMS coil. The latter two methods also permit real-time tracking of the TMS coil relative to the subject's brain (as visualized on a computer screen) during the TMS, to check whether the stimulation remains on spot.

Efficacy of TMS for auditory–verbal hallucinations

The first study using rTMS to improve auditory hallucinations was reported in 1999 by Hoffman and colleagues. They studied the effects of 1 Hz TMS over the temporoparietal cortex in three patients with schizophrenia and chronic, medication-resistant Auditory–Verbal Hallucinations (AVHs). The TMS condition was compared with sham stimulation using a blinded, crossover design. All three patients demonstrated greater improvement in hallucination severity following active stimulation compared to sham stimulation. This preliminary finding was followed up with an additional nine patients; a within-subjects analysis comparing active versus sham rTMS found that the former resulted in significant improvements in AVHs relative to sham stimulation (Hoffman *et al.*, 2000). The largest study to date was published five years later (Hoffman *et al.*, 2005) and utilized a parallel-group design with 27 patients in the active TMS group and 23 patients in the sham group. Right-handed patients experiencing auditory hallucinations at least five times per day were randomly allocated to receive either rTMS or sham stimulation. A total of 132 min of rTMS was administered over 9 days at 90% motor threshold. Hallucination change score (this scale is described under the section 'Measurement of hallucination severity') was more improved for rTMS relative to sham stimulation, as was the Clinical Global Impression scale (CGI). The CGI is a 7 point scale that requires the clinician to assess how much the patient's illness has improved or worsened relative to a baseline state at the beginning of the intervention. Hallucination frequency was significantly decreased during rTMS relative to sham stimulation and was a moderator of rTMS effects.

A meta-analysis of studies using rTMS as a treatment for auditory hallucinations supported the efficacy of TMS in reducing hallucinations (Aleman; Sommer & Kahn, 2007). Fifteen studies were identified that reported empirical data regarding rTMS treatment of auditory hallucinations. Of these, 10 studies fulfilled inclusion criteria and were included in the treatment effect analysis. For the 10 studies that were included, the total N was 216. Most studies used highly similar techniques and treatment settings. Patients were characterized by medication-resistant hallucinations, i.e., no clinical improvement after at least two different anti-psychotics. Typically, active rTMS was delivered over the left temporoparietal cortex (the left temporoparietal cortex is generally defined as the position halfway between the T3 and P3 electrode positions of the International 10–20 system, following Hoffman *et al.*, 2003), between 80 and 100% motor threshold is commonly used, and all studies used a frequency of 1 Hz. All studies included a sham rTMS control condition or control group. In sham rTMS, the coil is rotated by 90° so that the magnetic field does not enter the brain. Length of stimulation varied between studies, but was mainly between 15 and 20 min. Finally, the length of treatment varied from 4 to 10 days. Results revealed a mean standardized gain effect size of 0.76 providing support for the efficacy of this treatment in reducing the severity of auditory hallucinations in schizophrenia. When only studies were included that used continuous stimulation during the TMS sessions (nine studies), the mean effect size increased to $d = 0.88$ and heterogeneity among studies disappeared. (One study inserted pauses of 1 min for every minute of stimulation, to prevent heating of the coil). In contrast to the effects obtained on hallucinations, rTMS did not improve positive symptoms in general. Thus, the observed effect was specific to auditory hallucinations. With regard to the duration of the treatment, the meta-analysis did not show larger effect sizes in studies that included more treatment sessions.

A study that was conducted after this meta-analysis reported modest effects of rTMS, which were also present in the placebo condition (Vercammen *et al.*, 2009). Although real TMS was statistically superior to placebo, this was only marginally so. This study compared the classical 1 Hz rTMS over the left temporoparietal cortex (located as in Hoffman *et al.*, 2003) to a bilateral condition in which rTMS was delivered over the left and right temporoparietal location. The rationale for stimulating the left and right hemisphere was based on neuroimaging studies that reported activation of both sites during hallucinations (see Allen *et al.*, 2008). In addition, the authors hypothesized that the bilateral rTMS might reduce emotional distress associated with hallucinations to a larger extent, as the right hemisphere has been implied to a stronger extent in emotional processing. Both active conditions were compared to a sham condition, in which a MagStim placebo coil was used. The trial involved random assignment of 36 patients with schizophrenia to the three conditions, which involved 12 sessions of 20 min 1 Hz rTMS at 90% of the motor threshold over 6 days of treatment. The bilateral condition was not superior to the left hemisphere condition, however.

Finally, a recent study used 20 Hz instead of 1 Hz to improve AVHs in schizophrenia patients (Montagne-Larmurier *et al.*, 2009). The high frequency was used in order to deliver a large number of pulses in a brief period. Eleven patients were studied, rTMS was delivered over only 2 days; they were then followed for 6 months. The target area was identified by fMRI as the highest activation cluster along the posterior part of the left superior temporal sulcus from the BOLD signal of each subject during a language task. The authors reported a significant reduction in global severity and frequency AVHs between baseline and post-treatment day 12. Auditory hallucinations were entirely relieved at 6-month follow-up in two patients. A major limitation of this study was the lack of a sham-control group. The use of fast rTMS at 20 Hz was surprising, as such high frequencies are generally considered to increase excitability of the cortex. However, a recent study in cats reported that TMS pulse trains elicited initial activation (approximately 1 min) and prolonged suppression (5 to 10 min) of neural responses, which was observable both for slow and for fast rTMS (Allen *et al.*, 2007).

A number of issues remain. First, although the effect sizes in the meta-analysis (Aleman *et al.*, 2007) went in a positive direction, some studies did not clearly support the therapeutic efficacy of rTMS on hallucinations (e.g., McIntosh *et al.*, 2004; Lee *et al.*, 2005; Saba, *et al.*, 2006). Future studies should investigate why certain patients respond to rTMS treatment, while others do not seem to improve. Indeed, there is evidence of individual differences regarding treatment effects. For instance, d'Alfonso, *et al.* (2002) observed individual differences in the onset of the improvement. Duration of treatment effects may vary widely. Hoffman *et al.* (2005) reported that mean duration of survivorship was 13.1 weeks; however, survivorship was defined conservatively as return of AVHs to 80% baseline severity or a switch or increase in their anti-psychotic medication, which was the case for 7/45 patients in the survivorship study. There are no studies that investigated the effect of a 'repeat course' of TMS, with the exception of three case reports. Poulet *et al.* (2006) found that a second course of rTMS again greatly improved hallucinations (50% reduction on the AHRS) in a patient that relapsed 10 months after the first course. However, a weekly maintenance stimulation protocol (1-Hz-1000 stimulations at 100% MT each Wednesday) was not effective. Thus, the authors rather consider a 10,000-pulse rTMS course on a 1-week-per-month basis instead of the described 1-day-per-week maintenance protocol. Fitzgerald *et al.* (2006) describe two cases in which rTMS were provided to patients upon relapse of hallucinations following initial successful rTMS treatment in a clinical trial. They conclude that a repeat course of rTMS resulted in a marked improvement in the symptoms experienced by these two patients.

Finally, Thirthalli *et al.* (2008) reported successful use of maintenance rTMS for 8 months in a patient with anti-psychotic-refractory auditory hallucinations.

Factors that may affect responder status include chronicity, beliefs associated with hallucinations (e.g., patients that ascribe the voices to be omnipotent might be less responsive), frequency of hallucinations, the degree that patients wish to give up their voices, and the use of benzodiazepine and anticonvulsant medications (which may limit TMS effects).

Location of stimulation

The diverging findings might be related, in part, to individual variations in terms of the functional anatomical locus of hallucination activity and/or speech processing areas. In all studies, the left temporoparietal area was stimulated, and in a few, also the right temporoparietal area. However, hallucinations involve a much larger network. For instance, although studies suggest the involvement of the left and right temporal/temporoparietal cortex (e.g., Silbersweig *et al.*, 1995; Dierks *et al.*, 1999; Lennox *et al.*, 1999; Shergill *et al.*, 2000), other brain regions have also repeatedly been implicated (see Allen *et al.*, 2008 for a review). These include the thalamus, basal ganglia, cerebellum, Broca's area, and right prefrontal cortex (Sommer *et al.*, 2008). Thus, in order to enhance efficacy, brain imaging methods might be applied to determine the functional locus of hallucination activity individually and to target these regions of interest with rTMS using a neuro-navigator. Patients are scanned whilst experiencing hallucinations (they press a button during hallucinations when in the scanner), and these activation maps are used to navigate to areas for TMS. This approach has been taken in two recent studies. First, Hoffman *et al.* (2007) used fMRI guided rTMS in 16 schizophrenia patients with resistant hallucinations and reported that delivering rTMS to left temporoparietal sites in Wernicke's area and the adjacent supramarginal gyrus was accompanied by a greater rate of AVH improvement compared with sham stimulation and rTMS delivered to anterior temporal sites. In another fMRI-guided TMS study, Sommer *et al.* (2007) compared the efficacy of fMRI-guided rTMS to conventional positioning of the coil using the 10–20 international system. Both groups improved to an equal extent. Further research is needed to establish whether fMRI guidance yields better results.

A limitation of fMRI guidance is that, in order to obtain reliable activation patterns, patients should hallucinate with several intervals in the scanner. That is, activation during hallucinations and during epochs without hallucinations should be compared. The problem here is that most patients do not hallucinate with such intervals of several minutes altered by non-hallucination periods. An alternative method would be to use language activation for fMRI-guided neuronavigation. Thus, activation during language tasks performed in the MRI scanner is used to identify auditory–verbal regions. This method has been used in a few previous studies (Schönfeldt-Lecuona *et al.*, 2004; Montagne-Larmurier *et al.*, 2009). A limitation of this approach may be that language areas do not necessarily overlap completely with the hallucination-relevant regions (which may include a stronger attentional and emotional component).

With the exception of Hoffman *et al.*'s fMRI-guided study, no studies have stimulated prefrontal sites. In a case study (Schreiber *et al.*, 2002) that applied rTMS for command hallucinations, a prefrontal site was also targeted. A schizophrenic patient with a 20-year history of auditory command hallucinations, responding poorly to conventional and novel neuroleptics, was treated with fast (10 Hz) rTMS administered to the right dorsolateral prefrontal cortex. This area was stimulated following documentation of right hypofrontality in pre-treatment single photon emission computed tomography. After 20 rTMS treatments, results for both Brief Psychiatric Rating Scale (BPRS) and Positive and Negative Syndrome Scale (PANSS) scores demonstrated a global improvement. Changes in other ratings scales (assessing depression, general mental state, and sleep) were minor and non-significant. Important to note is that there were no changes in the content, intensity, and frequency of hallucinations as a result of rTMS treatment. At follow-up, 6 weeks after the rTMS treatment ended, all scores (apart from PANSS) returned to pre-rTMS treatment baseline.

Number of stimuli and sessions

Another important issue concerns the duration of treatment, or the total number of pulses delivered to the brain area. Studies differ considerably in this regard. For example, Chibbaro *et al.* (2005) stimulated for 4 days, 15 min every day (a total of 3600 TMS pulses per patient), whereas Vercammen *et al.* (2009) stimulated for 6 days, 40 min a day (in two daily sessions; 14,400 TMS pulses per patient). It is conceivable that a longer duration of treatment, and a higher number of total TMS pulses, would relate to a better outcome. This has been suggested to be the case for rTMS treatment of depression (Gross *et al.*, 2007). However, the available data for hallucination trials do not unambiguously support this suggestion (Aleman *et al.*, 2007). Indeed, the Vercammen *et al.* (2009) trial did not report stronger effects than the Chibbaro *et al.* (2005) trial. On the other hand, the trials that have been published up to now are all small (*N* does not exceed 25 per group), and as a myriad of other factors may affect outcome, the statistical power to conduct a moderator analysis might be lacking. This underlines the need of larger, multicenter trials, as have been conducted for TMS in depression (e.g., O'Reardon *et al.*, 2007).

Cognitive changes

A number of studies have included neuropsychological testing in the design of the trial, to quantify possible changes in cognitive functioning. These studies report that there was no evidence of neurocognitive impairment associated with rTMS (D'Alfonso *et al.*, 2002; Fitzgerald *et al.*, 2005; Hoffman *et al.*, 2005). In the study by D'Alfonso *et al.* (2002), neuropsychological measures were included that were primarily aimed at auditory and verbal functions: An auditory imagery test in which subjects were asked to mentally compare acoustic characteristics of everyday sounds; the Rey Auditory–Verbal Learning Test (verbal memory); the Token Test, short form (verbal comprehension); and tests of verbal fluency and phoneme detection. The following nonverbal measures were also included: Judgment of Line Orientation, Line Bisection Test, Benton Visual Retention Test, and the

Test for Facial Recognition, short form. Of the neurocognitive measures, only the auditory imagery test revealed a significant performance difference between baseline and post-test; performance was significantly better at post-test. Fitzgerald *et al.* (2005) also included a neuropsychological battery in their study, comprising the Hopkins Verbal Learning Test, Verbal Fluency, Digit Span (forwards and backwards), Brief Visuospatial Memory Test-Revised, and the Visuospatial Digit Span. No differences between TMS and sham groups were observed on these tests. The Hoffman *et al.* (2005) study included the following neuropsychological measures: The California Verbal Learning Test (CVLT), Controlled Oral Word Association Test, and Animal Naming, which assess semantic processing and clustering of verbal information; the Digit Recall Task (nondistraction and distraction conditions), WRAT-R Reading Test, Trail Making Test (A and B versions), Grooved Pegboard (dominant and nondominant), Digit Symbol Task, and Temporal Orientation. A comparison of performance for the full neuropsychological battery following the treatment phase relative to baseline did not reveal any significant differences for patients randomized to rTMS versus sham stimulation.

Little is known as to which cognitive mechanisms are being altered in effective rTMS treatment. In the only study to date to have examined this issue, Brunelin *et al.* (2006) examined cognitive mechanisms and found that effective rTMS treatment coincided with improvements in source monitoring functioning, which has been argued to be an important mechanism in hallucinations (cf. Bentall, 1990). Alternatively, rTMS could alter connectivity in language processing pathways, and for example, restore a disbalance in connectivity between language production centres in the frontal lobe and speech perception areas in the temporparietal region (cf. Hoffman *et al.*, 2007). However, no other studies have examined other cognitive mechanisms underlying effective rTMS treatment in (auditory) hallucinations.

Side effects and safety

TMS has few side effects, the most frequent ones being scalp discomfort during stimulation and headache after stimulation. The headache usually disappears within a couple of hours after stimulation; analgesics are effective in treating the headache. TMS has a low rate (about 5%) of discontinuation due to adverse effects (most commonly headache) and has no systemic side effects typical with oral psychopharmacotherapy (such as sexual side effects, weight gain, nausea, constipation, or dry mouth). A recent paper extensively reviews safety issues and updated application guidelines (Rossi *et al.*, in press).

Little is known about the long-term effects of TMS, although there are no indications that there are any undesired side effects. Consequences for brain function deserve more investigation. An MRI study in healthy subjects indicated no structural brain changes in humans after high-dose rTMS (Niehaus *et al.*, 2000). In patients, Hoffman *et al.* (2005) and D'Alfonso *et al.* (2002) did not find any indication of negative effects of active rTMS on cognition. However, more studies are needed that examine possible side effects in the context of rTMS treatment.

Interactions may occur between type of medication and effectiveness of rTMS. In Hoffman *et al.* (2000), not all patients showed robust improvements after active rTMS and one factor contributing to this variable response was suggested to be concurrent anticonvulsant drug treatment, which seemed to reduce rTMS effects. In addition, symptoms prompting administration of anticonvulsant drugs (e.g., mood liability) were suggested to be negative predictors of rTMS response. Studies examining the effects of rTMS have also exclusively focused on auditory hallucinations and have not looked at the effects of rTMS in hallucinations from other modalities. One would presume that there is no change in these (i.e., non-auditory) hallucinations as the brain area stimulated in typical rTMS studies is targeted at auditory–verbal processing areas.

Measurement of hallucination severity

It is notoriously difficult to measure such a subjective experience, as is a hallucination. Hoffman *et al.* (2003) have pointed out that severity of AHs depend on several factors, including frequency, loudness, verbal content, affective charge, and attentional salience. Moreover, dimensions critical for determining symptom severity can be different for different patients and often do not covary between or within patients. Therefore, Hoffman *et al.* (2003) proposed a composite, patient-specific targeted symptom scale (hallucination change scale). The scale is anchored at baseline using the narrative description of AHs provided by the patient for the prior 24 h, which is assigned a score of 10. For subsequent assessments, the hallucination change scale ranges from 0 to 20 (with a score of 20 corresponding to hallucinations twice as severe as baseline). The strength of this measure is that it approaches clinical judgment as made in daily practice. A limitation may be that different clinicians may arrive at different values for the same patient, due to the subjective nature of rating the experience. In any case, it will be important that the interviewer performing the ratings should be blind for the treatment condition. A widely used scale in rTMS studies is the auditory hallucinations rating scale (Hoffman *et al.*, 2003), which is a 7-item scale measuring frequency, reality, loudness, number of voices, length, attentional salience, and distress level. This is a self-report scale, a drawback of which might be that the patient cannot always evaluate inner experiences in a consistent way. Most studies report composite scores to measure improvement, making it difficult to say exactly which aspects of hallucinations are improved after rTMS treatment. However, in the few studies who do attempt to identify which hallucination characteristics are modified after rTMS treatment, improvement is usually attributed to reductions in hallucination frequency (cf. Hoffman *et al.*, 2005). Some studies have used the Psychotic Symptom Rating Scales (PSYRATS; Haddock *et al.*, 1999), which are semi-structured interviews designed to assess the subjective characteristics of hallucinations and delusions. The Auditory Hallucinations Subscale (AHS) has 11 items: for frequency, duration, controllability, loudness, location; severity and intensity of distress; amount and degree of negative content; beliefs about the origin of voices; and disruption. The PSYRATS has been shown to have good inter-rater reliability, retest reliability, internal consistency, and sensitivity to change (Drake *et al.*, 2007).

Blinding

A serious problem in rTMS treatment studies regards the issue of blinding. Most studies report that they were single-blinded, and some even claim to be double blind. However, even when a placebo coil is used, the person delivering the TMS can be easily aware of the condition. That is, the distinction between real and sham TMS is readily made on the basis of muscle twitches in the face, scalp area, or extremities (when the coil is moved over the motor cortex). The same holds for the patient: Real TMS gives a particular sensation on the scalp (similar to tapping of the scalp with a finger), whereas sham does not produce these sensations or only to a very weak extent. Researchers are working on new placebo coils, such as the 'Real Electro-Magnetic Placebo' (REMP) device, which can simulate the scalp sensation induced by the real TMS while leaving both the visual impact and acoustic sensation of real TMS unaltered (Rossi *et al.*, 2007). The use of such coils will improve the methodological rigour of TMS studies.

Conclusion

It seems safe to conclude that rTMS has shown some promise for the treatment of hallucinations. Several studies have reported significant improvement in hallucination severity after a course of rTMS, and this has been confirmed meta-analytically. However, due to the small sample sizes, large placebo effects and other methodological difficulties, including location of stimulation and the chronicity of the groups studied, strong conclusions cannot be reached at this point. Future research should definitely include larger groups, in a multi-centre effort. Finally, it is important to note that the majority of rTMS studies included treatment-resistant patients. Given the favourable side effect profile of TMS, it is conceivable to extend its use to less chronic patient groups. For example, first-episode patients with primary auditory hallucinations could benefit from rTMS, maybe even without needing medication. We are aware, however, that this might be a small group. On the other hand, TMS could also be used as an adjunctive for those patients that use medication but still complain about the hallucinations. Indeed, given the fact that TMS primarily seems to reduce the *frequency* of hallucinations (Hoffman *et al.*, 2005), and not so much other aspects of hallucinations, it might be effective to combine it with cognitive therapies, so that people learn to cope with their hallucinatory propensity and may reduce distress due to hallucinations. Whether the use of MRI-based neuronavigation will improve the efficacy of TMS should also be determined in the coming years.

References

Aleman, A., Sommer, I.E., & Kahn, R.S. (2007). Efficacy of slow transcranial magnetic stimulation in the treatment of resistant auditory hallucinations in schizophrenia: A meta-analysis. *J Clin Psychiatry*, **68**, 416–21.

Allen, E.A., Pasley, B.N., Duong, T., & Freeman, R.D. (2007). Transcranial magnetic stimulation elicits coupled neural and hemodynamic consequences. *Science*, **317**, 1918–21.

Allen, P., Larøi, F., McGuire, P.K., & Aleman, A. (2008). The hallucinating brain: A review of structural and functional neuroimaging studies of hallucinations. *Neurosci Biobehav Rev*, **32**, 175–91.

Baeken, C., De Raedt, R., Van Hove, C., Clerinx, P., De Mey, J., & Bossuyt, A. (2009). HF-rTMS treatment in medication-resistant melancholic depression: Results from 18FDG-PET brain imaging. *CNS Spectrums,* **14**, 439–48.

Barker, A.T., Freeston, I.L., Jalinous, R., Merton, P.A., & Morton, H.B. (1985). Magnetic stimulation of the human brain. *J Physiol (Lond.)* **369**, 3.

Bentall, R.P. (1990). The illusion of reality: A review and integration of psychological research on hallucinations. *Psychol Bull,* **107**, 82–95.

Brunelin, J., Poulet, E., Bediou, B., *et al.* (2006). Low frequency repetitive transcranial magnetic stimulation improves source monitoring deficit in hallucinating patients with schizophrenia. *Schizophr Res,* **81**, 41–45.

Chibbaro, G., Daniele, M., Alagona, G., *et al.* (2005). Repetitive transcranial magnetic stimulation in schizophrenic patients reporting auditory hallucinations. *Neurosc Lett,* **383**, 54–7.

Cho, S.S., & Strafella, A.P. (2009). rTMS of the left dorsolateral prefrontal cortex modulates dopamine release in the ipsilateral anterior cingulate cortex and orbitofrontal cortex. *PLoS One,* **4**(8), e6725.

D'Alfonso, A.A.L., Aleman, A., Kessels, R.P.C., *et al.* (2002). TMS of auditory cortex in schizophrenia: effects on hallucinations and neurocognition. *Journal of Neuropsychiatry and Clinical Neurosciences,* **14**, 77–79.

Dierks, T., Linden, D.E., Jandl, M., *et al.* (1999). Activation of Heschl's gyrus during auditory hallucinations. *Neuron,* **22**, 615–21.

Drake, R., Haddock, G., Tarrier, N., Bentall, R., & Lewis, S. (2007). The psychotic symptom rating scales (PSYRATS): Their usefulness and properties in first episode psychosis. *Schizophr Res,* **89**(1–3), 119–22.

Fernandez, E., Alfaro, A., Tormos, J.M., *et al.* (2002). Mapping of the human visual cortex using image-guided transcranial magnetic stimulation. *Brain Research Protocols,* **10**, 115–24.

Fitzgerald, P.B., Benitez, J., Daskalakis, J.Z., *et al.* (2005). A double-blind sham-controlled trial of repetitive transcranial magnetic stimulation in the treatment of refractory auditory hallucinations. *J Clin Psychopharmacol,* **25**(4), 358–62.

Fitzgerald, P.B., Benitez, J., Daskalakis, J.Z., De Castella, A., & Kulkarni, J. (2006).The treatment of recurring auditory hallucinations in schizophrenia with rTMS. *The World Journal of Biological Psychiatry,* **7**(2), 119–22.

Fitzgerald, P.B., Laird, A.R., Maller, J., & Daskalakis, ZJ. (2008). A meta-analytic study of changes in brain activation in depression. *Human Brain Mapping,* **29**(6), 683–95.Erratum in *Human Brain Mapping,* **29**(6), 736.

Gross, M., Nakamura, L., Pascual-Leone, A., & Fregni, F. (2007). Has repetitive transcranial magnetic stimulation (rTMS) treatment for depression improved? A systematic review and meta-analysis comparing the recent vs. the earlier rTMS studies. *Acta Psychiatr Scand,* **116**, 165–73.

Haddock, G., McCarron, J., Tarrier, N., & Faragher, E.B. (1999). Scales to measure dimensions of hallucinations and delusions: The psychotic symptom rating scales (PSYRATS). *Psychol Med,* **29**(4), 879–89.

Hallett, M. (2000). Transcranial magnetic stimulation and the human brain. *Nature,* **406**(6792), 147–50.

Herbsman, T., Avery, D., Ramsey, D., *et al.* (2009). More lateral and anterior prefrontal coil location is associated with better repetitive transcranial magnetic stimulation antidepressant response. *Biol Psychiatry,* **66**(5), 509–15.

Hoffman, R.E., Boutros, N.N., Berman, R.M., *et al.* (1999). Transcranial magnetic stimulation of left temporoparietal cortex in three patients reporting hallucinated 'voices'. *Biol Psychiatry,* **46**, 130–32.

Hoffman, R.E., Boutros, N.N., Hu, S., Berman, R.M., Krystal, J.H., & Charney, D.S. (2000). Transcranial magnetic stimulation and auditory hallucinations in schizophrenia. *Lancet,* **355**, 1073–5.

Hoffman, R.E., & Cavus, I. (2002). Slow transcranial magnetic stimulation, long-term depotentiation, and brain hyperexcitability disorders. *Am J Psychiatry*, **159**, 1093–102.

Hoffman, R.E., Hampson, M., Wu, K., Anderson, *et al.* (2007). Probing the pathophysiology of auditory/verbal hallucinations by combining functional magnetic resonance imaging and transcranial magnetic stimulation. *Cerebral Cortex*, **17**, 2733–2743.

Hoffman, R.E., Hawkins, K.A., Gueorguieva, R., *et al.* (2003). Transcranial magnetic stimulation of left temporoparietal cortex and medication-resistant auditory hallucinations. *Arch Gen Psychiatry*, **60**, 49–56.

Hoffman, R.E., Gueorguieva, R., Hawkins, K.A., *et al.* (2005). Temporoparietal transcranial magnetic stimulation for auditory hallucinations: Safety, efficacy and moderators in a fifty patient sample. *Biol Psychiatry*, **58**, 97–104.

Lee, S.H., Kim, W., Chung, Y.C., *et al.* (2005). A double blind study showing that two weeks of daily repetitive TMS over the left or right temporoparietal cortex reduces symptoms in patients with schizophrenia who are having treatment-refractory auditory hallucinations. *Neurosci Lett*, **376**(3), 177–81.

Lennox, B.R., Park, S.B., Jones, P.B., & Morris, P.G. (1999). Spatial and temporal mapping of neural activity associated with auditory hallucinations. *Lancet*, **353**, 644.

McIntosh, A.M., Semple, D., Tasker, K., *et al.* (2004). Transcranial magnetic stimulation for auditory hallucinations in schizophrenia. *Psychiatry Res*, **127**(1–2), 9–17.

Montagne-Larmurier, A., Etard, O., Razafimandimby, A., Morello, R., & Dollfus, S. (2009). Two-day treatment of auditory hallucinations by high frequency rTMS guided by cerebral imaging: A 6 month follow-up pilot study. *Schizophr Res*, **113**(1), 77–83.

Niehaus, L., Hoffman, K.T., Grosse, P., Roricht, S., & Meyer, B.U. (2000). MRI study of human brain exposed to high-dose repetitive magnetic simulation of visual cortex. *Neurology*, **54**, 256–8.

Neggers, S.F., Langerak, T.R., Schutter, D.J., *et al.* (2004). A stereotactic method for image-guided transcranial magnetic stimulation validated with fMRI and motor-evoked potentials. *Neuroimage*, **21**(4), 1805–17.

Nowak, D.A., Hoffman, U., Connomann, B.J., & Schonfeldt-Lecuona, C. (2006). Epileptic seizure following 1 Hz repetitive transcranial magnetic stimulation. *Clin Neurophysiol*, **117**, 1630.

O'Reardon, J.P., Solvason, H.B., Janicak, P.G., *et al.* (2007). Efficacy and safety of transcranial magnetic stimulation in the acute treatment of major depression: a multisite randomized controlled trial. *Biol Psychiatry*, **62**, 1208–1216.

Poulet, E., Brunelin, J., Bediou, B., *et al.* (2005). Slow transcranial magnetic stimulation can rapidly reduce resistant auditory hallucinations in schizophrenia. *Biol Psychiatry*, **57**, 188–91.

Poulet, E., Brunelin, J., Kallel, L., *et al.* (2006). Is rTMS efficient as a maintenance treatment for auditory verbal hallucinations? A case report. *Schizophr Res*, **84**, 183–184.

Rossi, S., Ferro, M., Cincotta, M., *et al.* (2007). A real electro-magnetic placebo (REMP) device for sham transcranial magnetic stimulation (TMS). *Clin Neurophysiol*, **118**(3), 709–16.

Rossi, S., Hallett, M., Rossini, P.M., & Pascual-Leone, A. (in press). The Safety of TMS Consensus Group. (in press). Safety, ethical considerations, and application guidelines for the use of transcranial magnetic stimulation in clinical practice and research. *Clin Neurophysiol*.

Saba, G., Verdon, C.M., Kalalou, K., *et al.* (2006). Transcranial magnetic stimulation in the treatment of schizophrenic symptoms: A double blind sham controlled study. *J Psychiatric Res*, **40**, 147–52.

Sack, A.T., Kohler, A., Linden, D.E., Goebel, R., & Muckli, L. (2006). The temporal characteristics of motion processing in hMT/V5+: Combining fMRI and neuronavigated TMS. *Neuroimage*, **29**(4), 1326–35.

Schönfeldt-Lecuona, C., Grön, G., Walter, H., *et al.* (2004). Stereotaxic rTMS for the treatment of auditory hallucinations in schizophrenia. *Neuroreport*, **15**(10), 1669–73.

Schreiber, S., Dannon, P.N., Goshen, E., Amiaz, R., Zwas, T.S., & Grunhaus, L. (2002). Right prefrontal rTMS treatment for refractory auditory command hallucinations – a neuroSPECT assisted case study. *Psychiatry Res*, **116**, 113–7.

Schutter, D.J. (2009). Antidepressant efficacy of high-frequency transcranial magnetic stimulation over the left dorsolateral prefrontal cortex in double-blind sham-controlled designs: A meta-analysis. *Psychol Med*, **39**(1), 65–75.

Shergill, S.S., Brammer, M.J., Williams, S.C., Murray, R.M., & McGuire, P.K. (2000). Mapping auditory hallucinations in schizophrenia using functional magnetic resonance imaging. *Archives of General Psychiatry*, **57**, 1033–8.

Silbersweig, D.A., Stern, E., Frith, C., *et al.* (1995). A functional neuroanatomy of hallucinations in schizophrenia. *Nature*, **378**, 176–9.

Sommer, I.E., Diederen, K.M., Blom, J.D., *et al.* (2008). Auditory verbal hallucinations predominantly activate the right inferior frontal area. *Brain*, **131**, 3169–77.

Sommer, I.E., Slotema, C.W., de Weijer, A.D., *et al.* (2007). Can fMRI-guidance improve the efficacy of rTMS treatment for auditory verbal hallucinations? *Schizophr Res*, **93**, 406–8.

Thirthalli, J., Bharadwaj, B., Kulkarni, S., Gangadhar, B.N., Kharawala, S., & Andrade, C. (2008). Successful use of maintenance rTMS for 8 months in a patient with antipsychotic-refractory auditory hallucinations. *Schizophr Res*, **100**(1–3), 351–2.

Vercammen, A., Knegtering, H., Bruggeman, R., *et al.* (2009). Effects of bilateral repetitive transcranial magnetic stimulation on treatment resistant auditory–verbal hallucinations in schizophrenia: A randomized controlled trial. *Schizophr Res*, **114**, 172–9.

Wassermann, E.M. (1998). Risk and safety of repetitive transcranial magnetic stimulation: Report and suggested guidelines from the International Workshop on the Safety of Repetitive Transcranial Magnetic Stimulation, June 5–7, 1996. *Electroencephalogr and Clin Neurophysiol*, **108**, 1–16.

Wassermann, E., Epstein, C., & Ziemann, U., (Eds). (2008). *Oxford handbook of transcranial stimulation*. Oxford: Oxford University Press.

Chapter 4

Individual Cognitive Behavioural Therapy of auditory–verbal hallucinations

Ben Smith, Brendan O'Sullivan, Philip Watson, Juliana Onwumere, Paul Bebbington, Philippa Garety, Daniel Freeman, David Fowler, and Elizabeth Kuipers

In this chapter, we consider individual Cognitive Behavioural Therapy (CBT) for hallucinations. We provide a review of the theoretical and empirical literature and outline the treatment strategies used. We detail a clinical case of individual CBT for auditory–verbal hallucinations, describing the change processes from the perspective of both client and therapist. In particular, we consider the role of illness perceptions in the maintenance and psychological treatment of hallucinations. We then reflect on future directions and limitations of the CBT strategies described.

Theory and empirical evidence

It is important to note that as cognitive behavioural therapies for psychosis have developed they have increasingly done so in tandem with theoretical developments in our understanding of psychotic phenomena. Cognitive behavioural models of psychosis (e.g., Garety *et al.*, 2001, 2007; Morrison, 2001; Birchwood, 2003) emphasize the central role of emotional dysfunction as a precursor, and consequence of psychosis. These influential models also suggest that cognitive appraisals and perceptions concerning the nature of psychotic symptoms (including hallucinations) will influence the maintenance or recurrence of symptoms through coping responses, emotional dysfunction, and cognitive processes such as reasoning biases.

Cognitive-behavioural treatments of hallucinations have generally focused on auditory hallucinations. In comparison, visual, olfactory, and tactile hallucinations have received little attention (Gauntlett-Gilbert & Kuipers, 2003). There is no real consensus on a cognitive model for auditory hallucinations, although most (e.g., Johns *et al.*, 2001; Morrison, 2001) assume that auditory hallucinations are associated with speech processing in some way and that some sort of misattribution of inner speech is implicated. Rathod *et al.* (2008) note that in cognitive models of schizophrenia hallucinations are conceptualized as an individual's own automatic thought perceived as originating outside his or her own mind. Auditory, visual, and somatic hallucinations are therefore seen as internal cognitive phenomena that have been externalized and often lead to problematic and powerful emotional and behavioural responses. Cognitive models propose that under stress, thoughts can transform through inner speech to hallucinations (e.g., a voice telling an individual 'You are no good at anything'). These hallucinations may then be maintained by safety behaviours (e.g., avoiding work) as well as by distressing explanations (e.g., 'The Devil is speaking to me' or 'I am going insane') (Rathod *et al.*, 2008).

Meta-analyses of randomized controlled trials (e.g., Zimmerman *et al.*, 2005) support the efficacy of CBT in the treatment of symptoms of schizophrenia that are refractory to antipsychotic medication. The most consistent effect of CBT has been the improvement of positive and negative symptoms, particularly persistent delusions (Drury *et al.*, 1996; Kuipers *et al.*, 1998; Tarrier *et al.*, 1999, 2004; Sensky *et al.*, 2000). Unfortunately, meta-analyses rarely report the specific effects on auditory hallucinations and tend to report only the effect on positive symptoms overall. We know, however, that auditory hallucinations are prevalent in over 60% of individuals diagnosed with schizophrenia (Slade & Bentall, 1988), are often the most common and the most distressing symptom, and are explicitly targeted by CBT.

Zimmerman *et al.* (2005) conducted a meta-analysis in which symptom reduction of positive symptoms was 35% greater in the CBT group than in controls. They also found that the success rate for reducing positive symptoms increased from 41% in controls to 59% with CBT (Zimmermann *et al.*, 2005). The authors report that the overall fixed effect model effect size (FEM ES; an aggregate of the effect sizes across the studies) of CBT on positive symptoms was 0.35, with greater effect during acute psychotic episodes (ES, 0.57) than in the chronic state (ES, 0.27).

Pfammatter *et al.* (2006) in their review of the meta-analyses themselves concluded that CBT led to substantial declines in general psychopathology (ES, 0.45) and persistent reductions in positive symptoms (ES, 0.47). Furthermore, in their review of psychosocial treatments, Patterson and Leeuwenkamp (2008) report that the effects of CBT have generally been found to be stable through time with effects lasting from 6 months to 2 years after the cessation of treatment (e.g., Drury *et al.*, 1996; Tarrier *et al.*, 1999; Sensky *et al.*, 2000; Bechdolf *et al.*, 2005; Startup *et al.*, 2005; Temple & Ho, 2005).

Wykes *et al.* (2008) explored the effect sizes of current CBT trials. Thirty-four CBT trials were used as source data for a meta-analysis and investigation of the effects of trial methodology. Wykes *et al.* (2008) reported that there were overall beneficial effects for the target symptoms (33 studies; effect size [95% confidence interval {CI}, 0.548]) as well as significant effects for positive symptoms (32 studies), negative symptoms (23 studies), functioning (15 studies), mood (13 studies), and social anxiety (2 studies) with effects ranging from 0.35 to 0.44. Importantly, trials in which assessors were aware of group allocation had a larger effect size (approximately 50–100%). Wykes *et al.* (2008) conclude that as in other meta-analyses, CBT had a beneficial effect on positive symptoms. However, they warn that psychological treatment trials that make no attempt to mask group allocation are more likely to have inflated effect sizes.

Turkington *et al.* (2008) specifically address the issue of the medium term durability of individual CBT interventions. They report a five-year follow-up study (*n* = 59) of individuals who participated in a randomized controlled trial of CBT and befriending (BF). In comparison to BF and usual treatment, CBT showed evidence of a significantly greater and more durable effect on overall symptom severity (number needed to treat = 10.36, CI: 10.21, 10.51) and level of negative symptoms (number needed to treat = 5.22, CI: 5.06, 5.37) at five-year follow-up. Turkington *et al.* (2008) argue that the initial cost of CBT for individuals with medication refractory schizophrenia may be justified in light of symptomatic benefits that persist over the medium term. Turkington *et al.* (2008) also note that CBT can be fully manualized (e.g., Kingdon & Turkington, 2005) with clear protocols for training and supervision (e.g., Kingdon & Turkington, 2003). Quality assurance in terms of therapists' adherence to therapy style and proposed interventions can also be independently rated (Haddock *et al.*, 2001; Rollinson *et al.*, 2008).

In their review, Wykes *et al.* (2008) note that evidence-based guidance in the United States and United Kingdom do include CBT for psychosis. In 2003, in the UK, the National Institute for Clinical Excellence (NICE) included CBT in its preferred list of treatments for schizophrenia. In the updated 2009 NICE guidelines, CBT for psychosis retains evidence for a small effect size and continues to be recommended in the UK in the 2009 guidelines. Wykes *et al.* (2008) also note that CBT is recommended in the Schizophrenia Patient Outcome Report Team guidance in the United States.

Theory and practice of treatment strategies

Individual cognitive behaviour therapy differs subtly in its emphasis across those involved in clinical research; however, the theoretical advances made by Birchwood and colleagues tend to influence much of the CBT in the UK today. Birchwood and Trower (2006) note that, like drug trials, the majority of CBT for psychosis trials have actually aimed to directly eradicate or ameliorate the symptoms of psychosis. They recommend a contrasting treatment in which their goal is not the eradication of symptoms per se, but rather the reduction of distress and dysfunctional behaviours that exacerbate and maintain symptoms.

In their cognitive model of hallucinations, Chadwick and Birchwood (1994) and Birchwood and Chadwick (1997) showed empirically that distressing affect and behaviour arising from hallucinations are not simply the result of the content or topography of voices, but reflect the voice hearers' appraisal of the meaning of the voices (also see Trower *et al.*, this volume). The hallucination is therefore seen as an activating event (A), which is then appraised by the individual in the context of their belief system (B) and which leads to emotions and safety behaviours (C). The authors argue that this forms a cognitive–emotional–behavioural mechanism that maintains the belief in the power/dominance of the voice.

The treatment approach outlined by Birchwood *et al.*, proposes that an increase in perceived control over hallucinations, for instance, or a reduction in distress associated with them may have an enormous impact on quality of life even if the frequency or volume of the hallucinations remains unchanged.

The focus of CBT for hallucinations according to Birchwood *et al.* is therefore to change fundamentally the nature of an individual's relationship with their voices, by challenging their power and/or omnipotence, thus reducing the motivation to act on them. Based on this approach Birchwood and Trower (2006) have also developed specific individual CBT strategies for command hallucinations (also see Meaden *et al.*, this volume).

This type of exposure and modification of the content of the beliefs underlying an individual's auditory hallucinations has also been described in detail by Haddock and colleagues (Haddock *et al.*, 1993, 1998; Bentall *et al.*, 1994). Their aim is, through exposure to hallucination content and insight into its relationship to current thoughts, for individuals to recognize that their experiences are internally generated and therefore potentially amenable to modification. Thoughts and beliefs relating to the hallucinations are then modified using standard cognitive-behavioural methods to modify the impact of the content.

Morrison (2002) describes a single case example of cognitive therapy for drug-resistant auditory hallucinations that clearly illustrates a series of key elements to the cognitive approach to treatment. We will briefly reconsider this case example here. Steven experienced auditory hallucinations and was very motivated to reduce the distress that they caused. It was therefore agreed in CBT that efforts would be made to reduce distress and increase control even if voice frequency was unchanged. In order to achieve this, the therapist worked hard, in the first instance, to establish a basic cognitive-behavioural principle— that the interpretation of events and the subsequent responsive behaviours are important in creating and maintaining distress, not simply the events themselves.

A simple formulation of Steven's voices allowed him to see that the interpretation of the voices was what caused the majority of his distress, rather than the voices themselves. Alternative explanations of voices were considered and weighed up in light of the available evidence. These were (1) that the voices were a higher power, (2) that the voices were a form of mental illness, and (3) that the voices were an unusual thought process. To aid this discussion, Steven was given a lot of information about how common it is to hear voices. He soon started to conclude that there may be some link between his thoughts (often salient, important concerns) and his voices. The content of Steven's voices was dealt with directly using discursive cognitive therapy, weighing up the evidence for the assertions that the voices made (e.g., you will never get a girlfriend). Self-focused attention was also addressed. By focusing on his environment (practiced and tested out using behavioural experiments), he was able to ameliorate and sometimes prevent his voices. Steven's scores on the PANSS positive subscale reduced from 25 pre-treatment to 11 post-treatment and from 25 on the PSYRATS hallucinations subscale to 17.

CBT in psychosis can also differ in emphasis according to the specific client group. Valmaggia *et al.* (2005) describe three phases of CBT used with young people experiencing psychosis for the first time. Therapy begins with an engagement phase in which a collaborative relationship between therapist and client develops. The therapist aims to establish a mutual goal of reducing distress (see Birchwood *et al.*, above). In the second phase, a shared case formulation is drawn up, based on a detailed assessment. The hope is to establish links between thoughts, emotions, and behaviours. With auditory hallucinations, cognitive therapy techniques are used to change the beliefs about the origin, power, and dangerousness of voices in line with Chadwick and Birchwood (1994). In the last phase of therapy, treatment gains are consolidated and attention is given to relapse prevention strategies. Valmaggia *et al.* (2005) show how theoretical ideas originally developed around schizophrenia can be applied with young people experiencing psychosis for the first time.

More recently, the specific idea of influencing illness perceptions in CBT for psychosis has been suggested (Watson *et al.*, 2006). As discussed above, the aim in CBT across many disorders including psychosis is to develop a less threatening alternative explanation for current distressing experiences. This aim may be particularly relevant for people with a diagnosis of schizophrenia, whose illness perceptions may be particularly negative (Watson *et al.*, 2006). Illness perception research across a range of disorders shows that negative perceptions can predict poor outcomes (Hagger & Orbell, 2003). Watson *et al.* (2006) suggest that CBT should focus on promoting and shaping positive appraisals in an attempt to enhance and maintain emotional well-being.

We suggest here that illness perceptions form an important group of appraisals relevant to those experiencing auditory hallucinations. These are beliefs relating to how individuals make sense of, and understand, their health status (see Lobban *et al.*, 2003). They are thus a form of meta-cognition.

Leventhal *et al.* (1984) first proposed that people faced with a health threat assume the role of an active problem solver, in that they formulate a cognitive representation of their illness. They argued that these representations cover five core constructs: identity (the symptoms and label associated with the illness), cause (the aetiological attribution of the illness), cure/control (the extent to which they perceive their condition to be amenable to cure or control), consequences (the personal, social, and financial consequences associated with the illness), and timeline (how long they believe their illness will last). These cognitions are held to influence the practical and emotional responses to a health threat.

To measure the illness perceptions that make up Leventhal *et al.*,'s model, Weinman *et al.* (1996) developed the Illness Perception Questionnaire (IPQ). The IPQ has recently been used to assess the role of illness perceptions in non-affective psychosis. Watson *et al.* (2006) analysed a group of 100 individuals diagnosed with non-affective psychosis assessed within 3 months of relapse. Illness perceptions explained 46, 36, and 34% of the variance in depression, anxiety, and self-esteem, respectively. Perceptions of a longer timeline and more negative consequences were positively and independently correlated with depression. Thus negative illness perceptions in non-affective psychosis were clearly related to emotional dysfunction, supporting previous research (e.g., Jolley & Garety, 2004; Lobban *et al.*, 2004). Of importance here is that cognitive behavioural models of psychosis (e.g., Garety *et al.*, 2001, 2007; Morrison, 2001; Birchwood, 2003) emphasize the central role of emotional dysfunction as a precursor, symptom, and consequence of the symptoms of psychosis.

Using the Personal Beliefs and Illness Questionnaire, Birchwood et al. (1993) reported that a perceived loss of control over psychosis predicted demoralization and depression. Iqbal et al. (2000) used the same measure to assess 105 individuals with schizophrenia. They concluded that post-psychotic depression results from negative appraisals of illness and that depression then leads to further pessimistic illness perceptions. Birchwood (2003) argued that the emotional dysfunction in psychosis is therefore, at least in part, a psychological reaction to the psychosis itself (e.g., fear, avoidance, and catastrophic thinking).

The interest in illness perceptions in psychosis is a recent development. Insight is the conventional way of conceptualizing how people with a psychiatric illness, and particularly schizophrenia, appraise their experience of it. It implies a degree of acceptance of the idea of illness. However, David (1998) has reported that standard measures of insight are only modestly associated with outcome. He also suggested that emotional dysfunction in schizophrenia may be related to individuals appreciating the negative personal and social consequences associated with having (or being labelled with) a severe mental illness. This assertion appears to be supported by the recent research evidence (e.g., Watson et al., 2006).

Importantly, illness perceptions have been shown to be amenable to manipulation. Challenging negative beliefs about the controllability of an illness and developing individualized 'recovery action plans' has been shown to promote improved outcome in non-psychiatric conditions (Petrie et al., 2002). It may therefore be possible to target such negative illness perceptions within existing psychological treatments for psychosis, such as CBT.

On the basis of the work of Birchwood et al., and Garety et al., we propose the following approach to cognitive behavioural treatment. Perceptions of controllability over an illness and perceptions of an illness's consequences can be assessed, 'challenged', and re-aligned in a more adaptive way. The introduction of new unbiased information on others' experiences of coping with psychotic phenomena (such as hallucinations) can reinforce the cognitive process of normalizing them and making them less threatening. We propose that this normalizing approach may lend itself especially well to individuals experiencing anomalous experiences such as auditory hallucinations.

Another strategy is to shift the focus of attention outside of oneself. This can reduce distress and depression and enhance vocational and recreational functioning in a range of conditions in psychosis. It can also provide a competition of cues to reduce attending to symptoms in isolation, thus eroding the strength of an illness identity. In addition to this, exposing oneself to external environments (e.g., family, the internet, therapists, etc.) allows the use of these sources of social support to act as a stress buffer, thus reducing the probability of relapse. Engagement with such sources of support can allow for disconfirmation of negative thoughts. This further allows for the suggestion of substitute activities to counteract maladaptive coping activities that may only have been serving to reinforce and maintain previous low mood and symptoms.

Techniques to encourage a reduction of extreme and biased thinking patterns are important where these are present. The development of a shared and acceptable formulation allows for a more balanced causal explanation. Without encouraging a polarized locus of control, a more balanced explanation can be proposed and accepted. Baseline causal models often include an explanation of 'chance'. New formulations can reinforce healthy, informed, and realistic causal models consisting of 'hereditary' and 'stress' explanations. Undoubtedly, such a multifaceted cognitive behavioural approach to treatment can contribute to a more positive illness outlook in terms of chronicity. We would expect reductions in anxiety and depression in tandem with an improved illness perception profile.

Post-CBT appraisals may reflect a more adaptive illness perception profile, suggesting a durable shift in beliefs about illness. As individuals presenting with schizophrenia are highly susceptible to relapse, interacting personal and environmental factors may induce a recurrence of symptoms. However, individuals who are aware of the likelihood of this and who have 'made sense' of their problem during therapy will arguably be better equipped to deal with such an episode and cope better during recovery.

An example of treatment

Changing illness perceptions in CBT for schizophrenia: a case example from both the client and therapist's perspective

There are no existing accounts of how to conduct CBT for auditory hallucinations with a particular emphasis on illness perceptions. Furthermore, there are no detailed accounts of CBT for auditory hallucinations written directly from the client's perspective. This intervention was conducted as part of the Psychological Prevention of Relapse in Psychosis (PRP) Trial (ISRCTN83557988), a randomized controlled trial of CBT and family intervention in psychosis (Garety *et al.*, 2008). It is an example of how illness perceptions can change and foster emotional and symptomatic change. We believe the account benefits from including the reflections of the client rather than those solely of the therapist as this allows greater insight into why and how things changed.

Presentation

Client perspective (Brendan O'Sullivan)

I had always seen schizophrenia as an illness and my voices as a symptom of that illness. Other people had always told me that talking about the voices would not change anything at all. I had relied on the medication for 18 years, but the voices still persisted.

On a normal day, I would stay at home alone and the voices would say 'Just kill yourself' over and over. I thought to myself 'There is no cure for me'. I would not tell anyone what was going on, and I would bottle it all up inside. I would think to myself 'No-one will understand anyway'. As this process went on, the voices got worse, I got more anxious and also started to feel helpless and hopeless. I started to think 'I am a failure to myself and to my family. I should have beaten this years ago'.

I very strongly believed that the voices meant I was odd, strange, mental, different, abnormal, and ill. The voice always sounded so horrific that it fixated me, and I could not focus on anything else. I was sure that if people knew I heard voices they would think of me as mental.

Therapist perspective (Ben Smith)

Brendan, a thirty-eight year old white-British man, reported that he frequently heard a voice telling him to kill himself. The voice was distressing, unusual, and had an inhuman quality, shouted and screamed at him on a daily basis sometimes for hours at a time. Brendan report neither any paranoid or delusional ideas nor any other type of auditory or other hallucination. He noted that his mood was severely depressed and that he did not see the future getting any better or brighter. He reported high levels of alcohol consumption, low motivation, and low activity levels and moderate levels of worry and anxiety.

Brendan had a formal psychiatric diagnosis of schizophrenia. He was receiving a weekly depixol injection (40 mg), olanzapine (15 mg) daily, procycladine (5 mg) twice daily, diazepam (5 mg) three times daily, and chlorpromazine (10 mg) daily. He lived with his wife and their three children in East London.

Specifically, Brendan reported the following at baseline (see Table 4.1).

Assessment measures

A number of established psychometric measures were used to formally assess Brendan's symptoms at three time-points and are reported in Table 4.2 . The Scale for the Assessment of Positive Symptoms (SAPS: Andreasen, 1984) is a 35-item, 6-point (0–5) rating instrument for the assessment of the positive symptoms of psychosis. The Psychotic Symptom Rating Scales (PSYRATS; Haddock *et al.*, 1999) is a 17-item, 5-point scale (0–4)

Table 4.1 Baseline cognitions

I am a waste of space
I am just going to get worse
There is no cure for me
*There is nothing I can do with the voices
I will have to suffer this until the day I die
I am a failure to myself and to my family
My family are ashamed of me and my illness
*I should have beaten the voices years ago
This is my fault
I am weird, abnormal, strange and mental
I am a coward
*One day the voices will come and never go
*The voices will never go
*The voices are incurable

*Hallucinations specific cognitions.

Table 4.2 Psychometric measures used to assess Brendan's symptoms at three time points[1]

	Baseline	12 months	24 months	
SAPS (AH)	5	0	3	(Max 5, Min 0)
PSYRATS (H)	37	0	18	(Max 44, Min 0)
BDI-II	31	2	1	(Max 63, Min 0)
BAI	20	0	0	(Max 63, Min 0)
RSES	38	10	11	(Max 40, Min 10)
BCSS (NSS)	13	0	–	(Max 24, Min 0)
IPQ (Means)				
Identity	1.0	0	0.5	(Max 3, Min 0)
Timeline	4.67	–	1.0	(Max 5, Min 1)
Consequences	4.57	–	3.43	(Max 5, Min 1)
Cure/control	4.0	–	4.83	(Max 5, Min 1)
Causes (endorsed)	Hereditary	–	Hereditary	
	Chance	–	Stress	
	Stress	–	–	

[1]SAPS, The Scale for the Assessment of Positive Symptoms (Andreasen, 1984)—Auditory Hallucinations subscale; PSYRATS, The Psychotic Symptom Rating Scales (Haddock *et al.*, 1999)—Hallucinations subscale; BDI-II, The Beck Depression Inventory-II (Beck *et al.*, 1996); BAI, The Beck Anxiety Inventory (Beck *et al.*, 1988); RSES, The Rosenberg Self-esteem Scale (Rosenberg, 1965); BCSS, The Brief Core Schema Scales (Fowler *et al.*, 2006)—Negative Self subscale; IPQ, The Illness Perception Questionnaire (Weinman *et al.*, 1996), with permission from Cambridge University Press.

multidimensional measure of delusions and auditory hallucinations. The Illness Perception Questionnaire (IPQ; Weinman *et al.*, 1996) consists of items measuring five core illness constructs: identity, cause, consequences, cure/control, and timeline. The measure used was a version of the original IPQ modified by Weinman and Garety for application in psychosis samples. The Beck Depression Inventory-II (BDI-II; Beck *et al.*, 1996) is a self-report 21-item, 4-point scale (0–3) for the assessment of depression. The Rosenberg Self-Esteem Scale (RSES; Rosenberg, 1965) is a self-report 10-item, 4-point scale (1–4) that assesses current levels of global self-esteem. The Brief Core Schema Scales (BCSS; Fowler *et al.*, 2006) is a 24-item, 5-point self-report rating scale (0–4) that assesses evaluative beliefs about the self and others. The negative self sub-scale is used here. Finally, the Beck Anxiety Inventory (BAI; Beck *et al.*, 1988) is a self-report 21-item, 4-point scale (0–3) for the assessment of anxiety. The assessors were blind to treatment allocation (CBT) at all assessment points.

Background information

Client perspective

The voices started when I was 20 years old. I was soon medicated with an anti-psychotic, told that I had a schizophrenic illness, and would need to take medication for the rest of my life. I was left feeling worthless and suicidal. I have ended up attempting suicide, always after drinking alcohol, on many occasions in direct response to the command 'Just kill yourself'. I have been on and off anti-psychotics for 18 years and been admitted to hospital many times. I consider this a 'failure cycle' as I repeatedly failed to cope with the illness and did not get better.

Therapist perspective

Both Brendan's father and brother had diagnoses of schizophrenia and his cousin had committed suicide during a psychotic episode. Recent correspondence in Brendan's medical notes described him as 'a revolving door medication-resistant chronic schizophrenic patient'. It was clear that Brendan was not always compliant with his anti-psychotic medication.

Initial formulation

In developing an initial formulation of the development and maintenance of Brendan's symptoms, it was helpful to draw on cognitive models of psychosis (e.g., Garety *et al.*, 2001, 2007; Morrison, 2001; Birchwood, 2003). It seemed that Brendan's negative cognitions about himself, his future, his voices, and his illness were triggering low and anxious mood and that when in those low mood states, he was vulnerable to hearing intrusive aggressive voices. The strategies adopted by Brendan of using alcohol or diazepam to cope with the voices were functioning to prevent change both in his mood state and his original negative cognitions. He perceived his continual failure to conquer the voices as confirmation of many of his predictions about himself, the illness, and the voices (e.g., 'I am a waste of space', 'the voices are incurable'). He was then left vulnerable to further negative rumination, low and anxious mood, voices, and possible suicidal thoughts. Memories of past suicide attempts intruded into his consciousness, feeding voice content, further low mood, and negative cognitions.

Formulation development

Client and therapist perspective

A key aspect of cognitive therapy in psychosis is the development of a collaborative formulation (e.g., Garety *et al.*, 2001, 2007; Morrison, 2000). An idiosyncratic model (Fig. 4.1) was developed collaboratively. We agreed that this model was a good summary of the important factors involved.

Treatment

Therapist perspective

The formulation suggested that low and anxious mood were precursors to, and the consequence of, the voices, and that negative thoughts and unhelpful behaviour fed directly into these mood states. Two general areas for intervention were therefore identified.

First, Brendan's thoughts and beliefs were reviewed, including his thoughts about voice hearing (cognitive work). Second, his coping behaviours were replaced (behavioural work). We agreed the following more detailed treatment plan.

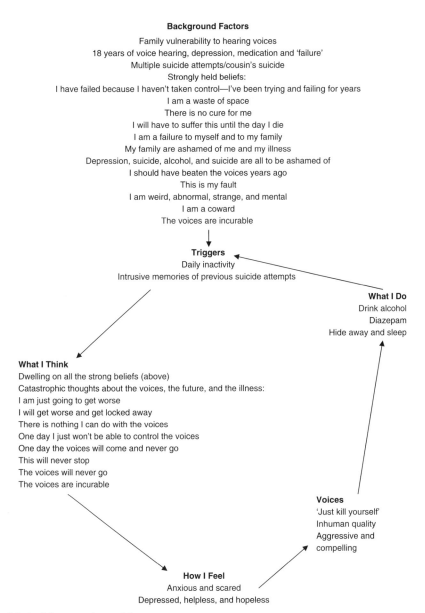

Fig. 4.1 An idiosyncratic model.

Voices To learn as much as possible about voices, who hears them, what they are and how people cope with them (for more on coping strategies, see Farhall, this volume).

Strongly held beliefs and thoughts To check that my strongly held beliefs and day-to-day thoughts that make me low, anxious, and vulnerable to voices are fair, even-handed, and stand up to some gentle scrutiny.

Behaviours   To continue to remain active and engaged in rewarding activities on a daily basis and to drop unhelpful coping behaviours such as diazepam and alcohol.

1. Voices

Client perspective

We found out that many other people (thousands in the UK) also hear voices (for more on normalizing hallucinations, see Garrett, this volume). We found out about the UK-based organization the Hearing Voices Network (HVN) and that people who hear voices can organize themselves into a network to help others (for more on self-help groups such as HVN, see May & Longden, this volume). We learnt that some people have recovered from hearing voices and that many professional, high-functioning people have heard or still hear voices. Voices are not simply a schizophrenic phenomena.

Therapist perspective

Brendan's current knowledge of voices was that they were symptoms of a schizophrenic illness that did not respond to medication. His beliefs about voices were also a key feature of the formulation (e.g., 'the voices are incurable'). It was therefore important to gather new information about voice hearing that would broaden his perspective and that may lead to a re-evaluation of his negative beliefs about hearing voices.

2. Strongly held beliefs and thoughts

Client perspective

A very important source of these harsh beliefs was my history of suicide. I felt deeply ashamed of this cowardly behaviour. I believed that suicide was wrong, shameful, cowardly, and gutless. I was sure that my family felt the same, as they never mentioned it. I believed that only really 'mad' people committed suicide and that it was a real sign of how ill I was. I blamed myself 100% for the attempts. I felt there were no excuses at all.

We discussed suicide in particular in detail. We found that suicide was far more common than I had thought. We also saw that most people (96% in one large study) who try to commit suicide do not have schizophrenia. It seemed that depression and alcohol played a big part in suicide.

I also decided to raise the issue of suicide with my parents and with my wife. It was really important to realize that the reason no one in the family mentioned suicide was not because they were so ashamed but because they knew that it upset me.

Therapist perspective

It was clear that 18 years of experiencing voices had impacted significantly on Brendan's beliefs. They were firmly held, longstanding, central to the formulation, and negative— hence they were up for review. Each of his beliefs was gently scrutinized to ensure that they were a fair reflection of the facts.

Cognitive change: Table 4.3 summarizes the key cognitions targeted and revised in therapy.

Table 4.3 Baseline and revised cognitions

Original thinking	Revised thinking
I am a waste of space	I am not a waste of space
I am just going to get worse	I have got better after all these years
There is no cure for me	*I can influence the voices
*There is nothing I can do with the voices	*I can do things to help the voices
I will have to suffer this until the day I die	Not necessarily—others recover, I can too
I am a failure to myself and to my family	My family are very proud of me
My family are ashamed of me and my illness	They are proud of me and not ashamed
*I should have beaten the voices years ago	I have been trying against the odds
This is my fault	This is only partly my fault
I am weird, abnormal, strange, and mental	I am like thousands of others - normal
I am a coward	I am not a total coward - I tried
*One day the voices will come and never go	*They have gone for the first time in 18 years
*The voices will never go	*They have gone
*The voices are incurable	*Others recover—So can I

*Hallucination specific cognitions.

3. Behaviours

Client perspective

It was clear that my long-term coping strategies of using alcohol and diazepam to cope with the voices were not working. I decided to try a new strategy borrowed from the HVN and say to myself 'Other people have learnt how to cope with this—I can too' and 'I am not alone—there are thousands of others out there'.

I started to read people's recovery stories and this gave me hope. This kept me busy and ready for the next session. I could also then dwell on the positive material I got from my research rather than my fears and worries. I started not to feel like such a 'freak', not so abnormal.

I had also decided to become more active so there was less time for moping about and getting low. These things (above) that I started to think and say in response to the voices helped them reduce in intensity.

Therapist perspective

Brendan's coping behaviours did not work. There was a notable lack of any cognitive strategy to deal with aggressive, negative voices. Brendan's negative and catastrophic beliefs about the voices meant that he did not have access to any positive statements or meanings with regard to the voices. The recovery stories and HVN information provided this new perspective from an informed source. Adopting a calm, positive self-statement of simply 'Other people have learnt how to cope with this so can I' reduced arousal, anxiety, and agitation and instilled hope. There was no available hearing voices group for Brendan to attend, so this option was not available to us.

Results

Outcome

Client perspective

After six months of CBT sessions, my voices had completely stopped. My mood had improved a lot and in collaboration with my psychiatrist, I began to slowly withdraw from all medications. At the end of 12 months of CBT sessions, I had not heard a voice in six months and not had an alcoholic drink in 12 months. I had been coping without my depot injection for six months and had been off all other medications for two months. I did not fully complete the IPQ measure at the end of CBT as I felt so well. The measure asks about illness and I did not feel ill anymore. I felt I was now in a phase of recovery. In agreement with my psychiatrist, I was discharged from all mental health services.

Therapist perspective and assessment measures

Twelve months after baseline assessment and having completed 20 sessions of CBT Brendan scored as indicated in Table 4.1. Brendan only completed the identity (symptom) section of the IPQ at 12 months and marked all symptoms as 'never'. This highlights that after CBT, he was reportedly symptom-free.

Follow-up

Client perspective

Four months after CBT sessions stopped, I experienced some severe health problems. These were investigated over a 2-week stay in hospital and I was told they could be life threatening. On returning home from an extended stay in the general hospital, I turned to alcohol to help cope with the intense health worries. I started to sit about at home and worry it could be cancer and soon got depressed.

My voices returned after a total absence of 10 months, and I was soon admitted (voluntarily) to hospital and prescribed a depixol (40 mg) depot injection and 15 mg olanzapine daily. I was thinking that 'I may as well just give up and not fight back'. There was no follow-up CBT available from my local mental health team.

Therapist perspective and assessment measures

Twenty-four months after baseline assessment and having had no contact with the research team since the 12-month assessment Brendan scored as indicated in Table 4.1.

It was clear that Brendan had experienced a relapse 8 months previously. Had he had access to follow-up CBT from his local mental health team, it is possible this could have been avoided. Brendan could have been helped to think less catastrophically about his physical illness and this may have meant he was less likely to revert to his old coping strategies (e.g., alcohol).

Reflections

Client perspective

It was very important at the beginning of the CBT sessions that we developed good rapport. The message of hope that I received was very important indeed. It was important that the therapist kept asking me what I thought. He wanted my opinion, which was a new idea to me. He was not just telling me what to do and how it was—I had to read things and say what I thought about them. As my mood lifted, I was able to get hold of my own strengths again. My experience also tells me that you actually have to work harder once the sessions have stopped than during them.

In my opinion, you cannot just leave it all to the therapist. You have to work with them and do your bit. You have to put in 100%. I told myself, no matter how bad you feel, you have to work at it. Once I did a little bit of homework, I got a boost. I was playing a part in my treatment for the first time, and I felt less helpless. I helped with my own recovery using strong will, hard work, and determination.

The information gathering was the key to me changing my beliefs. What changed for me in CBT was my attitude towards my voices and illness. In the past, I isolated myself and was isolated by the treatment I received, which meant I had no way of getting this new information.

At baseline, I would have described myself as suffering with schizophrenia. I saw this as a 'no-hope' situation and as a life sentence. Now, I would not describe myself as suffering with an illness. Looking back, I would not say that I was schizophrenic. I would say that I was someone who used to hear a lot of voices, was depressed, and anxious. However, I do understand that from a psychiatric perspective, I would have been described as schizophrenic. For me, schizophrenia meant no hope and that is why I now reject that term.

I feel I am in recovery from a very real illness. I do not think that voice hearing itself is an illness, but it can lead to a severe mental illness if you do not deal with it properly. My beliefs about the illness changed—I started to believe that it could change. CBT changed my view of the illness from harmful to less harmful. There is now a lot less fear attached to the illness in my mind.

I remain vulnerable to voices when I am under pressure, depressed, scared, or if I drink. I know where I stand. I am optimistic about the future. I am very proud of what I have achieved and so are my family. I now think of myself as one of many who hear voices, not someone who is schizophrenic and ill.

My depression is still not a problem despite a return of some of the voices. I do not feel under any pressure to stay well—I simply feel determined to stay well myself. The alcohol is the biggest obstacle to recovery. With it, I cannot treat myself with CBT. I cannot access my strengths.

Therapist perspective

The focus of CBT was on the mediators of Brendan's negative voices. These were hypothesized to be his negative self-beliefs, depressive cognitions, depressive behaviours, and negative illness perceptions. Significant cognitive, emotional, and behavioural change occurred in the key mediating areas and, it can be argued, had a positive mediating impact on voices. The reduction of distress may have then exerted a further beneficial influence on the frequency of voices as suggested by Trower *et al.* (2004).

Recent cognitive models of psychosis and Leventhal *et al.,*'s illness representation theory provided a sound theoretical framework from which to guide and assess treatment and outcome in individual CBT with Brendan. Targeting discrete illness perceptions through the use of established CBT techniques was a valuable approach.

For example, in the present case study, perceptions of Brendan's controllability over his illness and his perceptions of his illness's consequences were assessed, challenged, and re-aligned in a more adaptive way. The introduction of unbiased information on others' experiences of coping with psychotic phenomena served to reinforce the cognitive process of normalizing his experiences, therefore making them feel less threatening.

Shifting the focus of Brendan's attention outside of himself served to enhance his vocational and recreational functioning. It also provided a competition of cues to reduce him attending to his symptoms in isolation, thus eroding the strength of his illness identity. In addition to this, exposing himself to external environments (e.g., his family, the internet, therapists, etc.) allowed him to use these sources of social support to act as a stress buffer, thus reducing the probability of relapse. His engagement with such sources of support allowed for disconfirmation of negative thoughts and further allowed for the suggestion of substitute activities to counteract maladaptive coping activities (e.g., alcohol) that were only serving to reinforce and maintain his low mood and symptoms.

Integrating techniques to encourage a reduction of extreme and biased thinking patterns allowed Brendan to make less demands of himself. The development of a shared and acceptable formulation allowed for a more balanced causal explanation. Without encouraging a polarized locus of control, a more balanced, plausible, and realistic explanation was proposed and accepted. Indeed, unlike his baseline causal model that included an explanation of 'chance' (i.e., an external attribution), his 24-month assessment was a healthy, informed, and realistic causal model consisting of 'hereditary' and 'stress' explanations. Undoubtedly, such a multifaceted cognitive behavioural approach to treatment contributed to a more positive illness outlook in terms of chronicity, as clearly reflected in Brendan's follow-up timeline assessment. It is interesting to note the clear reduction in anxiety and depression in tandem with an improved illness perception profile between Brendan's pre-CBT assessment and his 24-month assessment.

Despite the return of Brendan's voices, his 24-month follow-up appraisal reflected an adaptive illness perception profile, suggesting a durable shift in his beliefs about his illness. Many individuals are highly susceptible to a return of voices; however, those who are aware of the likelihood of this and who have engaged in the therapy model discussed above will arguably be better equipped to deal with such a return.

The role of family as an important and emotionally salient information-gathering source and emotional support was also significant. It is possible that there was a synergy between in session conversations and between session family conversations, which enhanced cognitive change, supported behavioural changes, and maintained mood once it had started to improve.

Discussion

In this chapter, we have considered individual CBT for hallucinations. We reviewed the theoretical and empirical literature and outlined the treatment strategies used. In particular and using a case example, we have considered the role of illness perceptions in the maintenance and psychological treatment of hallucinations.

The case supports the hypothesis that illness perceptions (as well as other key cognitive appraisals) may provide useful intervention targets for manipulation in CBT for psychosis. If changing illness perceptions can significantly impact on depression and anxiety and greater emotional dysfunction is predictive of symptom severity (e.g., Smith *et al.*, 2006), then manipulating illness perceptions may directly influence illness outcome.

However, at present in the UK, inadequate numbers of trained CBT providers and problems with treatment resources create limitations. CBT is also not effective for all individuals and did not prevent relapse over the next two years in a recent randomized controlled trial ($N = 301$), although depression improved (Garety *et al.*, 2008). Questions also remain as to whether CBT for schizophrenia is effective cross-culturally (Rathod *et al.*, 2008) and much of the research currently derives from the USA and UK.

An awareness of the role played by illness perceptions and other appraisals within the context of a multi-factorial psychological model is likely to lead to improvements in interventions for those with psychosis and more specifically hallucinations. Future directions for CBT research will need to aim to develop more theoretically focused interventions to determine specific mechanisms mediating change, in order to develop improved treatment.

We conclude that CBT should emphasize that having a diagnosis of schizophrenia does not necessarily equate to a lifetime of uncontrollable symptoms. Steps can be taken to improve coping and reduce the impact of symptoms. Enhancing perceptions of controllability and working with beliefs about the impact of present/future perceived consequences and length of illness are important treatment strategies.

Acknowledgements

This work was supported by a programme grant from the Wellcome Trust (No. 062452). Many thanks to Ayse Dirik and Sarah Hutchinson for their help in researching this chapter.

References

Andreason, N.C. (1984). *The scale for the assessment of positive symptoms* (SAPS). Iowa: University of Iowa.

Bechdolf, A., Kohn, D., Knost, B., Pukrop, R., & Klosterkotter, J. (2005). A randomized comparison of group cognitive-behavioural therapy and group psychoeducation in acute patients with schizophrenia: outcome at 24 months. *Acta Psychiatr Scand*, **112**(3), 173–179.

Beck, A.T., Steer, R.A., & Brown, G.K. (1996). *BDI-II Manual.* San Antonio: The Psychological Corporation.

Beck, A.T., Epstein, N., Brown, G., & Steer, R.A. (1988). An inventory for measuring clinical anxiety: psychometric properties. *J Consult Clin Psychol,* **56**, 893–897.

Bentall, R. P., Haddock, G., & Slade, P. D. (1994). Psychological treatment for auditory hallucinations: from theory to therapy. *Behaviour Therapy,* **58**, 51–66.

Birchwood, M., Mason, R., Macmillan, F., & Healy J. (1993). Depression, demoralization and control over psychotic illness: a comparison of depressed and non-depressed patients with a chronic psychosis. *Psychol Med,* **2**, 387–395.

Birchwood, M., & Chadwick, P. (1997). The omnipotence of voices: testing the validity of a cognitive model. *Psychol Med,* **27**, 1345–1353.

Birchwood, M. (2003). Pathways to emotional dysfunction in first-episode psychosis. *Br J Psychiatry,* **182**, 373–375.

Birchwood, M., & Trower, P. (2006). Cognitive therapy for command hallucinations: not a quasi-neuroleptic. *Journal of Contemporary Psychotherapy,* **36**, 1–7.

Chadwick, P.D.J., & Birchwood, M. (1994). The omnipotence of voices: a cognitive approach to auditory hallucinations. *Br J Psychiatry,* **164**, 190–201.

David, A.S. (1998). The clinical importance of insight. In: Amador, X.F., David, A.S. (Eds) *Insight and psychosis.* New York: Oxford University Press. 332–351.

Drury, V., Birchwood, M., Cochrane, R., & MacMillan, F. (1996). Cognitive therapy and recovery from acute psychosis: a controlled trial. Impact on psychotic symptoms. *Br J Psychiatry,* **169**, 593– 601.

Fowler, D.G., Freeman, D., Smith, B., *et al.* (2006). The brief core schema scales (BCSS): psychometric properties and associations with paranoia and grandiosity in non-clinical and psychosis samples. *Psychol Med,* **36**, 749–759.

Garety, P.A., Kuipers, E., Fowler, D., Freeman, D., & Bebbington, P.E. (2001). A cognitive model of the positive symptoms of psychosis. *Psychol Med,* **31**, 189–195.

Garety, P.A, Bebbington, P., Fowler, D., Freeman, D., & Kuipers, E. (2007). Implications for neurobiological research of cognitive models of psychosis: a theoretical paper. *Psychol Med,* **37**(10), 1377–1391.

Garety, P.A., Fowler, D.G., Freeman, D., Bebbington, P., Dunn, G., & Kuipers, E. (2008). A randomised controlled trial of cognitive behavioural therapy and family intervention for the prevention of relapse and reduction of symptoms in psychosis. *Br J Psychiatry,* **192**, 412–423.

Gauntlett-Gilbert, J., & Kuipers, E. (2003). Phenomenology of visual hallucinations in psychiatric conditions. *J Nerv Ment Dis,* 191(3), 203–205.

Hagger, M., & Orbell, S. (2003). A meta-analytic review of the common-sense model of illness representations. *Psychol and Health,* **18**(2), 141–184.

Haddock, G., Bentall, R.P., & Slade, P.D. (1993). Psychological treatment of auditory hallucinations: two case studies. *Behav Cogn Psychother,* **21**, 335–346.

Haddock, G., Tarrier, N., Spaulding, W., Yusupoff, L., Kinney, C., & McCarthy, E. (1998). Individual cognitive-behaviour therapy in the use of hallucinations and delusions: a review. *Clin Psychol Rev,* **18**, 821–838.

Haddock, G., McCarron, J., Tarrier, N., & Faragher, E. (1999). Scales to measure dimensions of hallucinations and delusions: the psychotic symptom rating scales (PSYRATS). *Psychol Med,* **29**, 879–889.

Haddock, G., Devane, S., Bradshaw, T., *et al.* (2001). An investigation into the psychometric properties of the cognitive therapy scale for psychosis (CTS-Psy). *Behav Cogn Psychother,* **29**, 221–234.

Iqbal, Z., Birchwood, M., Chadwick, P., & Trower, P. (2000). Cognitive approach to depression and suicidal thinking in psychosis: 2. Testing the validity of a social ranking model. *Br J Psychiatry,* **177**, 522–528.

Johns, L.C., Rossell, S., Ahmad, F., *et al.* (2001). Verbal self-monitoring and auditory verbal hallucinations in patients with schizophrenia. *Psychol Med*, **31**, 705–715.

Jolley, S., & Garety, P.A. (2004). Insight and delusions: A cognitive psychological approach. In: Amador, X.F., David, A.S. (Eds). *Insight and psychosis. 2nd Edition*, New York: Open University Press.

Kingdon, D., & Turkington, D. (2003). *The case study guide to cognitive behaviour therapy of psychosis*. London: Wiley.

Kingdon, D., & Turkington, D. (2005). Cognitive therapy of schizophrenia. Guides to individualized evidence-based treatment. New York: Guilford Press.

Kuipers, E., Fowler, D., Garety, P.A., *et al.* (1998). The London–East Anglia randomised controlled trial of cognitive behaviour therapy for psychosis III: follow-up and economic evaluation at 18 months. *Br J Psychiatry*, **173**, 61–68.

Leventhal, H., Nerenz, D.R., & Steele, D.F. (1984). Illness representations and coping with health threats. In: Baum, A., Singer, J. (Eds). *Handbook of psychology and health. Volume IV*, Hillsdale: Erlbaum.

Lobban, F., Barrowclough, C., & Jones, S. (2003). A review of the role of illness models in severe mental illness. *Clin Psychol Rev*, **23**, 171–196.

Lobban, F., Barrowclough, C., & Jones, S. (2004). The impact of beliefs about mental health problems and coping on outcome in schizophrenia. *Psychol Med*, **37**, 1165–1174.

Morrison, A.P. (2001). The interpretation of intrusions in psychosis: an integrative cognitive approach to hallucinations and delusions. *Behav Cogn Psychother*, **29**, 257–276.

Morrison, A.P. (2002). Cognitive therapy for drug-resistant auditory hallucinations: a case example. In A.P. Morrison (Ed). *A casebook of cognitive therapy for psychosis*. London: Routledge.

NICE (2003). *Schizophrenia: full national clinical guidelines on core interventions in primary and secondary care*. London: Gaskell Press.

NICE (2009). *Schizophrenia: full national clinical guidelines on core interventions in primary and secondary care*. London: Gaskell Press.

Patterson, T.L., & Leeuwenkamp, O.R. (2007). Adjunctive psychosocial therapies for the treatment of schizophrenia. *Schizophr Res*, **100**, 108–119.

Petrie, K.J., Cameron, L., Ellis, C.J., Buick, D., & Weinman, J. (2002). Changing illness perceptions after myocardial infarction: an early intervention randomised controlled trial. *Psychosom Med*, **64**, 580–586.

Pfammatter, M., Junghan, U.M., & Brenner, H.D. (2006). Efficacy of psychological therapy in schizophrenia: conclusions from meta-analyses. *Schizophr Bull*, **32**, (Suppl 1), S64–S80.

Rathod, S., Kingdon, D., Weiden, P., & Turkington, D. (2008). Cognitive-behavioral therapy for medication-resistant schizophrenia: a review. *J Psychiatr Pract*, **14**(1), 22–33.

Rollinson, R., Smith, B., Steel, C., *et al.* (2008). Measuring adherence in CBT for psychosis: a psychometric analysis of an adherence scale. *Behav Cogn Psychother*, **36**, 163–178.

Rosenberg, M. (1965). *Society and the adolescent self-image*. Princeton: Princeton University Press.

Sensky, T., Turkington, D., Kingdon, D., *et al.* (2000). A randomized controlled trial of cognitive-behaviour therapy for persistent symptoms in schizophrenia resistant to medication. *Arch Gen Psychiatry*, **57**, 165–172.

Slade, P.D., & Bentall, R.P. (1988). *Sensory deception: a scientific analysis of hallucination*. London: Croom Helm.

Smith, B., Fowler, D., Freeman, D., *et al.* (2006). Emotion and psychosis: links between depression, self-esteem, negative schematic beliefs and delusions and hallucinations. *Schizophr Res*, **86**, 181–188.

Startup, M., Jackson, M.C., Evans, K.E., & Bendix, S. (2005). North Wales randomized controlled trial of cognitive behaviour therapy for acute schizophrenia spectrum disorders: two-year follow-up and economic evaluation. *Psychol Med*, **35**(9), 1307–1316.

Tarrier, N., Wittkowski, A., Kinney, C., McCarthy, E., Morris, J., & Humphreys, L. (1999). Durability of the effects of cognitive behavioural therapy in the treatment of chronic schizophrenia: 12 month follow-up. *Br J Psychiatry*, **174**, 500–504.

Tarrier, N., Lewis, S., Haddock, G., *et al.* (2004). Cognitive-behavioural therapy in first episode and early schizophrenia: 18-month follow-up of a randomised controlled trial. *Br J Psychiatry*, **184**, 231–239.

Temple, S., & Ho, B.C. (2005). Cognitive therapy for persistent psychosis in schizophrenia: a case-controlled clinical trial. *Schizophr Res*, **74**(2–3), 195–199.

Trower, P., Birchwood, M., Meaden, A., Byrne, S., Nelson, A., & Ross, K. (2004). Cognitive therapy for hallucinations: randomised controlled trial. *Br J Psychiatry*, **184**, 312–320.

Turkington, D., Sensky, T., Scott, J., *et al.* (2008). A randomised controlled trial of cognitive-behaviour therapy for persistent symptoms of schizophrenia: a five year follow-up. *Schizophr Res*, **98**, 1–7.

Valmaggia, L.R., Van De Gaag, M., Tarrier, N., Pijnenborg, N., & Sloof, C.J. (2005). Cognitive behavioural therapy for refractory psychotic symptoms of schizophrenia resistant to atypical antipsychotic medication: Randomised controlled trial. *Br J Psychiatry*, **186**, 324–330.

Watson, P.W.B., Garety, P.A., Weinman, J., *et al.* (2006). Emotional dysfunction in schizophrenia spectrum psychosis: the role of illness perceptions. *Psychol Med*, **36**, 761–770.

Weinman, J., Petrie, K., Moss-Morris. R., & Horne, R. (1996). The illness perception questionnaire: a new method for assessing the cognitive representation of illness. *Psychol and Health*, **11**, 431–445.

Wykes, T., Steel, C., Everitt, B., & Tarrier, N. (2008). Cognitive behaviour therapy for schizophrenia: effect sizes, clinical models and methodological rigor. *Schizophr Bull*, **34**, 523–537.

Zimmermann, G., Favrod, T.J., Trieub, V.H., & Pominib, V. (2005). The effect of cognitive behavioral treatment on the positive symptoms of schizophrenia spectrum disorders: a meta-analysis. *Schizophr Res*, **77**, 1–9.

Chapter 5

Group Cognitive Behaviour Therapy for psychosis

Louise Johns and Til Wykes

Introduction

Rationale

There is accumulating evidence that Cognitive Behavioural Therapy (CBT) delivered on a one-to-one basis is efficacious for individuals with psychosis and persistent positive symptoms (Pilling *et al.*, 2002; Tarrier & Wykes, 2004; Zimmerman *et al.*, 2005; Wykes *et al.*, 2008; see Smith *et al.*, this volume). However, given the shortage of trained therapists and the recommended length of treatment (NICE, 2003, 2009), individual CBT for psychosis (CBTp) is unfortunately not widely available in health services. An alternative approach is to deliver CBTp in a group format, which allows more people to be treated. This form of therapy still requires high levels of therapeutic skills in cognitive therapy, together with skills in facilitating groups.

There is some evidence that CBT for other mental health conditions can be provided in groups and can be as effective as CBT provided in individual sessions. In a review of group CBT, Morrison (2001) found that for social anxiety and depression, group treatment seemed to provide as much improvement as individual therapy. Intensive group CBT, i.e., longer group sessions over shorter treatment periods, produced slightly less improvement than longer therapies. However, this loss of effect size was offset by the greater number of patients treated over the same period and the advantage in cost-effectiveness. Morrison (2001) reported that individual therapy seemed to provide the better therapeutic option for one condition, obsessive-compulsive disorder, which may be related to the difficulty of doing exposure and response prevention in a group format.

Group treatment for psychosis is not a new idea. Consumer groups such as the Hearing Voices Network in the UK have been providing such support and advice for many years, based on the pioneering work of Romme and colleagues in the Netherlands (Romme & Escher, 1989). Their normalizing perspective proposed alternative strategies for dealing with voices other than attempting to suppress them with medication. They argued that the most important factor was people's reactions to the voices, rather than the experience of hearing voices per se. However, they suggested that before developing effective coping strategies, voice hearers need first to accept their experience of voices. An important step in this process involves talking about the voices. Since talking about their voices can make people feel vulnerable and stigmatized, dialogue can be easier with other voice hearers. Discussion among voice hearers gives people the opportunity to share similar experiences, using a common language, and to learn from one another. Self-help groups also reduce the isolation encountered by voice hearers and may also improve self-confidence.

Self-help groups, as the name implies, tend to be user led, and the focus is on open discussion and mutual communication between voice hearers (see May & Longden, this volume). Despite the ostensible benefits of these groups, to our knowledge, no formal research has been conducted to evaluate their success. More structured CBT groups have been developed and run by clinical psychologists, either focusing on auditory verbal hallucinations (voices) or addressing positive psychotic symptoms more generally, including voices. These groups have been evaluated, with promising results.

Evaluations of group CBT for auditory hallucinations

Before reviewing the evidence, it is worth pointing out that assessing the effects of the therapy is not always a simple matter, as different outcomes will be valued by different groups. Health service professionals may emphasize the reduction of specific symptoms measured on a scale, health service managers will emphasize the effects on use of psychiatric services, patients will want reductions in distress, and their relatives may wish to see the patient happier and leading a better quality of life. Most evaluations have used a variety of outcome measures and the issue of appropriateness of such measures will be discussed later in the chapter.

Most published evaluations of group CBT for voices have shown beneficial effects, although many studies are uncontrolled in that they have just investigated a cohort of patients at the beginning and end of treatment (Gledhill et al., 1998; Chadwick et al., 2000a; Perlman & Hubbard, 2000; Trygstad et al., 2002; Lecomte et al., 2003). Previous work by Slade (1990) suggests that merely asking people to monitor their voices, irrespective of the specific treatment, is likely to decrease their occurrence. Therefore, studies that make comparisons with a waiting list period, or better still a separate group that receive no treatment or an alternative treatment, are required to show clinical efficacy. However, uncontrolled studies do provide evidence of the feasibility and acceptability of this form of treatment. Most people in these studies reported that they were able to talk about their voices in the group after the first two or three sessions, and there are no reports of problems in facilitating the groups. The majority of the patients improved in either their distress, the frequency of their voices, or some change in their beliefs about the voices; however, few statistical tests were carried out. For instance, Perlman and Hubbard (2000) reported that seven out of nine clients reported improved symptom control. In the largest of these uncontrolled studies, Chadwick et al. (2000b) showed significant reductions in conviction of beliefs about the omnipotence of voices and improved control over voices.

Positive effects of group CBT for voices have also been reported by more rigorous studies using controlled designs. Wykes et al. (1999) used a waiting-list control design to evaluate their group treatment for voices. Twenty-one patients with schizophrenia and treatment-resistant, distressing auditory hallucinations were referred to a group programme consisting of six weekly sessions. The therapy followed a manualized protocol that emphasized individual power and control over voices as well as coping strategies. Sessions lasted for an hour and followed a semi-structured format. Each session dealt with a particular theme (described in more detail in *Treatment details*): sharing of information about the voices, models of psychosis, models of hallucinations, effective coping strategies, improving self-esteem, and an overall model of coping with voices. The outcome measures were varied and included measures of symptoms (Auditory Hallucinations Rating Scale: PSYRATS; Haddock *et al.*, 1999, Expanded Brief Psychiatric Rating Scale: BPRS-E; Ventura *et al.*, 1993) as well as self-report insight (IS; Birchwood *et al.*, 1994) and Beliefs About Voices Questionnaire (BAVQ; Chadwick and Birchwood, 1995), a self-report coping strategies assessment and measures of mood and self-esteem. These measures were completed at referral (week 0), pre-intervention (week 6), post-intervention (week 12), and 3-month follow-up (week 24). There were significant changes on the three main outcome measures (PSYRATS, BPRS-E, IS) following treatment compared to the waiting list period, showing improvements in voice frequency, severity, and insight. Changes on the PSYRATS and IS were maintained at follow-up. The other measures revealed reductions in perceived power of voices and distress, as well as increases in the number and effectiveness of participants' coping strategies. There was also an improvement in self-esteem following the group, which was maintained at follow-up.

The previous study investigated the effects of group CBT on people who had experienced psychosis over a number of years, so a follow-up study with a similar design was carried out by Newton *et al.* (2005) with young people with recent-onset auditory hallucinations. Participants were included if the onset of their voices was before the age of 18 years and they had been experiencing distressing voices that had not responded to medication for less than 3 years. The rationale was that an intervention during a 3-year critical period after onset might make the voices more amenable to treatment. The main outcome measures were similar to those in the Wykes *et al.* (1999) study and were administered at the same time points. This early intervention produced a significant reduction in auditory hallucinations over the total treatment phase (weeks 6–24), but not over the waiting period. The study also reported a trend for increased perceived control over the voices over the total treatment phase, which was significantly associated with reductions in distress about voices. However, the study did not find a significant reduction in general psychopathology or an increase in self-esteem after treatment. The authors suggested this might be because the young people had higher self-esteem and lower general psychopathology at baseline compared with the adult sample of Wykes *et al.* (1999).

A recent study used a waiting-list control design to evaluate group Person-Based Cognitive Therapy (PBCT) for distressing voices (Dannahy *et al.*, submitted). Thirty patients with schizophrenia and treatment-resistant, distressing voices entered one of six 8-session PBCT groups. The group sessions lasted ninety minutes and were facilitated by two experienced therapists. PBCT (Chadwick, 2006) is a third wave Cognitive-Behavioural Therapy, which emphasizes acceptance of self and voices to reduce distress and perceived voice control and to enhance social functioning. The primary outcomes were subjective distress and perceived voice control, which were measured using visual analogue scales. In addition, subjective well-being and functioning was measured using the Clinical Outcomes in Routine Evaluation (Evans *et al.*, 2000) and relating to the voice was assessed using the Voice and You (VAY; Hayward *et al.*, 2008) and the Southampton Mindfulness Questionnaire (SMQ; Chadwick *et al.*, 2008). Participants were assessed four weeks and one week prior to therapy, within a week of therapy ending, and one month after therapy. There were significant benefits following the group in terms of distress and perceived voice control, which were maintained at follow-up. Participants also became less dependent on their voices and showed significant gains in social functioning.

Two Randomized Controlled Trials (RCTs) have evaluated the efficacy of group CBT compared with treatment as usual, one intervention specifically for voices (Wykes *et al.*, 2005) and one for persistent positive symptoms (hallucinations and/or delusions) (Barrowclough *et al.*, 2006). Both studies were methodologically rigorous and contained a relatively large sample of participants who were randomized to two treatments—active versus treatment as usual. Wykes *et al.* (2005) evaluated the effectiveness of group CBT on social functioning and severity of hallucinations. Eighty-five participants with a diagnosis of schizophrenia who were experiencing distressing auditory hallucinations (rated on the Positive and Negative Symptoms Scale: PANSS; Kay *et al.*, 1987) were randomly allocated to group CBT ($N = 45$) or treatment as usual ($N = 40$). The patient group had severe levels of hallucinations that were not only distressing but interfered with their everyday life. The group therapy was the same as that reported in Wykes *et al.* (1999). Each CBT group typically included 6–8 participants. The therapists were drawn from local services and then trained on the treatment protocol. Many but not all were experienced in providing individual CBT. The two main outcomes were social functioning as measured by the Social Behaviour Schedule (SBS; Wykes & Sturt, 1986), which is completed from information provided by a key worker, and the severity of hallucinations as measured by the total score on the hallucinations scale of PSYRATS. Secondary outcomes were self-esteem and effective coping strategies. Assessments were carried out at baseline, 10 weeks (post therapy), and 36 weeks (six months following therapy). There was a significant improvement in social functioning (at 6-month follow-up) but no general effect of the group CBT on severity of hallucinations. However, there was a large cluster effect of therapy group, such that hallucinations were reduced in some but not all of the groups. Improvement in hallucinations was associated with receiving therapy early in the trial and having very experienced therapists (extensive CBT training, which included expert supervision for a series of individual cases for at least a year following initial training). There was some evidence that people in the CBT group enhanced their self-esteem and acquired more coping strategies, although these improvements did not reach statistical significance.

Barrowclough *et al.* (2006) evaluated the effectiveness of group CBT for schizophrenia using a longer, more formulation-based group intervention (addressing maintenance formulations of participants' presenting problems). One hundred and thirteen patients with persistent positive symptoms of schizophrenia were randomly assigned to receive group CBT ($N = 57$) or treatment as usual ($N = 56$). The group intervention ran for 6 months, with 18 sessions covering the following themes: CBT approach to psychosis; what is CBT; identification of main problems (delusional beliefs and voices were the main focus); formulating problems in terms of thoughts, feelings, and behaviours; negative thinking patterns and thought monitoring; thought challenging; behavioural strategies: experiments and action plans; stress, arousal, and medication; staying-well plans; follow-up and revision. Sessions lasted 2 hours including breaks and followed a detailed plan and timetable contained in the therapy manual. Ten CBT groups were conducted in total, with about six clients in each group (4–7). The primary outcome was improvement in positive symptoms as measured by the Positive Symptom Sub-Scale of the PANSS. Assessments were completed at baseline, post-treatment (6 months), and at follow-up (12 months). There was no significant difference between the group CBT and treatment as usual on the primary positive symptom measure either at the end of treatment or at 1-year follow-up. Similarly, group CBT did not appear to affect secondary outcomes of general psychopathology, global and social functioning, and mood. However, the group intervention did lead to reductions in feelings of hopelessness and improved self-esteem at the 12-month follow-up. The authors discussed possible reasons why their trial failed to replicate the effect on positive symptoms reported by Wykes *et al.* (1999) and concluded that it could not be accounted for in terms of inferior quality of therapy. In the current trial, a number of the therapists had worked on previous CBT trials for psychosis that had good symptom outcomes, high standards for training and supervision were adhered to, and measures of treatment fidelity showed no significant deviations from the treatment protocol. The limited treatment effects could reflect the outcome measures, or the group attendees and focus of the sessions. These are discussed further in *Discussion* part of the chapter.

Three further RCTs have evaluated the efficacy of group CBT when compared with an active control intervention. Bechdolf *et al.* (2004) compared a group CBT intervention with a psychoeducational (PE) group programme, on the following outcomes: relapse, symptoms, and compliance with medication. Eighty-eight in-patients with schizophrenia were randomized to receive either 16 sessions of group CBT ($N = 40$) or 8 sessions of group PE treatment ($N = 48$), in addition to routine hospital care. Sessions of both interventions were delivered to groups of eight patients within a therapy envelope of 8 weeks and were led by a CBT trained psychiatrist or clinical psychologist. The sessions were carried out while the patients were in hospital and continued when they were discharged during the treatment period. Sessions of both interventions followed a semi-structured format and lasted between 60 and 90 min, with a 5–10 min break. The group CBT treatment was based on the approach of Tarrier *et al.* (1990, 1993) and involved the following elements: assessment and engagement (sharing information about voices and delusions) ; models of psychosis; improving self-esteem; formulation of key-problems; interventions directed at reducing the severity and the occurrence of key problems; relapse prevention and keeping well. The PE programme covered symptoms of psychosis, models of psychosis, effects and side-effects of medication, maintenance medication, early symptoms of relapse, and relapse prevention. The approach was primarily didactic but also included formulation, guided discovery, and motivational interviewing. Assessments were conducted at baseline, post-treatment, and 6-month follow-up. The re-hospitalization rates were lower for the CBT group than the PE group during the follow-up period. Both forms of group therapy led to significant improvement in symptoms (for all PANSS subscales) at post-treatment and follow-up, but there were no significant differences between CBT and PE on any of the PANSS subscales. The authors suggested possible reasons for this, including the patient sample, which had relatively low positive symptom scores at baseline, and the CBT intervention, which addressed other issues such as self-esteem and relapse prevention, which may have reduced the impact of the therapy on psychotic symptoms. In addition, although the PE programme is reported to be mainly didactic, it seems to include cognitive-behavioural strategies of formulation and guided discovery. In a 24-month follow-up study, Bechdolf et al. (2005) found no significant group differences in terms of re-admission, symptoms, or compliance with medication.

A recent RCT evaluated the efficacy of group CBT for voices in comparison with group Supportive Therapy (ST) (Penn et al., 2009). Sixty-five out-patients with schizophrenia and treatment-resistant auditory hallucinations were randomly assigned to receive either group CBT or group ST for 12 one-hour weekly sessions. Each group contained one or two therapists and between 4 and 7 clients. The group CBT was a manual-based treatment based on the protocol of Wykes et al. (1999, 2005) and targeted reduction of the distress associated with auditory hallucinations. Group-enhanced ST is a manual-based intervention focusing on emotional support and counseling of non-symptom-related problems, in order to improve social integration (Penn et al., 2004). Therapists were randomly assigned to either group CBT or group ST and trained in the intervention in the 3 months prior to the first group session. A clinical psychologist reviewed the audio taped group therapy sessions and conducted weekly supervision with therapists to maintain treatment fidelity. The primary outcomes were beliefs about voices, assessed using the BAVQ-R (Chadwick et al., 2000), and severity of auditory hallucinations, measured using the PSYRATS hallucinations scale. Secondary outcomes included psychotic symptoms, self-esteem, social functioning, insight, depression, and hospitalization. These were measured respectively using the PANSS and PSYRATS delusions scale, the Rosenberg Self-Esteem Scale (Rosenberg, 1965), the Social Functioning Scale (Birchwood et al., 1990), the Beck Cognitive Insight Scale (BCIS; Beck et al., 2004), and the Beck Depression Inventory II (BDI-II) (Beck et al., 1996). Participants were assessed at baseline, post-treatment, 3 month, and 12-month follow-up. Contrary to predictions, group CBT did not result in a reduction in voice distress or intensity, as measured by the BAVQ-R and the PSYRATS. However, group CBT was associated with lower general and total symptom scores on the PANSS through 12-month follow-up. The authors suggested that clients might have used CBT strategies to manage the consequences of persistent auditory hallucinations (i.e., general symptoms such as anxiety and depression) rather than the voices themselves.

Unexpectedly, enhanced ST had a specific impact on auditory hallucinations: participants in the ST group rated their voices as less malevolent and were less likely to resist the voices, both after treatment and at follow-up. The authors were unsure how group ST produced this effect, but suggested that interventions combining CBT and ST elements might be promising for the treatment of medication-resistant psychotic symptoms.

Another recent study compared the effectiveness of group CBT and social skills training for recent onset psychosis (Lecomte *et al.*, 2008). Participants were aged between 18 and 35 and had current persistent or fluctuating psychotic symptoms. One hundred and twenty-nine participants were randomized to one of three conditions: group CBT, group Social Skills Training (SST) for symptom management, or a wait-list control group. They received 24 sessions of either treatment, twice a week, for 3 months. The therapists all had experience working with individuals with psychosis but minimal or no experience in delivering the group interventions; they received 2 days of intensive training in the treatment they were to offer. The CBT was based on individual CBT for psychosis, but adapted to a group format and tailored for first episodes (described in Lecomte *et al.*, 2003). SST focuses on skills needed to live in the community and includes teaching skills such as symptom management and relapse prevention. This study used the Symptom Management (SM) module (Liberman *et al.*, 1988). Videotapes of sessions were watched by supervisors and independent raters. The dependent variables were symptoms, measured using the BPRS-E (overall, positive and negative symptoms), and psychosocial variables of self-esteem, coping with stress and symptoms, decreasing substance use, insight, and improving social support. Assessments were carried out at baseline, post-treatment (3 months), and 6-month follow-up (9 months). Both treatments led to improvements in positive and negative symptoms compared with the wait-list control group, and the CBT group also resulted in lower overall symptoms. In addition, CBT impacted positively on self-esteem, coping skills, and social support, although the effect on coping diminished at follow-up.

Summary

The evaluations of group CBT for voices indicate mixed effects. In the earlier uncontrolled or waiting-list controlled studies, there was evidence that beliefs about voices could change. The studies of Wykes *et al.* (1999), Chadwick *et al.* (2000), and Newton *et al.* (2005) all found that beliefs about the powerfulness of voices were affected. Furthermore, the Wykes *et al.* study was able to show that changes in beliefs about voices led directly to reductions in levels of distress. However, in the more rigorous studies, fewer significant effects were found. Group CBT did reduce the severity of auditory hallucinations, but only if the therapy was provided by experienced CBT therapists (Wykes *et al.*, 2005). In addition, the rigorous trials have shown that these groups can improve participants' social functioning and self-esteem, and reduce their hopelessness. There is less evidence for a specific effect of group CBT when the treatment is compared with another psychological intervention (Bechdolf *et al.*, 2004; Lecomte *et al.*, 2008; Penn *et al.*, 2009). Group CBT seems to be as effective as individual CBT for psychosis. The meta-analysis of

Wykes *et al.* (2008) compared individual and group CBTp in relation to the outcome for the target symptom of therapy, and there was no difference between individual and group CBTp, with both having a modest effect size. However, overall, the evidence base for group CBT for psychosis is still limited, and there is currently more evidence to support the provision of CBT as an individual-based therapy (NICE, 2009).

Treatment details

The manuals developed for the treatment trials in the UK (Wykes *et al.*, 1999, 2005; Barrowclough *et al.*, 2006) will be described here, together with some modifications that have been made (Newton *et al.*, 2005; Penn *et al.*, 2009).

Voices group protocol (Wykes *et al.*, 1998)

The main aims of the therapy are to provide people in the group with an opportunity to learn new coping skills, to help participants feel less isolated, and to raise self-esteem. The session content is based on different approaches that have previously been shown to be successful: coping strategy enhancement (Tarrier *et al.*, 1990, 1993; see Farhall, this volume), normalization approaches (Romme & Escher, 1989; Kingdon & Turkington, 1991; see Garrett, this volume and Romme & Escher, this volume), and elements of CBT described by Fowler *et al.* (1995). All the sessions centre around three underlying principles:

- Therapy focuses on the normalizing rationale and a continuum of voice experiences. It is emphasized that hearing voices is something that many people experience and does not mean that somebody is 'mad'.
- It is suggested that the experience of hearing voices is best viewed as something that can be coped with, using any one of a number of coping strategies.
- There is a focus on the improvement of self-esteem.

There are seven group sessions, and each one has a specific goal.

Sessions 1–3

The first three sessions revolve around engaging clients in a dialogue about their voices and encouraging the exchange of information. A film of the BBC's Horizon programme 'Hearing voices' is used as a way of presenting other people's descriptions of their voices so that it is possible to start a dialogue of how group members' voices are the same or different. The therapists then help the group to discuss different models of voices. The vulnerability-stress model is easy for group members to accept, and the therapist should ensure that each member contributes to this sort of formulation, for example, by indicating instances of different types of stressor associated with the exacerbation of the voices. Medication is always described by the therapist as providing a protective layer to a sensitive person.

Session 1: The issues dealt with include sharing of information among group members about their voices. Therapists emphasize the similarities between group members' experiences and introduce a normalizing rationale and the continuum of unusual experiences.

Session 2: Therapists explore models of psychosis viewed in the film: medical, psychological, and both combined. They also discuss whether medication is helpful and other treatments for voices, for example, whether talking about voices, is helpful.

Session 3: Group participants' models of hallucinations are explored, specifically their physical attributes (Where do the voices sound like they come from?) and psychological attributes (What do you think causes the voices?). Explanatory themes are also explored, including the malevolence and powerfulness of the voices and consequences of ignoring the voices.

Sessions 4–7

These sessions focus on means of coping with voices and their effectiveness. Therapists should state that they realize many group members have been using coping strategies and have been coping with their voices on their own for a long time. Their resourcefulness and capabilities should also be acknowledged. Therapists then take an active role in drawing together the different coping methods by categorizing them and also suggesting new strategies. For homework, participants are asked to try new strategies for dealing with their voices. Unsuccessful attempts are discussed and evaluated, but the successful coping methods should be stressed. The emphasis is on the ability to control the experience and the effect of this mastery on mood. Medication and recreational drugs are raised in session 5 as things people might use to manage their voices. Session 5 also touches on the stigma of mental illness and voice hearing. Session 6 concentrates on how self esteem might affect coping with voices and this is explained through playing a game to raise group participant's self esteem. The last session is used to build a model of the experience of voices that is acceptable to all participants and includes coping as well as stressors. All clients leave with a copy of this model, which they should all feel they own and expresses their own difficulties.

Session 4: Methods of coping with voices are explored, together with their effectiveness. New strategies are introduced such as distraction (listening to music, watching television, and talking to somebody), engaging with the voices (telling them to go away), humming or singing, activities that increase self-esteem or positive mood, etc. Therapists should acknowledge that coping strategies can require a lot of effort and that different coping strategies are appropriate for different occasions.

Session 5: The majority of the session, following a review of the coping homework, is spent on discussing issues associated with stigma and labelling. Further homework is provided for clients to try additional strategies for dealing with the voices.

Session 6: In this session, therapists concentrate on eliciting information on how mood and self-esteem affect voices and then play a game to show that each group participant has personal attributes that are valued by others in the group.

Session 7: After feeding back the success of new coping strategies, the final session draws up a model of voices within the stress vulnerability context. It is very important for group members to 'own' the model and for their words to be used in the model. This is followed by a discussion of how members experienced the group and a review of the key learning points.

Adaptation for in-patients

Since in-patients may only be in hospital for a short period, the Wykes *et al.* (1998) group protocol has been adapted for use with this client group. There are three sessions in total, each lasting 50 min. Only 15 min of the film are shown at the beginning of the first two sessions. Otherwise, the content of the overall content is the same but with less detail being discussed in each session.

Adaptation for adolescent voice-hearers

Only a few adaptations of the Wykes *et al.* (1998) treatment protocol seem to be necessary for a young people's group (Newton *et al.*, 2005). An aide-memoire can be introduced at the beginning of each session to facilitate discussion. A more child-centred approach may be needed by therapists to encourage people to join in and say more (for example, asking participants to take turns to write on the flip chart, rather than speaking, if they are shy).

Adaptation by Penn and colleagues

Penn *et al.* (2009) modified the Wykes *et al.* (1998) manual in the following ways: (1) emphasizing coping skills rather than cognitive restructuring, (2) de-emphasizing self-esteem work, and (3) expanding the protocol from 6 to 12 sessions. Their group CBT sessions cover the following themes: Session 1, Introduction to treatment; Sessions 2–3, Psychoeducation; Sessions 4–5, Content of auditory hallucinations (i.e., what are the themes of clients' voices, such as whether they are benevolent or malevolent); Sessions 6–7, Behavioural analysis of auditory hallucinations; Sessions 8–9, Increasing and decreasing strategies for auditory hallucinations (i.e., identifying situations that increase and decrease hallucination severity); and Sessions 10–12, Coping strategies for auditory hallucinations. The initial sessions focus on building rapport among the group members and therapists and pointing out to participants that many other individuals have experiences similar to their own. Current theories of psychosis and commonly used treatments are explained. CBT techniques, such as self-monitoring and coping strategies, are central to the intervention. Self-monitoring is employed by asking participants to monitor their thoughts and actions prior to, during, and after auditory hallucinations. This allows participants to identify any patterns that may be present and encourages a functional analytic approach to their experiences. Individuals then begin to utilize coping strategies when they experience voices and are asked to monitor the effectiveness of these strategies. Over the course of treatment, multiple coping strategies are tried, and participants are encouraged to continue using the strategies that allow them to feel more control over their voices and that reduce the amount of distress they experience.

Group CBT for schizophrenia (Barrowclough *et al.*, 2001)

This is a longer and more formulation-based group intervention, which addresses participants' presenting problems rather than voices per se. However, the treatment manual was developed for clients with persistent positive symptoms, and the person's target problem was often a delusional belief or hallucination. In the RCT, two therapists conducted each session, and at least one therapist per group had training in CBT meeting the British Association for Behavioural and Cognitive Psychotherapies accreditation standards, plus experience in using CBT with people with psychosis. All therapists were provided with an initial training programme, and supervision sessions occurred monthly.

Main content of the sessions

The group intervention comprises 18 sessions, the content of which is outlined below.

Session		Content
Pre-group visit		Assessment, engagement, reassurance, information, how to get to group
Session 1		Introduction, video, initial problem list, thoughts, feelings, and behaviours
Session 2		What is CBT, example from therapist, showing link between thoughts, feelings, and behaviours
Session 3		Identifying main problem, mini-formulations
Session 4	One individual Session about here	Introduce problem monitoring; share mini-formulations and ways of intervening
Session 5*		Negative thinking patterns and thought monitoring
Session 6, 7, 8		Thought challenging
Session 9, 10, 11		Behavioural strategies: experiments and actions plans
Sessions 12 & 13		Stress, arousal and medication
Sessions 14 & 15**		Staying well plan
Session 16, 17, and 18		Emergency keeping well plan and follow ups

*With client's permission, contact care coordinator and give brief resume of progress.

**Arrange meeting with client and care coordinator to discuss a 'handover' plan.

Problem focus

A target problem for each participant is highlighted as soon as possible (with a maximum of two problems). This problem is then monitored on a weekly basis. Therapists should ensure that positive symptoms are considered as candidates for the problem list. The group attempts to deal with heterogeneity of problems by bringing all problems back to the cognitive model. Mini-formulations of problems include triggers, thoughts, feelings, and behaviours.

General format and structure for all sessions

Each session lasts 2 hours, including 15 min for breaks and 10 min for completing questionnaires. The session plan includes setting the day's agenda, reviewing homework, introducing the main topic, applying the topic to individuals' own experiences, problem formulations in small groups, discussion and comparison of group members' experiences, setting homework, and eliciting feedback on the session. The agenda is referred to as a plan and is written up at the beginning of the session on a flip chart as follows:

- Review of the week
- Feedback from last session
- Review of homework
- Introduction of today's main topic (didactic bit)
- Small group discussion/work on topic
- Large group discussion with feedback from small groups
- Set homework
- Feedback from today's session

As can be seen, each session is structured to have a

- Didactic component—e.g., negative thinking patterns,
- Small group discussion—breaking up into small groups (possibly on the basis of homogeneity, which might be sex of clients, similarities of symptoms) and performing a task arising from the didactic part (e.g., identifying individual negative thoughts), and
- Larger group discussion—therapists will facilitate feedback from small groups, using individual examples to help reinforce the CBT model.

Discussion

Group CBT for auditory hallucinations uses a range of therapeutic techniques that are not novel, but which have been adapted and applied in a group setting. The strategies used will overlap with those described in the chapters on individual CBT, coping strategies, psychoeducation, and appraisals. The process of suggesting and practising new coping skills recognizes and builds on clients' own natural coping strategies (Farhall *et al.*, 2007). It also overlaps with Coping Strategy Enhancement (CSE; Tarrier *et al.*, 1990, 1993), which identifies coping strategies already being used by clients and develops further strategies in response to any psychotic symptom, including auditory hallucinations. The focus on beliefs about voices, particularly those around power and control, is based on the work of Chadwick and Birchwood (1994). Unlike idiosyncratic explanations of voices, these appraisals are more easily discussed in a group setting, since most voice hearers who are in touch with services report voices that are powerful and difficult to control.

Advantages and disadvantages of group CBT for auditory hallucinations

Before reviewing the advantages and disadvantages of the group approach, it is worth mentioning a couple of issues in relation to CBT for voices, which apply to both individual and group sessions. One concerns the perceived safety of discussing voices: clients sometimes report that talking about their voices can be frightening because they might receive a backlash from the voices afterwards. In addition, clients may not attend sessions if their voices are particularly intense or if the voices instruct them not to do so. It is helpful if therapists acknowledge these potential difficulties at the outset of treatment and discuss with clients possible ways of dealing with them.

Advantages

There are some definite benefits to the provision of group CBT. People experiencing voices often report loneliness as a result of the voices. The experience can sometimes impair concentration so that conversation with others is difficult. Moreover, the pejorative nature of the voices not only reduces self-esteem but also can encourage social isolation by suggestions about negative actions or intentions of others. Groups may be able to reduce these effects and combat the feelings of isolation that voice hearers report. Groups have a built in social support, which can enable people to practise their social skills in a 'safe' environment. These benefits have been measured in the improvements in social functioning noted in some trials (e.g., Wykes *et al.*, 2005).

Group treatment for voices is also appealing because the anomalous experiences reported by different people with voices are very similar to each other in form even if the explanations of their cause are different. These anomalous experiences are also relatively frequent, and so it is easy to describe them. The group approach enables people to

- Share experiences of voices, which may facilitate testing and re-framing of experiences (this is particularly important as within the group, there will be a wide variety of explanations for the same unusual perception),
- Identify common factors that increase and decrease their experiences (such as finding out when the voices are worst or least frequent), and
- Share natural coping strategies to increase the coping repertoire (instead of the therapist having to make suggestions, the other members of the group can share their own effective strategies),

The group also provides a forum for discussing new information, which can enhance participants' understanding of the voices. It may also help to reduce clients' anxiety through the presentation of a normative view of hallucinations (i.e., that many people have similar experiences).

Qualitative studies have investigated the experiences of adults participating in hearing voices groups and their findings are consistent with reports from quantitative studies, indicating that people benefit from discussing their experiences with other voice-hearers (Chadwick *et al.*, 2000; Jones *et al.*, 2001; Martin, 2000). In a study of the experiences of young people who attended group CBT for voices, themes that emerged from the analysis of the qualitative data included (1) a safe place to talk, (2) normalizing and destigmatizing, (3) learning from and helping others, and (4) the role of the facilitators, in managing the group, positioning the participants as experts in voices, and using psychological techniques (Newton *et al.*, 2007).

Disadvantages

Some of the disadvantages relate to broader difficulties of running group therapy and others relate more specifically to group intervention for hallucinations. General difficulties include

♦ Individual differences in understanding and rates of change, which means that some people can be left behind while others get bored with any repetition,

♦ The possibility that an individual can monopolize or disrupt the group,

♦ A reluctance to discuss experiences or beliefs within the group because they are embarrassing or personal, and

♦ Inconsistent or poor attendance by some members, which requires an assertive approach to attendance such as reminders and even lifts to the group.

More specific issues include

♦ The possibility that listening to others' experiences of voices can be distressing to some members, especially if these are more severe or chronic than their own and

♦ The risk that confrontation can take place between attendees, particularly when discussing different explanations of the same phenomenon.

The group protocol developed by Wykes *et al.* (1998) is limited in its ability to deal with the content of clients' voices because of the small amount of time available for each individual problem. This limitation can be overcome to some degree by using a group format in which clients divide into small groups with therapists to discuss problems in more detail (Barrowclough *et al.*, 2001). Alternatively, the group could be thought of as a starting point from which some can graduate to longer more personal and individual therapy.

Factors influencing outcome

Appropriate outcome measures

When evaluating improvement following group CBT, the primary outcome of the treatment trials has been reduction in voices or positive symptoms, as measured by the PSYRATS or PANSS. However, only one RCT observed a reduction in hallucination severity following treatment (Wykes *et al.*, 2005), and this was associated with therapist expertise. It could be argued that voices are difficult to alter in a group setting and that a group approach is limited in this regard. However, individual CBT does not necessarily lead to reductions in severity of voices (Tarrier *et al.*, 1998) and indeed symptom reduction may not be the most appropriate target for CBT for psychosis (Birchwood & Trower, 2006). More apposite questions might be whether clients feel less isolated and socially stigmatized following treatment or whether they feel better about themselves and able to do more. These factors do seem to be influenced by group CBT, as shown by improvements on some of the secondary outcome measures used in the treatment trials (Wykes *et al.*, 2005; Barrowclough *et al.*, 2006). A further question might be whether group CBT for voices helps attendees to accept their voices. This has been suggested by Romme and Escher (this volume) to be an important step in coping with voices, and there is emerging evidence that approaches that incorporate acceptance into the therapy lead to reductions in the impact of persisting psychotic symptoms (Bach & Hayes, 2002; Gaudiano & Herbert, 2006).

Focus of the group CBT

Given that the outcome measures for group CBT tend to be the same as those used to evaluate individual CBT for psychosis, the question still remains as to why some group treatments failed to reduce psychotic symptoms (e.g., Barrowclough et al., 2006). One factor that might be relevant is the focus of the group sessions. Wykes et al. (2005) point out that a disadvantage of group work for people with complex problems is that it lacks the flexibility to respond to diverse problem presentations. They suggest that group CBT for psychosis might be more effective if there is homogeneity of symptom experience. Hence, in their study, the group focused on the common experience of hearing voices. This has the advantage that different group members report experiences that are similar in form, even if they have different beliefs about their cause. In addition, the voices are fairly frequent and easy to describe. In contrast, anomalous experiences associated with delusions can be varied and may no longer even be present. Consistent with this view, Barrowclough et al. (2006) found that negative feedback from their group members included issues that affected group dynamics, such as participants being dissimilar in terms of age or gender. They suggest that these factors might be addressed in clinical practice by selecting group participants on the basis of homogeneity of symptoms and demographic characteristics.

It is possible that the observed effect of group CBT on social functioning (Wykes et al., 2005) was due to the group's focus on the topic of voices. Wykes et al., noted that group participants were engaged in the process of group discussion about an important part of their experience—their voices. They proposed that this chance to practice their social skills as well as the opportunity to test out abnormal beliefs that had previously reduced their social contact had an impact on their social functioning outside the group. Alternatively, the effect on social functioning may just be the result of attending a group, regardless of the focus of the sessions. For example, Castelein et al. (2008) found that a facilitated peer support group for people with psychosis had a positive effect on social network and social support compared with a waiting-list control condition. This peer support group involved 16 sessions twice a week over eight months. Participants decided the topic of each session, and they discussed daily life experiences in pairs and within the group.

Therapist expertise

It is important at a clinical and service level whether expertise in the provision of CBT influences outcome following group CBT for auditory hallucinations. The majority of therapists in the treatment trials were clinical psychologists or psychiatrists, with considerable training and expertise in CBT. However, in the RCT of Wykes et al. (2005), not all the therapists were experienced in providing individual CBT. In a small, unpublished study, the transfer of skills necessary to run the voices group in this trial was tested using nurses who were offered 8 hours of training (4 of these hours being spent in groups themselves). Rating scales of CBT skills were used, as well as ratings of the use of the protocol (Ehntholt, 2000). The results showed that, following training, the skills of the nurses were equivalent to those of the experienced therapists (83% vs. 85%). In addition, the novices tended to stick to the protocol more often than the experts (96% vs. 78%). This study suggests that the skills can be transferred to novice therapists. However, the results of the RCT showed that the effectiveness of this skill transfer on the voice hearers was limited (Wykes *et al.*, 2005). In particular, groups facilitated by novice therapists did not lead to improvement in clients' hallucinations.

The study by Lecomte *et al.* (2008) also demonstrated that it is possible to train mental health workers to deliver a group CBT intervention. None of the therapists in that study had previous CBT training, but they all performed satisfactorily as group therapists, with the aid of a structured manual, on most of the therapeutic aspects measured. Furthermore, the group interventions delivered by these therapists did result in positive effects on participants' symptoms and other psychosocial outcomes. Greater improvements might have been observed with more experienced therapists, but the study wanted to examine whether CBT for psychosis could be made accessible in settings which have limited resources for extensive mental health training.

The feasibility of group CBT

For therapies to be adopted in health services, they need to be acceptable to clients. Both uncontrolled and controlled studies suggest that people who use the voices groups are not only satisfied with them but feel that they have gained benefit from attending. The therapeutic skills should also be transferable to a variety of health care professionals to increase delivery of the therapy. As described above, training staff to deliver the manualized group intervention is possible, although further training in CBT may be required for greater therapeutic effectiveness.

Maximizing attendance

Within the treatment trials, attendance to the group CBT programmes has generally been good. Wykes *et al.* (2005) reported that 79% of clients attended for at least five of the seven sessions, and 60% attended at least two-thirds of the sessions in the study by Barrowclough *et al.* (2006). Penn *et al.* (2009) defined therapy completion as attendance to at least six therapy sessions (out of a total of 12). Fifty-one participants (78%) completed six or more sessions, and participants attended an average of 8.3 sessions of CBT and 7.9 sessions of ST. This may be a reflection of the efforts taken in the trials to encourage participants to attend, and it is possible that attendance rates are lower in routine clinical practice.

It is very important to make sure that everything possible is done to ensure attendance at the first session, since this may be the biggest hurdle to overcome. Where possible, transport should be arranged to bring clients to the first session. A discussion of how group members will continue to make their way to sessions is highlighted at the first meeting. Alternatives include members helping each other, e.g., meeting at the bus stop, enlisting support workers to help clients, or arranging taxis if necessary. For subsequent sessions, it is helpful to telephone each client one or two days before to troubleshoot any difficulties that may be envisaged in getting there that week. When non-attendance occurs, there are problems of helping clients who miss sessions to catch up while not being overly repetitive or getting behind schedule for those who have attended. Barrowclough *et al.* (2006) suggest that clients who miss sessions can be offered a limited number of individual sessions (maximum 2) with the client perhaps coming half an hour earlier to the group for this purpose.

Group participants

As discussed above, the similarity of group participants seems to be important for successful group CBT, both in terms of demographic characteristics and psychotic symptoms. In addition, certain client characteristics have been found to predict group alliance among individuals with schizophrenia (Johnson *et al.*, 2008). Group alliance refers to how clients rate their relationship with the group, and was examined during the RCT by Penn *et al.* (2009). The results showed that stronger group alliance was predicted by a higher level of insight within the group, a lower individual level of autistic preoccupation, and a lower individual level of social functioning. Stronger group alliance was associated with fewer sessions missed and higher therapist ratings of treatment engagement.

Conclusions

There is evidence from controlled trials supporting the efficacy of group CBT for hallucinations in reducing symptoms and improving social functioning and self-esteem, although the evidence base is much less than that for CBT for psychosis provided on an individual basis (NICE, 2009). One advantage of group as opposed to individual CBT is that it is a relatively short therapy, which might be easily implemented in health services, although therapists need to be adequately trained and skilled in both CBT and facilitating groups. Group treatment may not be suitable for everyone and individual CBT should also be available for those whose experiences are too disturbing to discuss, except in a more supportive individual relationship. Although it has not been tested, group CBT for voices could add to the therapeutic effects of individual CBT by introducing participants to new ways of thinking about their experiences. A hearing voices group may be useful either prior to individual therapy, for clients to begin talking about their experiences, or as an adjunctive to individual therapy. It may possibly help to reduce the duration of individual treatments or even increase the effectiveness of individual CBT. In itself, even if group CBT does not have a consistent effect on the severity of hallucinations, it is a useful service provision that offers emotional and practical support to this stigmatized and isolated client group.

References

Bach, P., & Hayes, S.C. (2002). The use of acceptance and commitment therapy to prevent the rehospitalization of psychotic patients: A randomized controlled trial. *J Consult Clin Psychol*, **70**, 1129–1139.

Barrowclough, C., Haddock, G., & Lobban, F. (2001). *Group Cognitive Behaviour Therapy for Schizophrenia: Treatment Manual.* Academic Division of Clinical Psychology, School of Psychiatry and Behavioural Sciences, University of Manchester, and Tameside and Glossop Community & Priority NHS Trust.

Barrowclough, C., Haddock, G., Lobban, F., *et al.* (2006). Group cognitive-behavioural therapy for schizophrenia: Randomised controlled trial. *Br J Psychiatry*, **189**, 527–532.

Bechdolf, A., Knost, B., Kuntermann, C., *et al.* (2004). A randomized comparison of group cognitive-behavioural therapy and group psychoeducation in patients with schizophrenia. *Acta Psychiatr Scand*, **110**, 21–28.

Bechdolf, A., Köhn, D., Knost, B., Pukrop, R., & Klosterkötter J. (2005). A randomized comparison of group cognitive-behavioural therapy and group psychoeducation in acute patients with schizophrenia: Outcome at 24 months. *Acta Psychiatr Scand*, **112**, 173–179.

Beck, A.T., Steer, R.A., & Brown, G.K. (1996). *Beck Depression Inventory-II.* Pearson Assessment.

Beck, A.T., Baruch, E., Balter, J.M., Steer, R.A., & Warman, D.M. (2004). A new instrument for measuring insight: The Beck Cognitive Insight Scale. *Schizophr Res*, **68**, 319–329.

Birchwood, M., Smith, J., Cochrane, R., Wetton, S., & Copestake S. (1990). The social functioning scale—The development and validation of a new scale of social-adjustment for use in family intervention programmes with schizophrenia patients. *Br J Psychiatry*, **157**, 853–859.

Birchwood, M., Smith, J., & Drury, V. (1994). A self-report insight scale for psychosis – reliability, validity and sensitivity to change. *Acta Psychiatr Scand*, **89**, 62–67.

Birchwood, M., & Trower, P. (2006). The future of cognitive–behavioural therapy for psychosis: Not a quasi-neuroleptic. *The Br J Psychiatry*, **188**, 107–108.

Castelein, S., Bruggeman, R., van Busschbach, J.T., *et al.* (2008). The effectiveness of peer support groups in psychosis: A randomized controlled trial. *Acta Psychiatr Scand*, **118**, 64–72.

Chadwick, P., & Birchwood, M. (1994). The omnipotence of voices: A cognitive approach to auditory hallucinations. *Br J Psychiatry*, **164**, 190–201.

Chadwick, P., & Birchwood, M. (1995). The omnipotence of Voices. 2. The Beliefs About Voices Questionnaire (BAVQ). *Br J Psychiatry*, **166**, 773–776.

Chadwick, P., Lees, S., & Birchwood, M. (2000a). The revised Beliefs About Voices Questionnaire (BAVQ-R). *Br J Psychiatry*, **177**, 229–232.

Chadwick, P., Sambrooke, S., Rasch, S., & Davies, E. (2000b). Challenging the omnipotence of voices: Group cognitive behaviour therapy for voices. *Behav Res Ther*, **38**, 993–1003.

Chadwick, P. (2006). *Person-Based Cognitive Therapy for Distressing Psychosis.* Chichester: John Wiley & Sons.

Chadwick, P., Hember, M., Symes, J., Peters, E., Kuipers, E., & Dagnan, D. (2008). Responding mindfully to unpleasant thoughts and images: Reliability and validity of the Southampton Mindfulness Questionnaire (SMQ). *Br J Clin Psychol*, **47**, 451–455.

Dannahy, L., Chadwick, P., Hayward, M., Turton, W., & Gashe, C. (submitted). Group Person-Based Cognitive Therapy for Distressing Voices: Pilot data from six groups. Submitted to *Journal of Behaviour Therapy and Experimental Psychiatry*.

Ehntholt, K. (2001). *Evaluation of a CBT Group Treatment for In-patients with Auditory Hallucinations: A Pilot Study.* DClin Psych Thesis, Kings College London.

Evans, C., Mellor-Clark, J., Margison, F., *et al.* (2000). CORE: Clinical outcomes in routine evaluation. *J Ment Health*, **9**, 247–255.

Farhall, J., Greenwood, K.M., & Jackson, H.J. (2007). Coping with hallucinated voices in schizophrenia: A review of self-initiated strategies and therapeutic interventions. *Clin Psychol Rev*, **27**, 476–493.

Fowler, D., Garety, P.A., & Kuipers, E. (1995). *Cognitive-Behaviour Therapy for Psychosis.* Chichester: John Wiley & Sons.

Gaudiano, B.A., & Herbert, J.D. (2006). Believability of Hallucinations as a potential mediator of their frequency and associated distress in psychotic inpatients. *Behav Cogn Psychother*, **34**, 497–502.

Gledhill, A., Lobban, F., & Sellwood, W. (1998). Group CBT for people with schizophrenia: A preliminary evaluation. *Behav Cogn Psychother*, **26**, 63–75.

Haddock G., McCarron, J., Tarrier, N., & Faragher, E.B. (1999). Scales to measure dimensions of hallucinations and delusions: The psychotic symptom rating scales (PSYRATS). *Psychol Med*, **29**, 879–889.

Hayward, M., Denney, J., Vaughan, S., & Fowler, D. (2008). The Voice and You (VAY): A person's assessment of the relationship they have with their predominant voice. *Clin Psychol Psychother*, **15**, 45–52.

Johnson, D.P., Penn, D.L., Bauer, D.J., Meyer, P., & Evans, E. (2008). Predictors of the therapeutic alliance in group therapy for individuals with treatment-resistant auditory hallucinations. *Br J Clin Psychol*, **47**, 171–183.

Jones, S., Hughes, S., & Ormrod, J. (2001). A group evaluation of a hearing voices group. *Clinical Psychology Forum*, **8**, 35–38.

Kay, S.R., Fiszbein, A., & Opler, L.A. (1987). The Positive and Negative Syndrome Scale (PANSS) for schizophrenia. *Schizophr Bull*, **13**, 261–276.

Kingdon, D.G. & Turkington, D. (1991). A role for cognitive behavioural strategies in schizophrenia. *Soc Psychiatry Psychiatr Epidemiol*, **26**, 101–103.

Lecomte, T., Leclerc, C., Wykes, T., & Wallace, C. (2003). Group CBT versus Group symptom management for treating psychotic symptoms of young individuals presenting with a first episode of schizophrenia—preliminary results. *Schizophr Res*, **60**, 324–324.

Lecomte, T., Leclerc, C., Corbière, M., Wykes, T., Wallace, C.J., & Spidel, A. (2008). Group cognitive behaviour therapy or social skills training for individuals with a recent onset of psychosis? Results of a randomized controlled trial. *J Nerv Ment Dis*, **196**, 866–875.

Liberman, R.P., Wallace, C.J., Eckman, T., & Wirshing, W. (1988). *Symptom Management Module–UCLA Social and Independent Living Skills.* Camarillo: Psychiatric Rehabilitation Consultants.

Martin, P.J. (2000). Hearing voices and listening to those that hear them. *Journal of Psychiatric Mental Health Nursing*, **7**, 135–141.

Morrison, N. (2001). Group cognitive therapy: Treatment of choice or sub-optimal option? *Behav Cogn Psychother*, **29**, 311–332.

Newton, E., Landau, S., Smith, P., Monks, P., Shergill, S., & Wykes T. (2005). Early psychological intervention for auditory hallucinations: An exploratory study of young people's voices groups. *J Nerv Ment Dis*, **193**, 58–61.

Newton, E., Larkin, M., Melhuish, R., & Wykes, T. (2007). More than just a place to talk: Young people's experiences of group psychological therapy as an early intervention of auditory hallucinations. *Psychology and Psychotherapy—Theory Research and Practice*, **80**, 127–149.

NICE (2003). *Schizophrenia: Full National Clinical Guideline on Core Interventions in Primary and Secondary Care.* London: Gaskell Press.

NICE (2009). *Schizophrenia; Core Interventions in the Treatment and Management of Schizophrenia in Adults in Primary and Secondary Care.* www.nice.org.uk/CG 82

Penn, D.L., Mueser, K.T., Tarrier, N., *et al.* (2004). Supportive therapy for schizophrenia: Possible mechanisms and implications for adjunctive psychosocial treatments. *Schizophr Bull*, **30**, 101–112.

Penn, D.L., Meyer, P.S., Evans, E., Cai, K., & Burchinal, M. (2009). A randomized controlled trial of group cognitive behavioural therapy versus enhanced supportive therapy for auditory hallucinations. *Schizophr Res*, doi: 10.1016/j.schres.2008.12.009.

Perlman, L.M. & Hubbard, B.A. (2000). A self-control skills group for persistent auditory hallucinations. *Cognitive and Behavioural Practice*, **7**, 17–21.

Pilling, S., Bebbington, P., Kuipers, E., *et al.* (2002). Psychological treatments in schizophrenia: I. Meta-analysis of family intervention and cognitive behaviour therapy. *Psychol Med*, **32**, 736–782.

Romme, M., & Escher, A. (1989). Hearing voices. *Schizophr Bull*, **15**, 209–216.

Rosenberg, M. (1965). *Society and the adolescent self-image.* Princeton: Princeton University Press.

Slade, P.D. (1990). The behavioural and cognitive treatment of psychotic symptoms, in R. P. Bentall (Ed.), *Reconstructing Schizophrenia* (pp. 234–253). London: Routledge.

Tarrier, N., Harwood, S., Yusopoff, L., Beckett, R., & Baker A. (1990). Coping Strategy Enhancement (CSE)—A method of treating residual schizophrenic symptoms. *Behavioural Psychotherapy*, **18**, 283–293.

Tarrier, N., Beckett, R., Harwood, S., Baker, A., Yusupoff, L., & Ugarteburu I. (1993). A trial of two cognitive-behavioural methods treating drug-resistant residual psychotic symptoms in schizophrenic patients. I. Outcome. *Br J Psychiatry*, **162**, 524–532.

Tarrier, N., Yusupoff, L., Kinney, C., *et al.* (1998). A randomised controlled trial of intensive cognitive behaviour therapy for chronic schizophrenia. *Br Med J*, **317**, 303–307.

Tarrier N. & Wykes, T. (2004). Is there evidence that cognitive behaviour therapy is an effective treatment for schizophrenia? A cautious or cautionary tale? *Behav Res Ther*, **42**, 1377–1401.

Trygstad L., Buccheri R., Dowling G., *et al.* (2002). Behavioural management of persistent auditory hallucinations in schizophrenia: Outcomes from a 10-week Course. *J Am Psychiatr Nurses Assoc*, **8**, 84–91.

Ventura, J., Green, M.F., Shaner, A., & Liberman, R.P. (1993). Training and quality assurance with the Brief Psychiatric Rating Scale—The drift busters. *Int J Methods Psychiatr Res*, **3**, 221–244.

Wykes, T., & Sturt, E. (1986). The measurement of social behaviour in psychiatric patients: An assessment of the reliability and validity of the SBS schedule. *Br J Psychiatry*, **148**, 1–11.

Wykes T., Hayward, P., & Parr, A-M. (1998). *Voices Group Protocol.* Department of Psychology, Institute of Psychiatry and South London and Maudsley NHS Trust.

Wykes, T., Parr, A., & Landau, S. (1999). Group treatment of auditory hallucinations: Exploratory study of effectiveness. *Br J Psychiatry*, **175**, 180–185.

Wykes, T., Hayward, P., Thomas, N., *et al.* (2005). What are the effects of group cognitive behaviour therapy for voices? A randomised control trial. *Schizophr Res*, **77**, 201–210.

Wykes, T., Steel, C., Everitt, B., & Tarrier, N. (2008). Cognitive behaviour therapy for schizophrenia: Effect sizes, clinical models, and methodological rigor. *Schizophr Bull*, **34**, 523–537.

Zimmermann, G., Favrod, J., Trieu, V., & Pomini, V. (2005). The effect of cognitive behavioural treatment on schizophrenia spectrum disorders: A meta-analysis. *Schizophr Res*, **77**, 1–9.

Chapter 6

Appraisals: Voices' power and purpose

Peter Trower, Max Birchwood, and Alan Meaden

What should the focus of treatment be in Cognitive-Behaviour Therapy (CBT; see Smith *et al.*, this volume)—the hallucinations as symptoms of the schizophrenic illness or the clients' distressed reaction to the hallucinations? Judging by a recent review of outcome studies on CBT for schizophrenia (Wykes *et al.*, 2008), the prevailing approach is to target the symptoms, an approach modelled on the traditional prescribing of neuroleptics to treat the symptoms (see Sanjuan *et al.*, this volume). The alternative and we believe more relevant approach for cognitive-behavioural as opposed to neuroleptic treatment (Birchwood & Trower, 2006) is to target the distress and associated behaviour directly. We know from research reviewed below that clients respond in a wide variety of ways to their voices, both emotionally and behaviourally. Some are greatly distressed and fright-ened, some become depressed, and others angry. Some may harm themselves or others, some become avoidant and withdrawn or try to get relief through substance or alcohol misuse, and others shout and swear at the voices. Yet others are reassured and amused and seek contact with their voices.

It is now well established that this diversity of reactions is largely a consequence of each individual's appraisal of their voice rather than simply being an integral part of a psy-chotic illness. Romme and Escher (1989; see Romme & Escher, this volume) originally showed in their classic study how a person's ability to cope with voices varied according to their appraisal of the voice.

The development of a cognitive model of voices

Building on the work of Romme and Escher, Benjamin (1989) and others, Chadwick and Birchwood (1994) observed that if clients appraised their voice as belonging to someone with power and authority, they would be likely to respond with a degree of anxiety and acceptance of that authority and compliance with it, whereas no such reaction would be likely if they thought the voice was self-generated. Given this mediating role of beliefs, Chadwick and Birchwood considered that Beck's cognitive model for depression—recently published at the time—could in principle be adapted and equally applied to voices, with similar implications for Cognitive Therapy (CT) (see also Beck & Rector, 2005). They conducted two studies aimed at investigating the clinical utility of a cognitive approach in systematically identifying and categorizing the types of belief people hold about their voices, and then, if successful, making these beliefs the target of treatment.

In the first study, the authors were able to identify in detail the behavioural, cognitive, and affective responses to persistent voices in 26 patients, demonstrating that highly disparate relationships with voices—fear, reassurance, engagement, and resistance—reflected key differences in beliefs about the voices. All patients viewed their voices as omnipotent and omniscient. However, beliefs about the voice's identity and meaning led to voices being construed as either benevolent or malevolent. Patients provided cogent reasons for these beliefs, which, interestingly, were not always linked to voice content; indeed, in 31% of cases, beliefs were incongruous with content, as would be anticipated by a cognitive model. This was a strong demonstration of cognitive mediation, since if beliefs about voices were at odds with voice content, it suggested that meanings were constructed by individuals rather than directly voice driven; and indeed, patients disclosed 'compelling' evidence for their beliefs, which only occasionally drew upon voice content.

Without fail, voices believed to be malevolent provoked fear and were resisted, and those perceived as benevolent were courted. However, in the case of imperative voices, the primary influence on whether commands were obeyed was the severity of the command (see Meaden *et al.*, this volume).

The second study illustrated how these core beliefs about voices may become a new target for treatment. The authors described the application of an adapted version of cognitive therapy to the treatment of four patients' drug-resistant voices. Where patients were on medication, this was held constant, while beliefs about the voices' omnipotence, identity, and purpose were systematically disputed and tested. Large and stable reductions in conviction in these beliefs were reported, and these were associated with reduced distress, increased adaptive behaviour, and, unexpectedly, a fall in voice activity. These changes were corroborated by the responsible psychiatrists. Collectively, the cases provided one of the early affirmative tests of the promise of CT as a treatment for auditory hallucinations.

In a subsequent study, Birchwood and Chadwick (1997) conducted a more rigorous test of their cognitive model, and found as predicted that beliefs about voices, and not voice activity per se, held the key to understanding the affect and behaviour they generate. In keeping with their first investigation (Chadwick & Birchwood, 1994), affect and behaviour showed no relationship with voice form or topography; only when key beliefs about voices' power and purpose were considered was affect and behaviour meaningful. Thus, malevolent voices were resisted and benevolent ones courted. Voices construed as benign were associated with a greater diversity of coping strategy than those considered malevolent or benevolent, including 47% who scored high on scales of resistance and engagement, which embodied strategies as diverse as 'I try to stop my voice' (resistance), 'I take my mind away from them' (resistance), 'I follow what they say' (engagement), and 'I listen to my voices' (engagement).

They concluded that coping behaviour (see Farhall, this volume) is not a serendipitous affair 'randomly assigned to hallucinators' as it were, but driven (and indeed constrained by) these core beliefs; in the absence of these externalizing attributions, a wider range of coping behaviours was observed. Affective responses to voices was in keeping with these key beliefs but showed no link to voice topography; similarly, the high level of depression in this sample of voice hearers was linked to these beliefs in addition to positive symptoms, a known correlate of depression in psychosis.

In a minority of cases—24%—voices followed directly from content, as judged by neutral raters. For example, in one, the voice identified itself as a neighbour who made threats that were explicitly contingent upon compliance with certain demands. It follows then that since voice content and beliefs are linked, albeit in a minority of cases, and as beliefs are closely related to coping, then in some instances coping will follow from content. The cognitive model would allow for this, as it does not imply the absence of a link between triggering events and beliefs, but one suggestive of cognitive mediation. However, the role of cognitive mediation was clear, as in nearly three quarters of individuals there was either no relationship with content or an inference from content was needed to 'establish' the belief.

To summarize, the cognitive model proposed that people's beliefs about voices would also shape how they felt and coped. Four empirical papers (Chadwick & Birchwood, 1994, 1995; Birchwood & Chadwick, 1997; Close & Garety, 1998) provided empirical support for this cognitive formulation of voices. These studies showed first that people who hear voices do indeed construct meaning from the experience. Specifically, four beliefs appear to be of particular importance. That is, identity (Who is the voice?), purpose (Why is the voice talking to me, not someone else?), omnipotence (How powerful is the voice?), and control. Second, there is evidence to suggest that beliefs play a mediating role. Voices believed to be malevolent are associated with resistance and high distress, in contrast to those believed to be benevolent, which are associated with engagement and lower distress or pleasure. Also, voices believed to be omnipotent are associated with more common and severe symptoms of depression. The cognitive conceptualization then has first shown that voices are a psychological problem when, and only when, they are associated with emotional or behavioural problems, and second it has yielded a CBT treatment option for drug-resistant voices.

Further aspects of the cognitive model of voices have been developed and made explicit in a number of ways by Birchwood and other colleagues since it was first proposed and evaluated. These developments will now be described.

The ABC format

The first development of the cognitive model of voices made clear its explanatory structure to advance both the theory and practice of the CBT approach. Chadwick *et al.* (1996) used the ABC format adapted from Rational Emotive Behaviour Therapy (REBT), where A is the activating event, B are the beliefs about the A, and C stands for the emotional and behavioural consequences of the beliefs, given the activating event. Structuring the model in terms of this format provided a number of novel insights:

◆ First, voice activity is shown to be an activating event (A)—an anomalous experience that activates the belief system (B).

- Second, the distress and behavioural disturbance is a consequence at C, and as such becomes the 'problem', the relief of which becomes the goal of treatment. This is in contrast to the traditional approach, which would most likely place voice activity as a symptom to be treated at C.
- Third, the model identifies the beliefs (B) as mainly responsible for the consequential distress at C, and hence the focus for CBT intervention.

So in sum, the voice at A triggers the beliefs at B, which are largely responsible for creating the problem emotions and behaviours at C, and therapy is targeted at B in order to achieve the goal of relief at C. This model contrasts with the traditional neuroleptic model that has been more commonly adopted in CBT approaches, in which the voice is the symptom at C, and change at B is targeted to relieve the symptom. The final insight then is that CBT should primarily be aimed at emotional and behavioural change at C via B, and not primarily aimed at symptom change.

Social Rank Theory

A second development of the cognitive model was the incorporation of Social Rank Theory (SRT). One of the novel insights that was implicit in the cognitive model was that the appraisals and consequent distress and behaviour may be understood in terms of the nature of patients' *relationship* with their voice, in particular their personification of it. The idea of a relationship helps to explain why the appraisals were particularly focused on power (omnipotence) and valence (malevolence/benevolence). SRT (Chance, 1988; Gilbert, 1992; Gilbert & Allan, 1998) is particularly suited to understanding these links as it provides a general theory of how humans respond under conditions of dominance and entrapment by another. The experience of voices exemplifies this type of relationship. Furthermore, clear evidence is emerging that these symptoms commonly reflect a core self-perception of low social rank; that is the person sees themselves as being in an inferior, subordinate, and stigmatized position not only to the voice, but also to other people, particularly family and peers and also the community at large.

SRT argues that various mental mechanisms developed as part of the evolution of group living and the development of social hierarchies. In these contexts, those with superior strengths/skills were able to threaten attack or intimidate those less able, and those in subordinate positions would defend themselves by fleeing or submitting. These two mechanisms that operate as 'attack the weaker and submit to the stronger' are played out internally in patients who hear hostile voices. Hence the attack voice is normally derogating and controlling (just as any hostile dominant would be to a subordinate), and the person experiences these internal signals as requiring submission or appeasement. However, the consequences of the low social rank that these strategies entail have severe consequences, in terms of low self-esteem, humiliation and entrapment, anxiety and depression, and submissive behaviour including complying with the demands of dominant others.

SRT can best be understood in the context of the evolutionary psychology perspective. In this approach, humans and other animals in socially ranked relationships compete for resources (e.g., access to food or sexual partners) and to control each other's behaviours (Price & Sloman, 1987) and must do different things according to whether they are likely to win or lose such conflicts (Gilbert, 2000). Competing for access to resources can include alliance building, garnering support (e.g., de Waal, 1996) and trying to be attractive to others (Gilbert, 1997). However, hostile dominant strategies involve control over subordinates, via vigilance to subordinate violations and challenges, which are punished with attacks and threats. These are designed to undermine the confidence of the subordinate so that he/she backs down, submits, or complies. Indeed, hostile attacks from dominants are stressful and can increase cortisol and reduce serotonin levels in subordinates (Sapolsky, 1990; Gilbert & McGuire, 1998). In humans, dominant individuals are also able to issue commands, which subordinates will often have to comply with or obey (Scott, 1990). Subordinates have their own strategies for gaining access to resources in these contexts (in the presence of hostile dominants). For example, low-ranking primates copulate out of sight of more dominant individuals (de Waal, 1996) and feign lack of interest in forbidden objects, i.e., deception (Byrne, 1995). However, they are punished if caught and they have to be able to defend themselves if picked on. Those animals who evaluate they are in inferior positions, and would lose a conflict, may defend themselves by compliance, avoidance, submitting, escaping, and/or defensive aggression (Marks, 1987; Dixon, 1998). Offensive and defensive strategies involve different brain pathways and mechanisms (Adams, 1979). To put it briefly, dominant individuals are orientated to exert control over resources (and subordinate behaviour) by a mixture of alliance building, detection of (vigilance to) violations, and issuing threats, while subordinates engage in vigilance to threats from above and make efforts at hiding if they do seek out resources, with a readiness to flee, submit, or back down if threatened. Humans appear to have the mechanisms to act in both ways (as a dominant and as a subordinate) depending on which social group role they are operating in (Plutchik & Conte, 1997). In humans, hostile-dominant and threatened-subordinate interactions are commonly played out verbally (e.g., issuing commands, orders, instructions) and/or delivering verbal attacks (e.g., negatively labelling the other, criticism, and shaming). The purpose of a verbal, shaming attack seems similar to those of a physical threat, i.e., to subordinate the other to the wishes/interests of the 'attacker'. In the clinical literature, families where these behaviours (hostile dominating-subordinating interactions) are common are known as high-expressed emotion families in which criticism (shaming-derogating), attention to violations of expected behaviour, and intrusion-control are common (Wearden et al., 2000). We suggest that just as these types of relationship (hostile attack, subordinate defence) can be played out between individuals, they can also be played out internally. In essence, people can have a high-expressed emotion relationship with themselves—getting angry and critical for violations and failures, and shaming and negatively labelling themselves (Driscoll, 1989). In other words, the evolved mechanisms for vigilance to violations, derogating subordinates, and issuing commands are directed at the self as object, and these internal, attacking signals in turn activate submissive defences (Gilbert, 2000). In the 'two chair psychotherapy technique', depressed people are asked to role-play their critical thoughts by expressing them from one chair and then to switch chairs and explore the feelings and self-beliefs to experiencing these 'attacks' (Greenberg *et al.*, 1993). After delivering an attack on themselves, the depressed person often responds to such attacks by agreeing with the substance of an attack (e.g., 'yes, it is true I am an inadequate, worthless person') and quite commonly will take up submissive postures in the feeling chair (Gilbert, 2000). Depressed people appear to experience their self-attacks as dominant, powerful, controlling, and shaming and stressful, can feel beaten down by them and have to submit to them. Indeed, Greenberg *et al.* (1990) suggested that it is the inability to defend oneself against one's own self-attacks that results in depression. Self-attacking and self-criticism can be understood then as acting as internally generated signals (hostile-dominant) that can provoke internally generated (subordinate) defences.

Applying this approach to voices, we noted earlier that people who hear voices often relate to them as if they were relating to real external others, i.e., there is a role relationship. We have seen that the voice(s) is commonly experienced as male and malevolent, as derogating and shaming, typically issues commands, is experienced as powerful and omnipotent, and 'knowing', i.e., knows of (can detect) shameful things and violations that the person would like to keep hidden (Chadwick & Birchwood, 1994). Indeed, attacking voices and experiences of thought broadcasting are often experienced as an inability to keep 'from view' (deception) one's own thoughts and experiences. In essence, malevolent voices appear to have many of the properties of a dominant hostile other (seeking out wrongdoing and deceptions, derogating and punishing, commanding and controlling).

Such signals activate coping attempts to defend against the attacks by (at times) not only efforts to resist and fight back (defensive aggression), but also by submission and desires to escape the (hostile dominant) malevolent voice(s). Interestingly, people who generally feel inferior and subordinate to others tend to have the same feelings about their voices. Birchwood *et al.* (2000) found that the more subordinate patients felt to others in general the more subordinate to, powerful and distressed they were to their voices. If self-attacking is the result of an interplay between (internal) hostile dominant mechanisms and subordinate coping mechanisms, it remains unclear why patients with depression know that their self-attacking is internally generated, but patients who hear psychotic voices do not.

In summary, we believe the expanded cognitive theory of voices, drawing on SRT, can be used to explain the nature of the relationship to the powerful voice. Indeed, research has shown that powerful voices evoke just these types of consequences in voice hearers. The findings from a number of studies can be seen to exemplify this view:

- Voice hearers construct the link between themselves and their voice as having the nature of an intimate interpersonal relationship and often one that is inescapable (Benjamin, 1989). In a cross-sectional study, Junginger (1990) found that recent compliance was more likely where the individual personified the voice (i.e., attributed it to an identity).

◆ As we have seen, over 85% of voice hearers saw the voice as powerful and omnipotent, whereas the hearer is usually weak and dependent, unable to control or influence the voice (Birchwood & Chadwick, 1997).

◆ More than two-thirds of voice hearers were at least moderately depressed, which was directly attributable to the interpersonal appraisal of power and entrapment by the voice.

◆ The greater the perceived power and omnipotence of the voice, the greater the likelihood of compliance (Beck-Sander *et al.*, 1997), though this relationship is not linear and is moderated by appraisal of the voice's intent and consequences of resisting.

◆ Voice hearers perceive the voice as omniscient, (e.g., know the person's present thoughts and past history, was able to predict the future, etc.); this was seen as evidence of the voices' power.

◆ Some voice hearers construed their voice as benevolent, others as malevolent and persecutory (Chadwick & Birchwood, 1994, Birchwood & Chadwick, 1997).

◆ Those with benevolent voices virtually always complied with the voice, irrespective of whether the command was 'innocuous' or 'severe' (Beck-Sander *et al.*, 1997), whereas those with malevolent voices were more likely to resist, and this resistance increased if the command involved major social transgression or self-harm (Chadwick and Birchwood, 1994). However, subjects predicted the malevolent voice would inflict harm whenever they resisted and, if they continued to resist, felt compelled to appease the voice by carrying out an alternative action (Beck-Sander *et al.*, 1997).

Social Rank Theory shows features in common between hallucinations and depression (Gilbert *et al.*, 2001), namely the effect of the dominant-subordinate schema on the nature of the relationship when the voice or 'other' is in the dominant role, triggering in the patient the 'involuntary subordination response'.

Given a reasonably sound empirical base for a social rank understanding of the relationship between voice hearer and voice, we next explored the idea that the same type of dominant-subordinate rank may characterize other key relationships, particularly parents and siblings, and possibly from childhood onwards. This would follow from social rank theory, which says that the appraisal of social subordination to another comes from a *general* process of social comparison serving the formation of social ranks (Gilbert & Allen, 1998). Moreover, social rank involves not only a comparison of relative strength and power, but also social attractiveness and talent; perceived belonging, or 'fit' with a social group, is also considered to be involved in the process of social comparison (Gilbert *et al.*, 1995).

We therefore predicted that those who perceive themselves to be entrapped in a subordinate and inferior position with regard to their voice will also perceive themselves that way in their significant social relationships. To test this, we carried out a study in which we examined whether the relationship with the voice is a paradigm of social relationships in general, in accordance with the prediction of social rank theory (Birchwood *et al.*, 2000). In a sample of 59 voice hearers, measures of power and social rank difference between voice and voice hearer were taken in addition to parallel measures of power and rank in wider social relationships. We found that subordination to voices was closely linked to subordination and marginalization in other social relationships. This was not the result of a mood-linked appraisal. Distress arising from voices was linked not to voice characteristics but social and interpersonal cognition.

This study confirmed our prediction—voice hearers who perceive their voices as higher in social rank and more powerful than themselves perceive a similar difference in social rank and power between self and others in their social world. Thus, the subordinate relationship is mirrored in other social relationships and suggests the operation of anomalous interpersonal schemata subserving both. We found evidence that the genesis of these schemata is often found in early caregiver relationships (Drayton *et al.*, 1998) and in social marginalization.

We can now with reasonable confidence assume that powerful voices (hallucinated relationships) and powerful others (actual relationships) have a common theme—they both generate social signals and stimuli (activating events) that trigger the involuntary subordination response and the dysfunctional cognitive, emotional, and behavioural consequences so far discussed. However, we can extend this still further and include important other social stimuli that can set the subordination response in train. Such activating events are the actual and/or perceived life events—the onset of psychosis, possible compulsory hospitalization, loss of roles and goals, and the stigma of schizophrenia. Rooke and Birchwood (1998) found that these can all lead to actual and/or perceived low social rank, particularly marked by loss of social attractiveness and talent, of belonging, or 'fit' with a social group. In a word, they can lead to marginalization and loss of a sense of self.

In summary, among the various signals and stimuli that communicate low social rank to the individual are the voices, the family milieu—specifically the relationship to the parents and siblings, such as is commonly found in high-Expressed Emotion (EE) environments—and psychosis-related life events which, in the context of the wider community, stigmatize and 'down rank' the individual.

Type and function of safety behaviours

The original account of the cognitive model particularly emphasized the role of beliefs in producing emotional distress, while Social Rank Theory drew out the meaning and function of the emotion and behaviour in terms of a dominant-subordinate relationship with the voice. However, the question arises as to why the appraisals and consequent distress and behaviour are maintained over such long periods of time and so resistant to remission. Therefore, a further elaboration of the cognitive model has recently been developed, which addresses this problem.

In terms of the ABC model, the focus here is on the suspected cycle of influence of the consequent behaviour (C) in maintaining the power and down-ranking inferential beliefs (B) about the activating voice (A). Behaviour is functionally integral with the

distressing emotion at C, so, for example, avoidance or escape behaviour is functionally associated with anxiety, both being generated by the threat beliefs. From the client's
point of view, such behaviours form part of their coping strategy, i.e., to avoid or escape
from the appraised threat. However, the question arises as to whether these 'safety-seeking'
behaviours, far from helping, actually maintain and exacerbate the problem (Salkovskis,
1991) by preventing disconfirmation of the power and self-downing beliefs about the
voice—a prediction that was made and tested in a recent study by Hacker *et al.* (2008).

The notion that safety behaviours are linked to distress in schizophrenia has been demonstrated by Freeman *et al.* (2001). They found that individuals with persecutory delusions used safety behaviours to mitigate threats from persecutors. Their findings suggest
that delusional distress is associated with delusional threat and that safety behaviour use,
particularly avoidance, was associated with anxiety. Freeman *et al.* (2007) replicated these
findings in a larger sample. The cognitive model would lead to the prediction that distress
and safety behaviour would follow from beliefs about the power and malevolence of the
persecutor, but this was not specifically tested by Freeman *et al.* (2001). Clearly, this would
be the prediction for voice hearers, and in the case of those who have command hallucinations, the prediction would be that these behaviours would include compliance or at
least appeasement. Hacker *et al.* (2008) therefore hypothesized that

- People who hear voices engage in safety behaviours, including but not limited to compliance, to reduce specific perceived threats from their voices, i.e., threat of physical
  harm, shame, and loss of control.
- Safety behaviours and voice-related distress are driven by an increased conviction in
  beliefs about voice omnipotence, and these associations cannot be accounted for by
  voice topography (e.g., content, loudness) or mood.
- The association of safety behaviours with voice-related distress is mediated by beliefs
  about voice omnipotence.

The authors (Hacker *et al.*, 2008) carried out a cross-sectional study of 30 individuals
with hallucinations, assessing voice content and beliefs with the Cognitive Assessment of
Voices Interview Schedule (Chadwick & Birchwood, 1994; Close & Garety, 1998), the
Beliefs About Voices Questionnaire Revised (Chadwick *et al.*, 2000), anxiety and depression
with the Hospital Anxiety and Depression Scale (Zigmond & Snaith, 1983), and the Safety
Behaviour Questionnaire (Freeman *et al.*, 2001).

First, three sources of threat were identified—fear of physical harm, shame, and loss of
control. More than half the sample scored 5 or more (on a 0–10 scale, 0 being no threat
and 10 very much so) on all three threats. Twenty-six of the 30 participants reported
using safety behaviours in the last month.

Examples of safety behaviours used included

- avoidance (77%), including food believed to be poisoned and of walking out in crowds
  for fear of 'demonic' attack;
- in-situation safety behaviour (70%), including hypervigilance, such as checking windows for persecutor and changing route or clothing (disguise and deception);

- escape (23%), including leaving home because the voices said they were coming;
- pre-emptive aggression (53%), including shouting back and pre-emptive assault such as hitting people believed to be under the power of the voices;
- compliance and appeasement (50%), including full compliance such as hitting others, smashing windows, and overt and covert appeasement;
- help seeking (40%) such as contacting a 'good alien' via telepathy; and
- rescue factors (10%) such as believing God was intervening.

Omnipotence and malevolence were significantly correlated with all three types of threat. The degree of safety behaviour use and voice-related distress were associated with voice omnipotence beliefs (mood or voice characteristics did not account for this relationship). The association of safety behaviour with increased distress was mediated by beliefs about voice omnipotence.

As Beck and Rector (2005) note, 'reliance on safety strategies by hallucinators tends to maintain the hallucinations. Unfortunately, the effort spent on avoiding or neutralizing the voices leads to a curtailment in the scope of activities, which, in turn, increases isolation and, for many, leads to a paradoxical increase in voice activity' (Beck & Rector, 2005, p. 594).

Assessment based on the cognitive model of voices

The current version of the cognitive model of voices integrates and makes explicit the themes from the theories and research reviewed earlier, namely the ABC format, social rank theory, and the type and function of safety behaviours (Fig 6.1).

In brief, voice activity at A is appraised within a dominant-subordinate schema at B, giving rise to power beliefs and negative self-evaluative core beliefs, which in turn elicit at point C emotional distress, and a number of safety behaviours, which maintain the beliefs by preventing their disconfirmation. The model informs and guides the assessment and formulation, and these in turn guide the intervention. In this chapter, we describe our recommendations for engagement, socialization into the model, assessment, and formulation. The intervention steps for voices in general and for command hallucinations in particular are outlined in Meaden *et al.*, this volume.

Engagement

Engaging and retaining individuals in a therapeutic alliance is fundamental to any form of psychological assessment, formulation, and therapy, and no less so for voice hearers. However, engaging individuals who hear voices can be especially difficult due to the very distracting and distress-invoking nature of hallucinations. Consequently, there are particular as well as general principles that need to be deployed in the development of a sound therapeutic alliance. Key aspects of these sessions include

- Establishing rapport and trust through empathic listening and positive regard, and flexibility about session arrangements (venues, times, shorter or longer sessions),

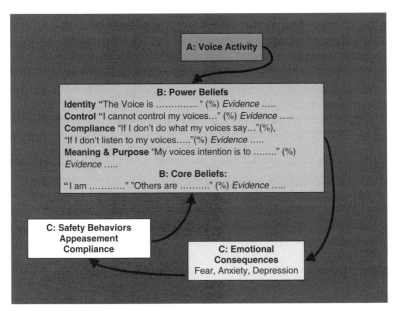

Fig. 6.1 The cognitive model of voices.

◆ Facilitating the client to give a detailed account of the experience of hearing voices and the beliefs the client has about their voices,

◆ Emphasizing a commitment to the client and the client's priorities, especially helping the client to reduce the distress and disturbance he experiences due to hearing voices,

◆ Monitoring and addressing beliefs that could threaten the engagement process; for example, the client may be concerned about the expectations and pace of therapy or about being sectioned when disclosing information about symptoms,

◆ Ensuring the client feels free to disagree, remain silent, or withdraw. The use of a symbolic 'panic button' gives the client control over the process of therapy, with the option to disengage at any point,

◆ Giving the client permission and reassurance to talk about their experiences, given that they may feel anxious or ashamed about doing so, such as thinking the therapist will label thinking it is 'crazy' to hear voices. The therapist needs to put the client at ease by giving explicit permission to talk openly about any issue,

◆ Awareness that the client may be reluctant to continue therapy due to their voices expressing anxiety about treatment or about the trustworthiness of the therapist. Anticipating that voices may comment adversely about the therapist will help the therapist develop strategies for keeping the client engaged.

Socializing the client into the 'cognitive' model

The idea of socializing the client into the cognitive model here is to begin the process of helping the client to distinguish between facts (voices) and beliefs (about the voices), that the beliefs are the main source of the distress, that the beliefs, unlike facts, can be true or false, and can and should be changed in order to overcome the distress. So, for example, it can be pointed out that it is a fact that the client hears a voice, which criticizes or makes commands, but it is a belief of the client—albeit held with high or even total conviction— that the voice is omnipotent, or must be obeyed in order to avoid being severely punished in some way. The choice of example must be carefully considered in the early stages of socialization. A good choice to start with would be a belief that the client has less than 100% conviction in and would be prepared to question. The value of this preparatory work at this early stage is to help the client gain some optimism for change, some insight into the direction and target of change, and to increase motivation to continue to work with the therapist over a sustained period. However, it is essential to continue the process of socialization and to ensure the client's understanding and commitment throughout the stages of assessment, formulation, and intervention.

Assessment and formulation

Assessment and formulation form the nub of stage 1, clearly preceding and giving direction to stage 2 intervention. However, in practice, assessment, formulation and intervention (as well as engagement and socialization) form a continuing reciprocal and iterative process. In these early sessions, the parameters of the 'power' belief system relating to the voice are identified and their role formulated, but this focus can, if necessary, be broadened in later sessions, and the early learning, developmental origins of the power beliefs, and core beliefs about the self and others can be explored, as suggested below.

The 'power' beliefs—the beliefs that define the client-voice power relationship—are identified and explored in the early sessions. These are

> *Power and control*—the belief that the voice is omnipotent, e.g., 'is much more powerful than me' and 'I do not have any control over the voice'.
>
> *Omniscience*—as part of the omnipotence belief, that the voice is all-knowing, e.g., 'knows everything that I am thinking', 'can predict the future', 'can shame me', and 'is always correct'.
>
> *Compliance, resistance, and appeasement*—also as part of the omnipotence belief, and characteristic of command hallucinations, e.g., 'The voice must be obeyed', 'If I resist the voice and don't fully comply, I must at least appease the voice', and 'If I don't obey or sufficiently appease the voice, the voice can inflict harm on me or shame me'.
>
> *Voice identity*—e.g., the belief that the voice is God or the devil.
>
> *Purpose and Meaning*—the belief that the voice is malevolent and wishes to punish the voice hearer or benevolent and has well meaning intentions.
>
> *Self and other*—the negative person evaluations, of both the self and others, e.g., 'I am a bad person and deserve to be punished', 'others (including the voice and other people) are bad and I do not deserve this punishment'.

The therapist uses these power belief concepts and the SRT framework to explore the client's beliefs about the voice. Assessment of these beliefs and more general assessment of the client's symptoms and behaviours are carried out mainly by interviewing the client and by means of the questionnaires and ratings listed below.

The therapist approaches the interview with the comprehensive ABC cognitive model of voices in mind as an interview guide, and in order to generate tentative hypotheses. However, the therapist keeps these hypotheses strictly to themselves in the initial interview and asks the client for an account of the problem entirely from their own point of view. Generally speaking, the therapist is expecting an AC account at this stage, but in the client's own words, where C is the client's experienced distress and A the voice, which the client is likely to believe is the cause of their distress, it is unusual for the client to have much, if any awareness, that the distress is mediated by B, the beliefs.

Having got a general account of the problems as experienced, the therapist asks the client to identify the emotional C, and if he gives more than one, make a note of all of them, but then focus on one, giving him the choice which one to start with. It is important to be sure to assess a specific *emotion*, such as anxiety, depression, shame, guilt, and not a thought and not a vague state such as upset. Then identify the action tendency—usually a safety behaviour at C that is associated with that particular emotion.

The therapist's next task is to help the client to identify the beliefs at B, particularly the power beliefs. This can be done in a direct way ('who do you believe the voice is?' 'If you don't do what the voice says, what will happen?') or by asking what connects A to C in their minds, i.e., what is it about the voice at A that makes them feel so afraid and avoidant or depressed and withdrawn at C. This is a particularly useful method as it is a gentle way of bringing to the client's mind that their appraisal at B mediates the voice activity at A with their distress and behaviour at C. A further method of identifying appraisals is by using measures, selecting the most relevant from those listed below (see the 'Assessment measures' section below).

The next step is to help the client to see that these power beliefs are the client's own beliefs *about* the voice and not an objective feature of the voice itself—hence B is separated from A. The therapist makes a careful distinction (for herself and the client) between the voice as an activating event, e.g., what the voice actually says, and the client's interpretation of the voice content. In this way, the process of socialization to the cognitive model, already started in the very first phase of engagement, is now elaborated.

Next, the therapist helps the client to see that it is the B (e.g., the belief in the power and malevolence of the voice) that leads to C, rather than the voice activity at A alone.

The therapist is then set to develop a formulation around the theme of the identity, malevolence, and power differential between client and voice, with the consequence of being shamed and exposed, or in the case of command hallucinations, of the need to comply, or appease if resisted, and the fear of punishment (including being shamed and exposed) if not obeyed or appeased. Having arrived at this formulation, the therapist's task is to tentatively propose it to the client (or preferably elicit it by Socratic questioning), with the aim of achieving a shared understanding.

If this shared understanding is achieved, therapist and client can then explore, perhaps at a later stage in therapy, the psychological origins of this power relationship, thus giving the client a convincing alternative formulation, which will further weaken the power of the voice. As this is as much an intervention as an assessment strategy, we describe its use later as part of stage 2. However, at this early stage, the therapist may well be reformulating in her own mind, ready to use this strategy at the appropriate time. We can illustrate this point from one of our cases, David. The therapist hypothesized that David's beliefs about his voice arose from the trauma of a childhood rape. The beliefs were construed as reactions to, and attempts to make sense of, the hallucinatory experience. Associated evaluative themes related, on the one hand, to the client's sense of worthlessness and sense that he deserved punishment and, on the other, to anger at the abuser, whom he saw as abusing this trust. The therapist kept this tentative reformulation in the back of her mind ready to use as an intervention strategy when the time was right. Thus, CBT for voices can be seen to involve a number of levels: initially working at the level of power, control, and identity beliefs and later progressing to work on beliefs about meaning and purpose and their relationship to the person's beliefs about themselves and others. The process of exploring and communicating the formulations—indeed the therapeutic process per se—involves utilizing the skills of collaborative empiricism and guided discovery long established in cognitive therapy (e.g., Beck *et al.*, 1979), and didactic and Socratic techniques in rational emotive behaviour therapy (e.g., Dryden & Neenan, 2004).

Assessment measures

An efficient way of identifying all aspects of the problem—voice activity, appraisals about the voice, and consequent emotions and behaviours, is the use of measures. Below we list those measures we use, both specific (some developed specifically for this problem) and general.

Beliefs About Voices Questionnaire-Revised (BAVQ-R; Chadwick *et al.*, 2000). This measures key beliefs about auditory hallucinations including benevolence, malevolence, and two dimensions of relationship with the voice: 'engagement' and 'resistance'. It, like its companion assessment the Cognitive Assessment Schedule, is usually completed on the most dominant and distressing voice.

The Cognitive Assessment Schedule (CAS; Chadwick & Birchwood, 1995) is used in conjunction with the BAVQ-R to further assess the individual's feelings and behaviour in relation to the voice and his/her beliefs about the voice's identity, power, purpose, or meaning and in the case of command hallucinations, the most likely consequences of obedience or resistance.

Voice Compliance Scale (VCS; Beck-Sander *et al.*, 1997). This is an observer rated scale to specifically measure the frequency of command hallucinations and level of compliance/resistance with each identified command. This was developed as a research instrument, but for ordinary clinical assessment, the clinician can obtain from the patient (or other informant like a relative) a description of all those commands and associated behaviours (compliance or resistance) within the previous 8 weeks where they felt compelled to respond. The clinician then classifies each behaviour using the following scale: neither appeasement nor compliant (1), symbolic appeasement, i.e., compliant with innocuous and/or harmless commands (2), appeasement, i.e., preparatory acts or gestures (3), partial compliance with at least one severe command (4), and full compliance with at least one severe command (5).

Voice Power Differential Scale (VPD; Birchwood *et al.*, 2000). This measures the perceived relative power differential between the voice (usually the most dominant voice) and the voice hearer, with regard to the components of power including strength, confidence, respect, ability to inflict harm, superiority, and knowledge. Each is rated on a 5-point scale and yields a total power score.

Omniscience Scale (OS; Birchwood & Chadwick, 1997). This scale measures the voice hearer's beliefs about their voices' knowledge regarding personal information. The scale is in effect a subscale of the BAVQ-R with some additional items.

Evaluative Beliefs Scale (EBS; Chadwick *et al.*, 1999). This scale measures global and stable negative person evaluations. It has three scales, Other–Self ('Other people think I am totally bad'), Self–Self ('I am totally bad'), and Self–Other ('Other people are totally bad'), each with six items measuring a sense of worthlessness, unlovability, helplessness/weakness, badness, failure, and inferiority. The client is asked to indicate their agreement with the statements on a 5-point scale ranging from 'agree strongly' to 'disagree strongly'. The scale has satisfactory psychometric validity and reliability.

In addition to these measures of the specific targeted beliefs, we also routinely include more general measures for symptoms and distress, including the following psychometrically sound and well-established scales:

Positive and Negative Syndrome Scale (PANSS; Kay *et al.*, 1987). This is a widely used, well established, and a comprehensive symptom rating scale measuring mental state.

Psychotic Symptom Rating Scales (PSYRATS; Haddock *et al.*, 1999) measure the severity of and distress associated with a number of dimensions of auditory hallucinations and delusions. The auditory hallucinations scales rate frequency, duration, location, loudness, beliefs regarding origin (external/internal), amount and degree of negative content, amount and intensity of distress, disruption to life, and controllability. The delusions scales rate amount and duration of preoccupation, conviction, amount, and intensity of distress and disruption to life. All scales are rated 0 (none) to 4 (extreme) and yield total scores for hallucinations and delusions.

Calgary Depression Scale for Schizophrenia (CDSS; Addington *et al.*, 1993) is specifically designed for assessment of level of depression in people with a diagnosis of schizophrenia. It is a quick, reliable observer rating scale that does not overlap with negative symptoms and measures depressed mood, hopelessness, self-depreciation, guilty ideas of reference, pathological guilt, morning depression, early wakening, elevated risk of attempted suicide, and observed depression.

Risk of Acting on Commands Scale (RACS; Byrne *et al.*, 2006). This rating scale was specifically designed by the authors to identify the level of risk of acting on commands and the amount of distress associated with the commands, and to help monitor change in such levels as therapy progressed.

Administering these measures may form part of the engagement process itself, demonstrating an accurate attunement to the complexity of the client's difficulties and reinforcing the message that the client and their concerns are being taken seriously. The measures are most commonly given during the initial assessment and thus aid in the planning and initial targeting of interventions. Specific measures can be used periodically as process measures to gauge the impact of interventions (particularly those assessing affect, beliefs, and behaviour) whilst more global measures of mental state and symptomatology may prove too intrusive to use repeatedly and may best be employed at the end of therapy and any follow-up.

A further aid to evaluation of therapy for command hallucinations is the CBT for command hallucinations therapy adherence protocol (Byrne *et al.*, 2006), which enables an assessment to be made of the extent to which the therapist adheres to principles and practice of CBT for command hallucinations and offers a useful guide as to the steps indicated for each stage of therapy. As such, the protocol serves as a useful training aid and fidelity marker if used in conjunction with audio or video taping of therapy sessions.

Assessment case example: Naomi

Naomi is a 24-year-old young woman who reported first hearing a voice when she was thirteen. She described having taken some unknown 'drugs' after which she experienced a voice talking to her for one day only. A year later, she said that she began to hear several voices, which were much louder and more distressing: she experienced these voices as frightening because of their nasty content. Following the onset of these voices, Naomi reported threatening someone with a knife, resulting in admission to a psychiatric hospital where she remained for the most part until the age of 17.

Naomi described a difficult childhood in which she witnessed physical violence between her parents. She was reportedly beaten by her mother and raped at seven years by an adult known to her. At the age of eight, Naomi said that she was referred to a child specialist because of her behaviour. She described how she had found it difficult to communicate: she would stare at the television and scream if her mother tried to talk to her. In addition, during early adolescence, Naomi reported that her parents separated and, subsequently, her mother had difficulties coping with her and her younger brother.

Naomi also said that, as a result of finding school work difficult, she misbehaved in secondary school and became an outsider from her peers after being suspended for assaulting a teacher. Naomi also said that her parents had been unable to help her, academically, because their education had been limited. By the age of 24, Naomi was living in supported housing with other young people with mental health problems.

During the initial assessment, Naomi described hearing 'hundreds' of voices, both male and female, with a female voice being the most dominant. She reported hearing the voices almost continuously, both inside and outside her head. She described them as extremely loud, often shouting, and said that their content was always unpleasant or negative. She said that the voices frequently commanded her to harm or kill herself (e.g., telling her to 'cut your wrists', 'jump out of windows', 'go in front of cars', 'eat what's in the toilet', 'put hot water on yourself') and that often they threatened to 'mash' her (i.e., kill her themselves). According to Naomi, the voices were also very critical of her, saying things like 'you are ugly' and 'you are no good'. Unsurprisingly, Naomi said that she found the voices very distressing.

Beliefs about power and control

According to the voice power differential scale (Birchwood *et al.*, 2000,) Naomi believed that the voices were more powerful than her, much more confident and superior to her and much more able to harm her than she was able to harm the voices. Although she rated being equally as strong and knowledgeable as the voices and rated 'we respect each other about the same'. Naomi believed that she had some control over the voices but only occasionally (i.e., the majority of the time they were uncontrollable). She believed that the voices were 50% more powerful than her because

- she had very little control over them,
- she was unable to stop them talking,
- of their attitude and their tone, and
- the voices made her do things, including harm herself.

The voices also appeared to possess extraordinary 'Omniscience':

- the voices could read her mind and commented on things she was thinking,
- they knew all about her, and her past, and
- they made predictions about the future.

Despite reporting little control over the voices, Naomi said that she was able to 'call up' the voices and have conversations with them.

Beliefs about compliance/resistance

Naomi reported that she had complied with some of the voices' commands to harm herself or others on several occasions in the past: including starting a fire, cutting her wrists and legs, taking an overdose, and throwing hot water over another person. At those times, Naomi reported feeling compelled to obey the voices out of fear: she had believed that if she resisted, the voices would harm her and would increase in frequency and in their aggressive, nasty tone. She also reported that she had felt pain in her body if she resisted the voices' commands. At the time of the assessment, however, Naomi reported being 100% convinced that she would *not* act on commands to harm herself, others, or property because she believed that it was wrong to do so. Nonetheless, Naomi said that she did comply with innocuous commands, such as 'tidy your room' and 'eat food', about two or three times daily. She believed that it was in her interest to comply with such commands and that their frequency decreased once she complied.

At the time of the assessment, Naomi was rated as 'high risk of acting on the voices' commands, with likely harm to self or others, and she was rated as 'reporting high levels of distress associated with the commands'.

Beliefs about identity

Naomi was unsure about the identity of the voices, although she said that sometimes she believed them to be the spirits of dead people.

Beliefs about meaning

Naomi reported being 100% convinced that the voices had been caused by taking some drugs when she was younger. She also believed that she was being punished for past misdeeds and that the nasty tone of the voices meant that they were trying to harm her in some way.

The intervention for Naomi is described in detail in Meaden *et al.*, (this volume), but in brief focused mainly on the issues highlighted in the assessment outlined here, particularly her beliefs about the voices' power and control, about compliance and resistance, and identity and meaning. The main compliance behaviours targeted for intervention were acting on commands to harm herself or others. The outcome for Naomi is also fully described in Meaden *et al.*, (this volume), but briefly there were positive changes pre- to post-therapy on all of the measures, although not all these changes stood up over the follow up period.

In summary, this chapter has described the origins and development of the cognitive model of voices in general and command hallucinations in particular, and its distinctive focus on distress and dysfunctional and dangerous behaviour rather than the symptoms per se, and the need to identify and modify the beliefs that specifically give rise to these consequences. We then showed how a formulation based on the model can be used as a guide to assessment of these beliefs and their role in perpetuating the problem when they give rise to safety behaviours as construed by the client. Finally, we describe the assessment steps and illustrate these with the case of 'Naomi'. The intervention based on this model, the formulation and assessment, is the focus of the chapter by Meaden *et al.*, in this volume, where we follow through with the case of Naomi and other case material.

Conclusion

Like any form of therapy, Cognitive Therapy for Command Hallucinations (CTCH) is not a complete panacea for all cases of command hallucinations, although we see no circumstances where it would be counterproductive or iatrogenic if skillfully carried out. However, there clearly are types of difficulties that would be resistant to change. One of the difficulties is where the client believes the voices are benevolent and not malevolent and where the compliance is voluntary rather than involuntary. This may be combined of course with a paranoid view that other people who are the target of the hostile commands are indeed conspiring against the client and the voices, are evil people, and deserve to be punished. Clearly, cognitive work needs to be undertaken with these beliefs before CTCH as described in this chapter could be applied. In other respects, however, there is no reason in our view why CTCH cannot be used in the majority of cases, and indeed, because of its distinctive focus on distress, usefully used in combination with or alongside other treatment approaches described throughout this volume, particularly those that emphasize a mindfulness approach.

References

Adams, D.B. (1979). Brain mechanisms for offense, defense and submission. *Behav Brain Sci*, **2**, 201–241.

Addington, D., Addington, J., & Maticka-Tyndale, E. (1993). Assessing depression in schizophrenia: the Calgary Depression Scale. *Br J Psychiatry Suppl*, **163** (suppl. 22), 39–44.

Beck, A.T., & Rector N.A. (2005). Cognitive approaches to schizophrenia: theory and therapy. *Annu Rev Clin Psychol*, **1**, 577–606.

Beck, A.T., Rush, A.J., Shaw, B.F., & Emery, G. (1979). *Cognitive Therapy of Depression*. New York: Guilford.

Beck-Sander, A., Birchwood, M., & Chadwick, P. (1997). Acting on command hallucinations: a cognitive approach. *Br J Clin Psychol*, **36**, 139–148.

Benjamin, L.S. (1989). Is chronicity a function of the relationship between the person and the auditory hallucination? *Schizophr Bull*, **15**, 291–310.

Birchwood, M., & Chadwick, P. (1997). The omnipotence of voices: testing the validity of a cognitive model. *Psychol Med*, **27**, 1345–1353.

Birchwood, M., Meaden, A., Trower, P., Gilbert, P., & Plaistow, (2000). The power and omnipotence of voices: subordination and entrapment by voices and significant others. *Psychol Med*, **30**, 337–344.

Birchwood, M., & Trower, P. (2006). The future of cognitive-behavioural therapy for psychosis: not a quasi-neuroleptic. *Br J Psychiatry Suppl*, **188**, 107–108.

Byrne, R. (1995). *The Thinking Ape: Evolutionary Origins of Intelligence*. Oxford: Oxford University Press.

Byrne, S., Birchwood, M., Trower, P., & Meaden, A. (2006). Cognitive behaviour therapy for command hallucinations. London: Routledge.

Chadwick, P., & Birchwood, M. (1994). The omnipotence of voices: a cognitive approach to auditory hallucinations. *Br J Psychiatry Suppl*, **164**, 190–201.

Chadwick, P., & Birchwood, M. (1995). The omnipotence of voices II: the beliefs about voices questionnaire. *Br J Psychiatry Suppl*, **166**, 773–776.

Chadwick, P., Birchwood, M., & Trower, P. (1996). *Cognitive therapy for delusions, voices and paranoia*. Chichester: Wiley.

Chadwick, P., Trower, P., & Dagnan, D. (1999). Measuring negative person evaluations: The evaluative beliefs scale. *Cognit Ther Res*, **23**, 549–559.

Chadwick, P., Lees, S., & Birchwood, M. (2000). The revised beliefs about voices questionnaire (BAVQ-R). *Br J Psychiatry Suppl*, **177**, 229–232.

Chance, M. (1988). *Social Fabrics of the Mind*. Hove: Lawrence Erlbaum Associates.

Close, H., & Garety, P. (1998). Cognitive assessment of voices: further developments in understanding the emotional impact of voices. *Br J Clin Psychol*, **37**, 173–188.

de Waal, F.M.B. (1996). *Good Natured: The Origins of Right and Wrong in Humans and Other Animals*. Cambridge, MA: Harvard University Press.

Dixon, A.K. (1998). Ethological strategies for defence in animals and humans: their role in some psychiatric disorders. *Br J Med Psychol*, **71**, 417–445.

Drayton, M., Birchwood, M., & Trower, P. (1998). Early attachment experience and recovery from psychosis. *Br J Clin Psychol*, **37**, 269–284.

Driscoll, R. (1989). Self-condemnation: a comprehensive framework for assessment and treatment. *Psychotherapy*, **26**, 104–111.

Dryden, W., & Neenan, M. (2004). *Rational Emotive Behavioural Counselling in Action*, London: Sage.

Freeman, D., Garety, P.A., & Kuipers, E. (2001). Persecutory delusions: developing the understanding of belief maintenance and emotional distress. *Psychol Med*, **31**, 1293–1306.

Freeman, D., Garety, P.A., Kuipers, E., Fowler, D., Bebbington, P.E., & Dunn, G. (2007). Acting on persecutory delusions: the importance of safety seeking. *Behav Res Ther*, **45**, 89–99.

Gilbert, P. (1992). *Depression: The Evolution of Powerlessness*. Hove: Lawrence Erlbaum.

Gilbert, P., Price, J., & Allan, S. (1995). Social comparison, social attractiveness and evolution: how might they be related? *New Ideas Psychol*, **13**, 149–165.

Gilbert, P. (1997). The evolution of social attractiveness and its role in shame, humiliation, guilt and therapy. *Br J Med Psychol*, **70**, 113–147.

Gilbert, P., & Allan, S. (1998). The role of defeat and entrapment (arrested flight) in depression: an exploration of an evolutionary view. *Psychol Med*, **28**, 584–597.

Gilbert, P., & McGuire, M. (1998). Shame, social roles and status: the psychobiological continuum from monkey to human. In *Shame: Interpersonal Behavior, Psychopathology and Culture* (ed. P. Gilbert & B. Andrews), pp. 99–125. Oxford: Oxford University Press.

Gilbert, P. (2000). Varieties of submissive behavior as forms of social defense: their evolution and role in depression. In *Subordination and Defeat: An Evolutionary Approach to Mood Disorders and their Treatment* (ed. L. Sloman and P. Gilbert), pp. 3–45. Mahwah: Lawrence Erlbaum.

Gilbert, P., Birchwood, M., Gilbert, J., *et al.* (2001). An exploration of evolved mental mechanisms for dominant and subordinate behaviour in relation to auditory hallucinations in schizophrenia and critical thoughts in depression. *Psychol Med*, **31**, 1117–1127.

Greenberg, L.S., Elliott, R.K., & Foerster, F.S. (1990). Experiential processes in the psychotherapeutic treatment of depression. In *Depression: New Directions in Theory, Research and Practice* (ed. C.D. McCann & N.S. Endler), pp. 157–185. Toronto: Wall and Emerson Inc..

Greenberg, L.S., Rice, L.N., & Elliott, R. (1993). *Facilitating Emotional Change: The Moment-by-Moment Process*. New York: Guilford Press.

Hacker, D., Birchwood, M., Tudway, J., Meaden, A., & Amphlett, C. (2008). Acting on voices: omnipotence, sources of threat, and safety-seeking behaviours. *Br J Clin Psychol*, **47**, 201–213.

Haddock, G., McCarron, J., Tarrier, N., & Faragher E.B. (1999). Scales to measure dimensions of hallucinations and delusions: the psychotic symptom rating scales (PSYRATS). *Psychol Med*, **29**, 879–889.

Junginger, J. (1990). Predicting compliance with command hallucinations. *Am J Psychiatry*, **147**, 245–247.

Kay, S.R., Fiszbein, A., & Opler, L.A. (1987). The positive and negative syndrome scale (PANSS) for schizophrenia. *Schizophr Bull*, **13**, 261–269.

Marks, I.M. (1987). *Fears, Phobias, and Rituals: Panic, Anxiety and their Disorders*. Oxford: Oxford University Press.

Plutchik, R., & Conte, H.R. (eds.) (1997). *Circumplex Models of Personality and Emotion*. Washington DC: American Psychological Association.

Price, J.S., & Sloman, L. (1987). Depression as yielding behavior: an animal model based on Schjelderup-Ebbe's pecking order. *Ethol Sociobiol*, **8**, 85–98.

Romme, M., & Escher, A. (1989). Hearing voices. *Schizophr Bull*, **15** (2), 209–217.

Rooke, O., & Birchwood, M. (1998). Loss, humiliation and entrapment as appraisals of schizophrenic illness: a prospective study of depressed and non-depressed patients. *Br J Clin Psychol*, **37**, 259–268.

Salkovskis, P. (1991). The importance of behaviour in the maintenance of anxiety and panic: a cognitive account. *Behavioural Psychotherapy*, **19**, 6–19.

Sapolsky, R.M. (1990). Adrenocortical function, social rank and personality among wild baboons. *Biol Psychiatry*, **28**, 862–878.

Scott, J.C. (1990). *Domination and the Arts of Resistance*. New Haven: Yale University Press.

Wearden, A.J., Tarrier, N., Barrowclough, C., Zastowny, T.R., & Rahill, A.A. (2000). A review of expressed emotion research in health care. *Clin Psychol Rev*, **20**, 633–666.

Wykes, T., Steel, C., Everitt, B., & Tarrier, N. (2008). Cognitive behaviour therapy for schizophrenia: effect sizes, clinical models and methodological rigor. *Schizophr Bull*, **34**, 523–537.

Zigmond, S., & Snaith, R.P. (1983). The Hospital Anxiety and Depression Scale. *Acta Psychiatr Scand*, **67**, 361–370.

Chapter 7

Cognitive Therapy for command hallucinations

Alan Meaden, Max Birchwood, and Peter Trower

Introduction

Working with people experiencing command hallucinations can seem daunting for many practitioners. Histories of risk behaviour and associated media coverage may lead clinicians to avoiding working with this group; seeing them perhaps as largely the domain of forensic services. In truth, such symptoms are common and individuals who experience them frequently seek help. In this chapter, we illustrate an evidence-based approach to working with command hallucinations based on our extensive clinical and research experience and findings.

The key feature that distinguishes command hallucinations from 'ordinary' hallucinations is that the voice is experienced or interpreted as commanding rather than commenting. These perceived commands range from making a harmless gesture (turning the lights off) to behaving in ways that are potentially injurious or lethal to self or others (stabbing another person, cutting ones wrists).

Command hallucinations occur at a high rate in both adult psychiatric and forensic patients but vary considerably from study to study (e.g., 18 to 89%), with a reported median rate of 53% across eight studies (Shawyer *et al.*, 2003). These authors further report a median prevalence of 48% for harmful commands in non-forensic patients, but again the range was considerable: from 7 to 70%. Forensic groups are likely to be higher, with 83% of voice hearers found to have so-called command hallucinations with 'criminal' content. Command hallucinations that command violence are held by some to be an increased risk factor for violence (Monahan *et al.*, 2001). At least partial compliance to these harmful commands was reported by Shawyer *et al.* (2003) in 31 % (median rate across studies) in community samples, but with a very wide range: 0–92% suggesting methodological difficulties in the studies reviewed. Compliance with voice commands has been found to be associated with identification of the voices as real people or identities, hallucination-related delusions, and emotional involvement with the voices (Erkwoh *et al.*, 2002). In a recent study, we found that acting on voices was predicted by the voice hearer's beliefs about the voice (Hacker *et al.*, 2008).

Cognitive Therapy for Command Hallucinations (CTCH) like all cognitive therapies for psychosis conceptualizes cognitive processes as central to understanding psychotic experiences and working with them. It also, perhaps uniquely, clarifies the psychological processes that underlie many of the risk behaviours tenuously linked to command hallu-cinations and offers a set of therapeutic principles for reducing such risk. This very clear explanatory model, in the ABC framework, is outlined in Trower, Birchwood, and Meaden (this volume). Therapeutic change is targeted at C, i.e., the focus is on voice-related distress and compliance behaviour, which is a consequence of dysfunctional beliefs at B. In this regard, our model owes much to Rational Emotive Behaviour Therapy (REBT) as first practiced in 1955 by Albert Ellis (Ellis, 2004). We have also adopted concepts from Social Rank Theory (Trower, Birchwood & Meaden, this volume) in deepening our understanding of the unique power some voices appear to have over the individuals who experience them. Understanding this power relationship holds the key to explaining the subordinate compliant behaviour individuals engage in. This overarching theme of power runs through all therapeutic efforts and is used both implicitly and explicitly in the thera-peutic relationship. The perceived need to obey seemingly powerful voices is crystallized in what we have termed the voice power schema (a set of inter-related voice beliefs). The target of therapy is to deconstruct these power schema and reduce distress and compliance behaviour and thereby risk.

CTCH is not an altogether novel enterprise. We have found evidence of an early account that illustrates the key features of our approach. John Percival (cited by Peterson, 1982), the son of English Prime Minister Spencer Percival (1762–1812), provides a vivid account of his experience. When 27 years old, John Percival started seeing visions and hearing voices that told him to do strange things. His behaviour became so erratic that a 'lunatic doctor' was called who strapped him to his bed and gave him broth and medi-cine. John describes his experiences, attempts to understand, and recover from them as follows:

'Those voices commanded me to do and made me believe a number of false and terrible things. I threw myself out of bed, I tried to twist my neck, and I struggled with my keepers. When I came to Dr. Fox, I threw myself over a style, absolutely head over heels, wrestled with the keepers to get a violent fall, asked them to strangle me, endeavoured to suffocate myself on my pillow, threw myself flat on my face down steep slopes … and upon the gravel walk, called after people as my mother, brothers, and sisters, and cried out a number of sentences, usually in verse, as I heard them prompted to me—in short for a whole year I scarcely uttered a syllable or did a single act but from inspiration.'

'On another occasion being desired to throw myself over a steep precipice near the river Avon—with the promise that if I did so, I should be in heavenly places or immediately at home; I refused to do so for fear of death and retired from the edge of the precipice to avoid temptation … but this last was not till after repeated experiments of other kinds and proved to me that I might be deluded.'

'For I was cured at last, and only cured of each of these delusions respecting throwing myself about, by the experience that the promises and threats attendant upon each of them were false. When I had fairly performed what I was commanded, and found that I remained as I was, I desisted from trying it…'

'I knew I had been deceived—and when any voice came to order me to do any thing, I conceived it my duty to wait and hear if that order was explained, and followed by another—and indeed I often rejected the voice altogether. And thus, I became of a sudden from a dangerous lunatic, a mere imbecile, half-witted though wretched being, and this as the first stage of my recovery.'

Unfortunately, not all individuals who experience these symptoms are able to develop such insights or to challenge their voices in this way. In CTCH, a therapeutic relationship is developed, which enables clients to understand and test out the false claims that their voices make and learn new coping strategies (cognitive, behavioural, and physiological) to resist their voice's commands and better manage their distress. The therapeutic relationship is further utilized to model power and the retaking of control.

Engaging, assessing, and agreeing the focus

We have put forward in some detail in Trower, Birchwood, and Meaden (this volume) our theoretical model—our cognitive model of voices, including the ABC structure and social rank theory—which guides our assessment and formulation for voices in general and also the practical steps involved in engagement and formulation. The model and the steps are, of course, applicable for people with specific command hallucinations, and the reader is referred to Trower, Birchwood, and Meaden (this volume) for these detailed guidelines. In this chapter, we will summarize these points but focus mainly on the interventions that follow from the model, though of course the entire process of engagement, assessment, formulation, and intervention does not proceed in a fixed sequence but flows in a flexible, integrated, and cyclical way.

Table 7.1 illustrates the key stages and interventions of CTCH, which guide our therapeutic endeavours and serve to maintain a clear focus that links to our standardized formulation templates, which we also illustrate in our key case examples below.

We have chosen two case studies reported by Byrne *et al.*, 2004 that best illustrate the process of CTCH and demonstrate its effectiveness, producing changes at C. Other brief vignettes are used throughout to further illustrate key points.

Two case studies

Our first illustrative case is Naomi, a 24-year-old-woman who began hearing voices at the age of thirteen. Soon after hearing voices, she threatened someone with a knife, resulting in admission to a psychiatric hospital. During therapy, Naomi reported a traumatic childhood characterized by physical violence, rape, and subsequent behavioural problems. She found school difficult, her behaviour making it hard to develop and maintain friendships. She was suspended from school on a number of occasions.

At assessment, Naomi described hearing hundreds of voices almost continuously (male and female), with a female voice being the most dominant. They were extremely loud, often shouting, and always unpleasant (e.g., 'you are ugly' and 'you are no good'). Her voices frequently commanded her to harm or kill herself (e.g., 'cut your wrists', 'jump out of windows', 'go in front of cars', 'eat what's in the toilet', 'pour hot water on yourself'), and threatened to 'mash' her (e.g., kill her themselves). Understandably, she found these voices very distressing.

Table 7.1 The key tasks at each stage of CTCH

CTCH Stage	Key Tasks
Assessment and engagement	1 Obtain a detailed account of the person's psychotic experiences and development of beliefs about voices.
	2 Anticipate and address engagement problems: voices commenting on therapist. Pass a message to the voice—therapist not trying to get rid of you but help with your distress.
	3 Introduce symbolic panic button (to model control early on and promote engagement).
	4 Normalize experiences: nosey neighbours, school bully analogies.
Socializing the client into the ABC model	1 Use lower conviction beliefs/ones that have changed in their level of conviction: the tooth fairy, favourite band.
	2 Explore the advantages and disadvantages of voice beliefs being true and false.
	3 Normalize the role of beliefs in everyday life: cat in the night versus a burglar and link to different likely affective responses.
	4 Reframe difficulties in 'ABC' terms.
Developing and sharing the formulation	1 Develop the formulation initially around the power schema (including evidence for each belief), compliance behaviours and distress.
	2 Hold back core belief and subordination schemas for later reformulation and advanced CTCH work.
Setting goals for therapy	1 Set goals around reducing distress and the use of safety/compliance behaviours.
	2 Draw on the clients own doubt: examples of when the voices got it wrong.
Promoting control	1 Reframe what the client is already doing – what increases and decreases the voices (triggers and cues).
	2 Introduce/teach new coping strategies e.g., switching voices on and off, developing boundaries.
	3 Reframe coping strategies as evidence of control and therefore as evidence of the power shift.
Reframing and disputing power beliefs	1 Draw on clients doubt and own concerns that beliefs may be wrong.
	2 Dispute omniscience of the voices: discredit the truth of what they say, their capacity to carry out threat, knowledge they have about the person and others and their ability to make predictions, question evidence, use logical reasoning.
	3 Dispute compliance beliefs: when acted against the voices with no consequences,
	4 Explore imagined consequences of disobedience.
Reducing safety behaviours	1 Identify discomfort intolerance beliefs.
	2 Use metaphors (e.g., Garlic and Vampires—holding up brick walls).
	3 Emphasizing benefits of resistance → Use graded approach to reduce safety behaviours and appeasement → Reality testing of beliefs→ behavioural experiment.

Assessment revealed that she believed the voices were more powerful than her but that she had some limited control over them. They also made predictions about the future and knew all about her past behavior. Naomi had complied with some of the voices' commands to harm her or others on several occasions, including starting a fire, cutting her wrists and legs, taking an overdose, and throwing hot water over another person. If she did not comply, Naomi believed that the voices would and could harm her, they would increase in frequency and in their aggressive, nasty tone. Naomi reported that she had felt pain in her body if she resisted the voices' commands.

Naomi's beliefs about her voices, her related distress and behavior, and core beliefs were formulated.

Our second case, Kevin, is aged 18 and lives with his mother and her partner. He too described a difficult childhood growing up in atmosphere of domestic violence, his father left the family when Kevin was 4 years old, and he was raised by his mother and maternal grandmother. At school, Kevin had difficulties with reading and writing and was regularly bullied by other children. Kevin initially developed OCD and was later admitted to the adolescent unit of a local psychiatric hospital with both symptoms of OCD and hearing voices. He reported that he would wash his hands in response to voices telling him to do so. During his last admission, his grandmother, whom Kevin had been especially close to, became ill and died (Fig. 7.1).

Kevin reported hearing two voices (one male, one female), with the male voice being most dominant. He heard the voices several times a day, but mostly at night. They were quite loud and derogatory towards him and others (e.g., 'you are ugly', 'your mother is evil'),

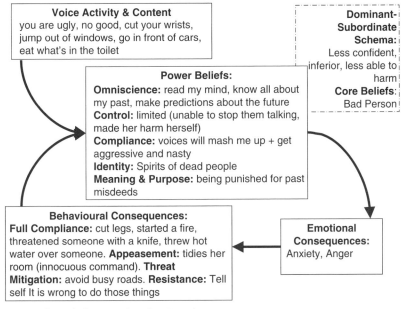

Fig. 7.1 CTCH formulation template for Naomi.

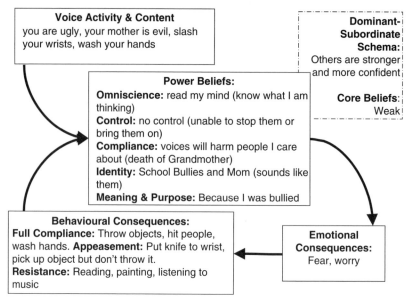

Fig. 7.2 CTCH formulation template for Kevin.

which he found very distressing. They also commanded him to harm himself and others (e.g., 'slash your wrists', 'hit that person'), as well as telling him to wash his hands frequently. Kevin felt scared and worried by the voices most of the time. He believed that the voices were more powerful and perceived himself to have no control over when they started or stopped. He had hit people on three or four occasions in the past (including his mother), in response to the voices. He also partially complied with commands to slash his wrists on one occasion in his teens, by taking a knife to his wrists but not cutting. He also reported partially complying with commands to throw things by picking up an object but not throwing it. If Kevin did not comply, at least partially, he believed that something bad might happen to him or his mother. The voices tended to decrease in loudness after he complied but also laughed at him. If he resisted, however, the voices got louder and made him feel more scared. Kevin's beliefs about his voices, related distress and behavior, and core beliefs were formulated as in Fig. 7.2.

Engagement

Engagement is the key to successful CTCH. Care co-coordinators (e.g., those responsible for planning and often delivering the care of clients), as well as the client, often require reassurance before proceeding. Trust must be established through empathic listening and addressing engagement beliefs (e.g., regarding expectations of and the pace of therapy, symptoms being exacerbated, or further restrictions being applied when disclosing information about commands and related behaviour). Time should be devoted to eliciting the client's theories about their voices, which will often have evolved into mini theories of the world and the clients (subordinate) place within it. This must be explored and understood sensitively and carefully, valuing the client's struggle and attempts to cope thus far. These theories and beliefs can subsequently be used to map out the person's power schema and to develop a CTCH case conceptualization, which guides the treatment process. Techniques and strategies adopted in CTCH at this stage include

- being flexible about session arrangements (shorter or longer sessions),
- the use of a symbolic 'panic button' (as described in Trower, Birchwood, and Meaden, this volume),
- giving permission for the client not to talk about their voices for brief periods, whilst asking permission to explore their concerns regarding this. This non-voice talk can be utilized at a later stage in developing coping strategies (see Farhall, this volume) and socializing the individual into the cognitive model,
- focusing on the emotional Cs for the client and reflecting these back in an empathic way,
- normalizing experiences (see Garrett, this volume) and actions using analogies of being bullied or having nosey neighbours,
- anticipating that the voice may attempt to discredit the therapist. The therapist may in turn raise their own social rank to battle the voices by noting their knowledge about voices, and
- remaining mindful of the clients emotional investment in their beliefs.

Kevin reported that the voices had criticized the therapist, saying 'it will all go wrong', and 'it's hopeless' saying about the therapist that they 'can't do anything'. Discussion revealed, however, that Kevin often disagreed with the voices, even though they did not like it and he felt scared for standing up to them. The therapist praised Kevin for his efforts and asked that he persevere despite the voices' negative responses.

Stephen had heard voices from an early age. He was slight in build and lived in an inner city area where he constantly felt in danger and was hypervigilant to sources of threat. Overall Stephen perceived himself as being of lower social rank compared to other people in general. He heard two male voices, one, very dominate, who he identified as a powerful school bully who had tormented him. This voice commanded him to dress and act in certain ways: shave your head, wear a leather jacket. If he complied he believed he would 'gain respect', whereas if he failed to comply he would be kept awake all night with taunts and insults, e.g., 'you are weak and useless'.

It was important to begin each session by asking Stephen about how the voices had reacted to the last therapy session. He reported that the voices had dismissed the therapist's efforts, saying 'don't listen to him, he knows nothing!' The voice had gone on to threaten Stephen, 'don't talk to him, he will poison you', and often kept him awake at night.

The therapist stressed his knowledge about working with others experiencing voices and noted that this was not an unusual reaction. The aim of improving Stephen's coping and control and reducing his distress were continually stressed as the main goals of therapy and not the elimination of the voices per se. The therapist asked that this be communicated to the voices. Stephen was able to continue with the sessions and his voices became less hostile about the therapy and the therapist.

Promoting control

Promoting a sense of control is an important practical and conceptual step in CTCH. It serves to consolidate initial engagement and build optimism for change. Crucially, it begins the process of undermining the perceived power of the voice and building evidence against the individual's own powerlessness.

We begin by reviewing and enhancing any existing coping strategies, emphasizing and valuing at the same time the client's strengths in coping with their voices so far. This can also serve to build discomfort tolerance, which is often helpful for those clients (as in the case of Stephen), where voices can sometimes carry out certain threats for non-compliance: keeping the person awake all night.

At the beginning of therapy, Kevin reported that the voices, he believed, had caused his grandmother's death by telling her to smoke heavily, causing her to develop cancer. With great care and sensitivity, the possibility that his grandmother had chosen to smoke was explored. Kevin became less convinced that the voices had caused his grandmother's death and so he could safely choose to ignore or defy them.

The process of promoting control involves developing or reinforcing a coping repertoire through clarifying the factors that increase or decrease the presence of voices. The aim is to bring some immediate relief and thereby underpin engagement. The therapist may introduce novel ideas that have been tried successfully by other voice hearers. The client is encouraged to decrease voice activity for short periods using these techniques. These periods can then be gradually lengthened and with growing confidence, the client can be helped to utilize their power to start the voices, thus increasing the sense of control further.

Naomi developed a variety of ways of coping with her voices, enabling her to have more control over them:

◆ Keeping occupied (regularly attending college, going out for a walk, shopping, tidying her room, cooking),

◆ Talking with or being in the company of trusted others,

◆ Reading a good book,

◆ Listening/dancing to music, and

◆ Watching an interesting TV programme or video.

By learning to ignore the voices as much as possible, and get on with other things, rather than engage in conversation with them, Naomi found that she was able to have more control over the voices and gain respite from them. This further reinforced her use of such coping strategies. Naomi observed that the voices sometimes began when she was stressed or worried about something. She found that relaxation and/or distraction techniques helped with this.

Coping strategies are often unique to that person and will depend upon the particular triggers or exacerbatory factors as in Naomi's case. However, we also usefully draw upon a number of commonly used strategies for promoting control:

◆ Watching/listening to the TV/Radio,

◆ Reading,

◆ Listening to music/radio through headphones,

◆ Humming/gargling,

◆ Following lyrics to favourite songs in one's head,

◆ Wearing ear plugs,

◆ Time-limiting contact,

◆ Only speaking to benevolent voices,

◆ Assertively addressing the voice, and

◆ Negotiating with voices.

A useful strategy in CTCH is to frame the voice and voice-hearer as being in a quasi-interpersonal relationship in which the client can develop boundaries. The aim of this is to help the client turn their attention to or away from the voice and therefore achieve some respite and have their own time. This enables the client to make their own decisions, rather than always listening to and waiting for the voice to initiate them. The voice is consequently seen as less powerful and the client can begin to set new boundaries by taking the stance that they are 'not always available' and will perhaps talk to the voice later. The person may subsequently come to view what the voices say as not as important as before and respond by saying 'I am not going to listen, I've got better things to do'.

Brian heard voices from the spirit world (which had previously been benevolent) saying *'lie on the railway lines'*, *'cut your hands off'*, *'kill yourself and come fly with us'*, and *'don't take medication'*. He often partially and sometimes fully complied with some of these commands. In the past, he believed that the voices had taken his legs away for non-compliance and they frequently kept him awake at night for not complying. Brian learned to develop boundaries with his voices by negotiating with them. He was subsequently able to get more sleep and was thus better able to cope with and develop a new understanding about his voices, recognizing their false claims and later their meaning and purpose.

CTCH formulation: Relocating the problem at B

As we outlined by Trower, Birchwood, and Meaden (this volume), case formulation is seen as an increasingly important activity in cognitive therapy. We have adopted a simple (at least seemingly so) template to aid reliability but also to enable a sustained focus on the key issues: voice related distress and compliance with commands. The cases of Naomi and Kevin illustrate the key information utilized in CTCH to promote change. Tightly defining and listing the power schema enables a sustained focus of therapy on power belief and their supporting evidence. We find the ABC formulation is a powerful tool capable of expressing and distilling most aspects of client's psychotic concerns and distress. Safety behaviours are broken down into full compliance, appeasement or partial compliance, and threat mitigation strategies (such as avoidance). All crucially prevent disconfirmation of compliance and other power beliefs. Clearly, formulating them in this way early on alongside resistance strategies enables the therapist to retain a clear focus. CTCH formulations also include core beliefs and social rank interpersonal schema. These are generally kept in the background to inform later reformulations at the advanced stages of CTCH.

The process of formulation may also involve separating out the various As, Bs, and Cs, mindful of the fact that there may be several As (e.g., derogatory comments, commands to harm self, commands to harm others), which may all lead to different or the same Bs (power schemas). The therapist must also carefully distinguish between the voice as an activating event (e.g., what the voice actually says) and the client's interpretation of the voice content. Specific examples or incidents are sought to tease out each A, B, and C. Each ABC chain can be then reframed and feedback to the client (thus beginning the process early on of socializing them into the model):

> 'So the voice said you are on your way (A) and you figured out it meant you were going to be killed (B) and that made you feel scarred (C)?'

Having arrived at this formulation, the therapist's task is to tentatively propose it to the client (or preferably elicit it by Socratic questioning), with the aim of achieving a shared understanding. If this shared understanding is achieved, therapist and client can then explore, perhaps at a later stage in therapy, the psychological origins of this power relationship, thus giving the client a convincing alternative formulation, which will further weaken the power of the voice. A key part of developing this shared understanding is locating the problems at C: agreeing that the behaviours and voice-related distress are to be targeted. This move enables the setting of the scene for developing subsequent therapy goals.

Relocating the problem at B is the next key stage. If clients do not accomplish this, then progress in disputing power beliefs and dropping safety behaviours will be compromised. A useful starting point is to help the client to distinguish between facts and beliefs. Beliefs, unlike facts, can be true or false, and can be changed, especially when they are unhelpful. In CTCH, voice occurrence is seen as a fact (A), but its power and the need to act on it is not—these lie at point B. A good choice to start with would be a belief that the client has less than 100% conviction in and would be prepared to question. Earlier non-voice-related talk can be valuable here; perhaps asking about a band that the person had once thought was the best but now has moved onto another artist. The value of this preparatory work at this early stage is to help the client gain some optimism for change and motivation to continue to work with the therapist.

Another strategy that can be introduced here is developing the rationale for questioning voice beliefs by considering the advantages and disadvantages of the beliefs being true or false. Once the client sees that they would be 'better off' if the beliefs were false, motivation to proceed with therapy will be further increased.

Agreeing and setting therapy goals in CTCH

The goals in CTCH are always to reduce distress and safety behaviour use. Implicitly, the stage of promoting control in CTCH begins the process of undermining the client's belief in the voices control over them. This is introduced as a recurring narrative in CTCH as evidence of the weakening perceived power of the voices, the clients' own increasing power, and, by implication, weakening other voice beliefs, since they may also be wrong. The next focus is to agree that the client's beliefs in the voice's power and omniscience should be questioned. Once agreed, the task is to clarify the evidence for these beliefs.

Brian's voices claimed credit for taking his legs away when an in-patients (an adverse drug reaction) reinforcing his belief in their power. They also appeared to know everything about him (omniscience), including bad and shameful things he had done.

Time should be devoted also to identifying the unhelpful use of safety behaviours and threat mitigation strategies. Unless these are clearly identified, progress in CTCH cannot be readily assessed or the validity of power schemas tested. In CTCH, safety behaviours may involve direct or partial compliance/appeasement with voice commands. Appeasement functions to reduce distress by in effect *buying off the voice*. The individual thus avoids punishment for non-compliance. Crucially, they also prevent disconfirmation of power schemas. The client must be helped to understand this in subsequent stages of CTCH. Dropping of these safety behaviours is therefore a clear target.

Kevin puts a knife to his wrist but does not actually cut his wrist. This buys him some temporary relief from the voices and they quieten down. He does not however learn that by ignoring the voice they cannot actually carry out their threats to harm people he cares about.

Threat mitigation strategies may also be used by the client. These are a further type of safety behaviour used by some clients and aim to reduce perceived threat.

Tony stays in his bed for many hours as he feels safe there, and he believes that if he does not leave his room during the day, then the voice cannot get him and 'chop him into pieces'. This threat mitigation, however, prevents him from ever learning that the voices cannot actually carry out their threats.

Disputing and reframing in CTCH

The overall aim of this phase of CTCH is to address the perceived power imbalance, which underpins compliance and distress. The specific aims are to

- reduce the perceived power of the voice and increase the perceived power of the voice hearer,
- reduce compliance, appeasement, and other safety behaviours and increase resistance,
- weaken the conviction that the client is being and will be punished or harmed, and
- weaken the conviction about the identity of the voice.

In CTCH, the therapist often has an end point in mind and aims to teach the client a particular point, i.e., 'so your voice tells lies'. We also employ the Socratic method exploring and questioning the client regarding their beliefs about their voices and allowing them to develop a new conclusion, hopefully one that is more helpful (e.g., 'my voice wouldn't tell lies, it only makes mistakes; my voice does not always tell the truth').

At different times and different stages of CTCH, both can be useful approaches and are skilfully mixed by the therapist to dispute power beliefs. Typically we

- begin by exploring the origin or source of the belief,
- tentatively and sensitively seek clarification, i.e., 'are you saying that the voice is all powerful and you have no control over it at all?'
- list and critically examine support, reasons, and evidence for the belief, i.e., 'it sounds like the devil (identity), I can't start or stop it (control), it knows all about me (omniscience)',
- develop and critically examine the implications and consequences of the belief: 'so you believe that you have to do what it says otherwise you will be punished?' and
- seek and fairly examine conflicting views (alternative points of view), i.e., 'so sometimes you can stop it or ignore it then (disputing control)?'

During this process, the therapist draws upon

- the client's own doubt, past or present,
- the client's own contradictory evidence and behaviour, and
- the client's own concerns about the possibility that their beliefs about the voices may be wrong.

Commonly, the client will tend to provide only supportive evidence, and help is often needed to build evidence against the belief. Disconfirming evidence can be built up from anything the client has noticed in the past that seemed to be inconsistent with what the voices said, including evidence that has been elicited during the course of therapy. By subsequently following a line of logical reasoning, further inconsistencies in the client's belief can be exposed.

Through Socratic questioning, Naomi realized that her voices said things that were contradictory. They made comments about her room being untidy, when it was clearly not, they also said 'you're ugly' one minute and 'you're beautiful' the next. Naomi concluded that she couldn't win with the voices, so she would just do what she wanted to do and agree with what she wanted to agree with.

We find that resistance to challenging evidence can be weakened by firstly rank ordering the evidence for and against each belief, from the most to least convincing. This evidence can then be questioned starting with the least convincing piece of evidence first, a disputation hierarchy.

Challenging omniscience

Discrediting the omniscience of the voices and revealing that they are fallible and make mistakes (just like everyone else) is an important strategy in down-ranking them and loosening their hold over the individual. Didactic techniques are often useful here.

Joe heard voices that told him that the end of the world was coming in the year 2000 (it did not!). Stephen's voice commanded him to shave his head and he would get respect from others (he did shave his head but did not experience more respect).

Key dispute: 'So, the voices make lots of claims about people but cannot back them up!'

Key dispute: 'So if they lie about this, what else are they lying about?'

Pre-therapy Kevin believed that he had to comply with the voices' commands because he feared that the voices might harm him or someone he cared about if he resisted. This belief was challenged in therapy. It was proposed that only something physical, like a knife or a bullet, can harm the physical body. Gradually, Kevin began to develop the belief that the voices were not physical objects, thus concluding that they could not do him any physical harm. It was also observed that the voices seemed to rely on Kevin to do what they said. The therapist subsequently explored what happened when Kevin chose *not* to act. Kevin began to realize that he had resisted the voices' commands many times without him or his family coming to any harm. He concluded that the voices could not physically make him comply and that they were powerless to act themselves.

Key dispute: 'So, they cannot do any harm to you or others; therefore, they cannot carry out their threats!'

Key dispute: 'They have not done anything when resisted', (Kevin did not use a safety behaviour and the feared consequences did not happen). 'The voices are therefore all mouth and no trousers'. In other words, the voices boast and make great claims about their abilities but are ultimately unable to carry them out.

Key dispute: 'If they are so powerful why do they need you to act for them?'

In some cases, the voices do carry out their threats: the voice does keep the person awake, abuses them by saying derogatory things about them, and shouts at them. This can be tricky in therapy as acting against the voices' commands or challenging their claims can result in the belief being reinforced when the voice does indeed punish them by keeping them awake or tormenting them. This requires careful assessment. The key question we ask here (drawing on REBT therapy and practice) is can the person stand or learn to tolerate it? Some examination of the longer-term benefits may be useful here in order to build motivation for the person to tolerate such unpleasant and distressing experiences. The use of coping strategies to manage these distressing episodes is often vital.

Key dispute: 'This is very difficult to bear but I can bear with it *and* I can use my coping strategies to cope'.

Having created uncertainty and weakened beliefs about omniscience, it becomes possible for the person to test out their compliance beliefs and begin to drop their use of safety behaviours.

Challenging compliance beliefs

Safety behaviours are adopted by the individual to reduce perceived threat and provide short-term relief. In this, they are effective and their value should be explicitly recognized. The therapist therefore needs to prepare the client for the task of reducing their use by noting that in the longer term, safety behaviours maintain beliefs about power and omniscience, prevent disconfirmation of the voices' ability to carry out their threats, and keep the client trapped in a subordinate position.

It is important to help the client identify the perceived consequences of carrying out a command compared with the perceived consequences of resisting it (e.g., short-term gains of reducing anxiety may be outweighed by long-term disadvantages: being sectioned, causing lasting harm to oneself or others). Safety behaviours have an important psychological function for the individual of appearing to prevent harm. They are the natural coping strategies, albeit dysfunctional ones. Consequently, clients are likely to be resistant to reducing them as this may increase their anxiety or make them feel that they have less ability to resist harmful commands. A systematic graded approach is likely to minimize both therapist and client anxieties.

Where catastrophic beliefs are identified, the therapist can explore the idea that obeying the command is a kind of safety behaviour, which is understandable as it reduces anxiety but prevents disconfirmation of the beliefs. Once the client grasps this principle, the beliefs can be challenged and empirically tested by the techniques described above.

We begin by constructing a treatment hierarchy and tackling those behaviours that are agreed to be less important. At the same time, we emphasize and encourage the use of coping strategies, being careful not to allow them to prevent disconfirmation of the belief. The use of a coping strategy is primarily to support the client in their efforts to drop the safety behaviour and resist the command.

Kevin's belief that he had to comply with the voices' commands was further addressed by asking him to consider the advantages and disadvantages of acting on their commands, particularly those with serious consequences to himself or others. Disadvantages of obeying included harming himself or others, the risk of getting into trouble with the police, and feeling very distressed. Socratic questioning also elicited the fact that the voices sometimes continued even after he had complied, and when they did stop, it was only for a short time. Advantages of resisting included not getting into trouble or putting himself in danger, feeling more in control, and no physical harm to himself or significant others. It was noted that Kevin often felt anxious initially; when resisting the voices' commands, however, this anxiety did gradually reduce, especially when he used a coping strategy taught to him by the therapist (a relaxation exercise). Kevin reached the conclusion that there were more advantages to resisting the voices' commands than complying with them.

Disconfirmation of voice beliefs and their claims in CTCH often involves using behavioural experiments. By carrying out or withholding safety behaviours, the compliance belief is explicitly tested. The usual procedure for devising such tests is adopted in CTCH. The clients predicted outcome must be clearly specified in order to avoid substitute delusional interpretations. Mental rehearsal may be helpful and afford the opportunity to test out potential barriers to carrying out the test. Initially, the client is encouraged to reduce the degree of appeasement and note that the feared outcome does not occur, hence weakening the belief.

Kevin resisted his voices' commands to wash repeatedly and observed that the feared consequence did not happen (his mom was not harmed that day). He concluded that the voices could not physically make him comply and that they were powerless to act themselves. Kevin concluded that just because the voices told him to do something did not mean he had to do it or that they had the power to make him. Kevin came to realize that he had the power to choose whether to comply or not.

Gradually, Kevin became less fearful that the voices could harm him if he resisted and he felt more able to choose when he complied or resisted. For example, he decided that it was OK to wash his hands once after going to the toilet or getting them dirty but no more than that. He also decided that he would resist any commands to harm himself or other people or to throw things. Kevin came to the conclusion that the voices were not as powerful as he had previously thought and that he was more powerful than he used to believe. He began to consider his relationship with the voices as more equal and his ability to stand up to the voices and to get on with his life in spite of them improved and he was able to continue attending college.

Consolidating the power shift

In this phase, we aim explicitly to raise the power of the individual in relation to both their voice and their interpersonal relationships more broadly. This has the potential to inoculate the client against interpersonal stressors and so potentially retain the benefits of CTCH. Raising awareness of the power shift is a useful step. Here, the client identifies evidence of their own mastery and control. Most of the preceding interventions are aimed at challenging the beliefs about the power of the voice, but these will also simultaneously and necessarily be proving that the client has mastery and control, not the voice. Through Socratic questioning, the client can be made aware of this. The following substitute beliefs can then be proposed (Table 7.2).

Table 7.2 Examples of powerful voice versus powerful self beliefs

Powerful Voice beliefs	Powerful Self beliefs
1 I must comply (at least partially) to prevent the voice harming me or others.	1 The voice cannot harm me or others, I can choose to resist or ignore its commands, it needs me to act for it.
2 I have no control over my voice.	2 I have learnt to have control over my voice by using the following coping strategies.
3 My voice is powerful and must be obeyed.	3 My voice is not so powerful, and I do not have to obey it.

Naomi came to believe that the voices were not as powerful as she had previously thought and that she was more powerful than she used to believe. She could now decide whether to agree with or believe what the voices said, and she could choose whether or not to act on what they said. Naomi developed a positive self-talk technique to help her in various situations telling herself 'I can do this!' or 'I can ignore them'. Gradually, she began to talk more positively about herself: she concluded that 'people who hear voices can get on with their lives despite the voices'. By the end of therapy, Naomi reported that she continued to hear the voices, but was able to ignore them or stand up to them.

Questioning the voice's command is a further strategy we employ in CTCH. This is an extension of the behavioural test and can be used once the client is feeling more in control and the power imbalance has begun to shift:

For example, Rebecca who had frequently tried to throw herself in front of moving cars learned to respond more assertively by saying: *'Why should I do that?'* and *'Why don't you do it yourself if you want to?'*

Such behavioural responses are designed to get the client to act against their dysfunctional power beliefs and in line with the new functional beliefs, thus further weakening the former and strengthening the latter.

Addressing broader power relationships

CTCH's integration of social rank theory carries with it the implication that individuals who are dominated by powerful voices are often subordinated to others (lower in their social rank) more generally and this is frequently reflected in their personal histories. Our extensive clinical and research work in this area (Birchwood *et al.*, 2000; Birchwood *et al.*, 2004) suggests that voice hearers construe themselves as being in an interpersonal relationship with their voices. This relationship is frequently characterized in terms of lower social rank and tends to be reflected in clients' other social relationships and personal histories. Addressing broader interpersonal power issues is therefore important, both to consolidate the shifting power balance with dominant voices and in potentially preventing relapses. Intervention here also serves to reduce potential distal As that may trigger or exacerbate voices or act as maintenance factors.

Mary is a particularly striking example of how powerful voices are mirrored in broader interpersonal power relationships. Mary heard the voice of her sister who put her down and threatened to steal her long-term partner. Her sister lived nearby and Mary felt that she was often putting her down, was more successful and attractive then her, and constantly tried to have sex with her partner. Mary had frequent arguments with both the voice of her sister (who laughed at her) and her actual sister who dismissed her accusations. Family therapy was offered subsequent to CTCH to both improve communication within the family and enable them to understand Mary's aggressive outbursts with them better.

Similar themes were evident with Kevin who heard the voices of bullies from his old school. Bullying also emerged as a common theme throughout his life; he reported having to cope with his neighbours' children throwing stones at him and being bullied at college. In therapy, ways of being more assertive were explored, and he was offered assert-iveness training at college.

Working with personal meaning

An important component of CTCH is to build upon shifts in the power balance and reduced distress. REBT theory posits that work at the core belief level is needed in order to effect longer-term changes. Clients may also not respond to interventions, which are targeted just at power beliefs. Sometimes, it is possible to reformulate the client's explana-tion for the origins of their voice in psychological or even neurological terms.

The therapist proposed to Kevin an alternative explanation for his experiences of voice hearing. It was proposed that the voices were in fact *memories* of his school bullies from the past. It was explained that the brain sometimes (if trauma is not properly processed) replays such memories at stressful times, causing Kevin to hear voices that *sound like* the bullies. We have found that voices that are more familiar or voices that are of particular importance for the person are more likely to be activated in this way. In Kevin's case, it was suggested that whenever he was feeling upset or angry he would be reminded of the bullies, which was likely to trigger those particular voices inside his head.

In addition, images of the bullies that seemed very real to Kevin were sometimes triggered at stressful times. As a consequence, Kevin believed that some of the bullies continued to live nearby. He was asked to describe the images in detail: he recalled that the boys in the images were 13 or 14 years old, wore school uniform, and they looked exactly as they had looked when Kevin was at secondary school. Through Socratic ques-tioning, it was proposed that today these boys would be 18 or 19 years old and, most likely, dressed differently. This was used as evidence to suggest that the images were vivid *memories* of the bullies from the past, rather than actual people in the present.

Kevin also reported sometimes experiencing images of the bullies punching and kick-ing him, as if in the present moment. However, there was never any evidence of fresh bruises afterwards, suggesting that Kevin was reliving unpleasant events from the past. Kevin came to believe that the voices and images of the bullies were memories from the past rather than real people in the here and now. This final deconstructing of the power schema enabled him to see the voices as even less powerful.

The evidence base for CTCH

The case vignettes described so far demonstrate that for some individuals, CTCH can bring about profound shifts in the way in which individuals appraise their voices, giving them greater control, an ability to desist from acting on their voices and lower their distress. These individuals also report an improved confidence in handling interpersonal situations and relating to others generally. We have also attempted to establish the effec-tiveness of CTCH in a larger trial with some promising results (Wykes *et al.*, 2007). In our first study (Trower *et al.*, 2004), we focused on measuring compliance behaviour and dis-tress in addition to standardized symptom measures. This was a single-blind intention to treat randomized controlled trial comparing CTCH against Treatment As Usual (TAU). The purpose was to evaluate whether by targeting power beliefs we could reduce compliance and/or appeasement and distress, and increase resistance as a primary outcome. Thirty-eight participants all reported two or more commands from their 'dominant' voice, at least one of which was a 'severe' command. Participants were considered at high risk of compliance on the basis of their compliance histories, use of the mental health act (1983) and hospital treatment.

The treatment group completed a median of 16 sessions and dropped in terms of compliance from 100% compliance (the selection criterion) over 12 months to only 14% compared to 53% for the TAU group. That this change was due to CTCH is validated by a change in conviction in power schemas, with the treatment group reporting a large and significant reduction in power beliefs, compared to the TAU group who showed no change. This effect was maintained at 12-month follow-up. When we statistically removed the effect of the power beliefs, the treatment effect disappeared, providing further evidence that it was belief change that was responsible for the reduction in compliance. Conviction in omniscience beliefs also fell significantly in the CTCH group but not in the TAU group and was again maintained at 12 months. Those receiving CTCH also showed a significant improvement in perceived control over voices, compared to TAU who again showed no change and was maintained at 12 months. Our other main target, voice-related distress, was also significantly impacted upon by CTCH in the treatment group at 6 months. By 12 months, depression had risen significantly in the TAU group but not in the CTCH group.

The data presented here suggests that CTCH, in the context of good quality and a high level of TAU services, exerts a major influence on the risk of compliance, reduces distress, and prevents the escalation of depression, compared to TAU alone. Depression is known to be high in this group from our previous research (Birchwood *et al.*, 2000), and confirmed in this study. This in itself may lead to further risk behaviour, especially suicide.

Limitations and future directions in CTCH

Our first trail study produced an effect size of major clinical significance. However, its sample size was small and was confined to one (though ethnically and economically diverse) part of the UK (the West Midlands). We are currently attempting to address these issues in a new three centre RCT, which we hope will replicate the study using different loci and different therapists, affording the opportunity to understand for whom CTCH is most effective and how durable any effects may be.

The durability of CBT for psychosis is of particular importance. There is a strand of psychiatric opinion that treatments for schizophrenia are only effective as long as they are active (McGlashan, 1988) and perhaps, therefore, a more theoretical and clinically relevant question might be 'how much further intervention is required to *maintain* the effect of treatment?' Longer-term funding of trials will be required to better establish treatment durability.

Finally, it should be evident by now that we do not make any claims regarding any reduction of symptoms (the A in cognitive terms) for CTCH. These often persist; though they may be reduced or even disappear in some individual cases. Our approach, we believe, is a true cognitive therapy: focusing on distress and behaviour.

References

Birchwood, M., Meaden, A., Trower, P., Gilbert, P., & Plaistow, J. (2000). The power and omnipotence of voices: subordination and entrapment by voices and significant others. *Psychol Med*, **30**, 337–344.

Birchwood, M., Gilbert, P., Gilbert, J., *et al.* (2004). Interpersonal and role-related schema influence the relationship with the dominant 'voice' in schizophrenia: a comparison of three models. *Psychol Med*, **34**, 1–10.

Byrne, S., Trower, P., Birchwood, M., & Meaden, A. (2006). *Cognitive therapy for command hallucinations: A social rank theory approach.* Hove: Brunner-Routledge**.**

Ellis, A. (2004). Why rational emotive behaviour therapy is the most comprehensive and effective form of behaviour therapy. *Journal of Rational Emotive & Cognitive-Behavior Therapy*, **22**(2), 20–38.

Erkwoh, R., Willmes, K., Eming-Erdmann, A., & Kunert, H.J. (2002). Command hallucinations: who obeys and who resists when? *Psychopathology*, **35**, 272–279.

Hacker, D., Birchwood, M., Tudway, J., Meaden, A., & Amphlett, C. (2008). Acting on voices: omnipotence, sources of threat, and safety-seeking behaviours. *Br J Clin Psychol*, **47**, 201–213.

McGlashan, T.H. (1988). A selective review of North American long-term follow-up studies of schizophrenia. *Schizophr Bull*, **14**, 515–542.

Monahan, J., Steadman, H., Silver, E., *et al.* (2001). *Rethinking risk assessment: the MacArthur study of mental disorder and violence.* New York: Oxford University Press.

Percival, J. A. (1838 & 1840). *Narrative of the treatment experienced by a gentleman, during a state of mental derangement; designed to explain the causes and nature of insanity, and to expose the injudicious conduct pursued towards many unfortunate sufferers under that calamity.* 2 Vols. London: Effingham Wilson. (*A Mad People's History of Madness.* (1982). Dale Petersen, Ed. Pittsburgh, PA: University of Pittsburgh Press.)

Shawyer, F., MacKinnon, A., Farhall, J., Trauer, T., & Copolov, D. (2003). Command hallucinations and violence: implications for detention and treatment. *Psychology, Psychiatry and the Law*, **10**(1), 97–107.

Trower, P., Birchwood, M., Meaden, A., Byrne, S., Nelson, A., & Ross., K. (2004). Cognitive therapy for command hallucinations: randomised controlled trial. *Br J Psychiatry Suppl*, **184**, 312–320.

Wykes, T., Steel, C., Everitt, B., & Tarrier, N. (2007). Cognitive behaviour therapy for schizophrenia: effect sizes, clinical models, and methodological rigor. *Schizophr Bull*, **10**(114), 1–15.

Chapter 8

Attention Training Technique and Acceptance and Commitment Therapy for distressing auditory hallucinations

Lucia R. Valmaggia and Eric Morris

As described in the previous chapters, the last two decades have seen a renewed interest in psychological interventions for auditory hallucinations. In this chapter, we describe two case studies illustrating how the Attention Training Technique (ATT) and Acceptance and Commitment Therapy (ACT) can be applied with people experiencing voices in the context of psychosis.

The chapter begins with an introduction describing the Attention Training Technique and Acceptance and Commitment Therapy, followed by two case examples. After the case examples, we will discuss the similarities and differences of the two approaches.

Attention Training Technique

ATT was first described by Adrian Wells in 1990, and it is a treatment technique that aims to alleviate psychological problems through both cognitive and metacognitive modification (Wells, 2007). ATT's theoretical basis lays in the Self-Regulatory Executive Function model (S-REF, Wells and Matthews, 1994), which proposes that self-regulatory processing is involved in appraising the personal significance of external events, body signals, and thoughts and therefore plays a crucial role in the formation of cognitions and beliefs (Wells & Matthews, 1996). The S-REF model suggests that a dysfunctional thinking style named cognitive attentional syndrome can lead to psychological disorders. *The cognitive attentional syndrome consists of perseverative thought in the form of worry/rumination, attentional strategies of threat monitoring, loss of cognitive efficiency/capacity, and coping behaviours that fail to provide corrective learning experiences and contribute to failures of self-regulation. Excessive and inflexible self-focused attention is a surface marker of the activation of this syndrome* (Wells, 2007). By enhancing the metacognitive control of attention, ATT targets the dysfunctional cognitive attentional syndrome and enables new functional self-regulation patterns and new, more functional, metacognitive beliefs to flourish.

ATT is a technique and as such should be embedded in a broader therapeutic framework such as metacognitive therapy (Wells, 1990) or Cognitive Behavioural Therapy (CBT). The case example below describes the use of ATT embedded in a CBT framework. CBT starts with an engagement and assessment phase characterized by a detailed assessment of the presenting problem. A detailed assessment of the auditory hallucinations experienced by the patients and of the associated distress and behavioural responses leads to a detailed formulation of the problem. The aim is to explore the relationship between thoughts and emotions and between thoughts and behavior. Depending on the formulation, specific techniques are then used aiming at a reduction of the symptoms and a reduction of the distress that accompanies the symptoms. The last phase of therapy focuses on consolidation of the achieved positive changes and on relapse prevention strategies.

ATT can be used as an intervention technique in the framework of CBT. The ATT protocol has been described by Wells (2000). Briefly, patients are asked to focus and maintain their attention on up to five different sounds in the room (such as ticking of a clock, the dishwasher, a dripping tap, etc.). Next, they are asked to switch their attention between different sounds. After that, they practice to divide their attention by listening to all the sounds at the same time. After a few weeks, once the patients can master their attention using neutral auditory stimuli, the auditory hallucination is approached as if it were another sound. Patients are asked to focus on the neutral sounds, then focus on the voices, then switch their attention between the voices and other sounds, and to divide their attention between the voices and other sounds. Patients are asked to practice ATT each day, twice a day for about 5–10 min at the time. As described above, the aim of the technique is not to be a distraction, but to modify the self-regulatory processes and to replace them with new processing configurations (Wells & Matthews, 1996).

Evidence for ATT

Preliminary data shows that ATT is effective in anxiety disorders (Wells, 1990; Wells, White, & Carter, 1997), hypochondriasis (Papageorgiou & Wells, 1998), and depression (Cavanagh & Franklin, 2000). The evidence for ATT with auditory hallucinations is limited to a case study (Valmaggia *et al.*, 2007), which describes the treatment of a patient with schizophrenia experiencing auditory hallucinations. Based on our clinical experience with patients suffering from hallucinations, ATT can be applied successfully with patients who experience intrusive voices similar to intrusive thoughts. These patients worry and ruminate about their voices and develop avoidant responses (Valmaggia *et al.*, 2007). Previous research suggested that ATT might be applied in a clinical setting (Ensum & Morrison, 2003), as it has been found that self-focused attention plays an important role in the mediation of auditory hallucinations (Morrison & Haddock, 1997a; Ensum & Morrison, 2003) and that attentional biases and ruminative processes are also reported in people hearing voices (Morrison & Haddock, 1997b; Johns *et al.*, 2001; Morrison *et al.*, 2002; Morrison, Wells, & Nothard, 2002).

Acceptance and Commitment Therapy

ACT is a contextual form of behaviour therapy that emphasizes mindfulness and acceptance in the service of helping people to live meaningful and vital lives. ACT is based upon functional contextual philosophy (Hayes, Strosahl, & Wilson, 1999) and relational frame theory (Hayes, Barnes-Holmes, & Roche, 2001), a modern behaviour analytic account of language. The ACT model considers that normal language processes play a significant role in human distress, through amplifying the salience, distress, and functional avoidance associated to private experiences.

ACT incorporates mindfulness and acceptance processes, and commitment and behaviour activation processes to help clients to reduce their struggle with unwanted private experiences and to act more consistently to their chosen life values (Luoma, Hayes, & Walser, 2008). The ACT model incorporates mindfulness as a component of a broader model that focuses on behaviour change. The model of treatment involves six interrelated processes: acceptance, defusion (decentring/distancing from literal meaning of private experiences), contact with the present moment, committed action, self as context, and values (Hayes, Strosahl, Bunting, Twohig, & Wilson, 2004). These treatment processes are used to help clients to develop greater *psychological flexibility*, which is defined as 'the opportunity for the client to persevere or change his/her behaviour in the service of attaining valued goals and outcomes (Bach & Moran, 2008). The desired outcome in ACT is psychological flexibility rather than direct symptom reduction (although this may happen secondary to changes in acceptance and committed action).

A way of considering the ACT approach is how it focuses on identifying and clarifying what the individual finds important for life meaning and vitality, and how therapy is about encouraging the person to behave more consistently to chosen life directions in the face of unwanted private experiences. ACT teaches the client to observe unwanted thoughts and feelings from a mindful, detached perspective and to experience a sense of self that transcends the content of moment-to-moment experience.

The ACT model is pragmatic in focus, suggesting principles of behaviour change but not seeking to explain the aetiology of a symptom or psychological problem.

Consistent with a pragmatic stance, what is considered 'true' in ACT is what is *workable*, rather than what may explain but not lead to changes in the problem (Hayes, Strosahl, & Wilson, 1999). Thus, the focus of ACT is about helping the client to change, rather than to gain insight (without a change in behaviour).

The style of therapy in ACT is to use metaphorical talk and exercises to foster a therapeutic context, rather than providing the client with direct instruction on coping methods or alternative explanations for experiences. This experiential learning approach is consistent with the literature about *rule governance* (cf., Hayes, 1989), which suggests that flexible, broad response repertoires are established and maintained when behaviour is contingency shaped, as opposed to the effects of rules, which can result in repertoires that are narrow and inflexible. This contingency-shaped learning helps the client to remain in contact with the present moment to learn from experience, rather than follow instructions that may result in the person developing further rigid and narrow response repertoires. Moreover, this approach reduces the effects of compliance to the therapist, increasing the chance that the client is making changes based upon the contingencies in their own lives, rather than simply trying to please the therapist.

The ACT therapist considers what normal language processes may be contributing to the distress and disability experienced by the client. The ACT model hypothesizes that due to the temporal and evaluative properties of language, people can engage in unworkable efforts to suppress or eliminate private experiences, and that through such efforts, these experiences may become more salient, exert greater influence, reinforcing a feedback loop of needing to be the target of avoidance (Hayes, Strosahl, & Wilson, 1999). The process-oriented focus of ACT suggests that the most efficient way to change this problem is to focus on the *control agenda* rather than attempting to fix or change the content of what is being controlled or avoided.

The ACT model considers that the problems with living that clients experience are in part due to the effects of *experiential avoidance* and *cognitive fusion*. Experiential avoidance is 'attempting to eradicate or resist contact with one's own unwanted thoughts, feelings, sensations, and other private events' (Bach & Moran, 2008, p.95). Cognitive fusion is the process 'when people are guided by the literal content of their thoughts rather than their direct experience with the world', which leads to behaviour that is inflexible, where people may persist in unworkable actions based on verbally construed rules, rather than being influenced by direct experience (Bach & Moran, 2008, p.97).

How does ACT view auditory hallucinations?

The ACT approach considers auditory hallucinations as similar to other private experiences, such as thoughts, emotions, urges, and memories, and as such can be the focus for efforts of control and avoidance. Consistent with its functional analytic account, the ACT model suggests that it is not the presence of auditory hallucinations *per se* that results in distress and disability, but rather it is when efforts to control, eliminate, or avoid this experience lead to diminished life meaning and poor functioning. ACT considers that it is the behavioural results of these control efforts that should be a focus for intervention, and the functional relationship that voices have be considered in the broader context of the person's values and life choices.

Evidence for the ACT approach

Evidence for outcomes and underlying processes theorized in the ACT model has been found across disorders and problems, including anxiety and mood disorders, chronic pain, and epilepsy (Hayes, Luoma, Bond, Masuda, & Lillis, 2006). There is emerging evidence to suggest that ACT is a promising intervention with psychosis, with two randomized controlled trials showing reductions in rehospitalization rates with in-patients (Bach & Hayes, 2002; Gaudiano & Herbert, 2006). Several correlational studies have found significant negative relationships between acceptance and mindfulness and distress/disability with voice hearing (Chadwick *et al.*, 2007; Shawyer *et al.*, 2007). More broadly, there is evidence that mindfulness is potentially a helpful intervention in reducing distress and increasing functioning for people who hear voices (Chadwick, Newman, Taylor, & Abba, 2005); similarly, mediational analyses of ACT with voice hearers suggests that the distress outcome is mediated by reductions in voice believability achieved by using mindfulness-based therapy (Gaudiano & Herbert, 2006).

Attention Training Technique—A case example 'Peter'

Peter is a 28-year-old man, and he has been hearing voices for the past 6 years. The voices started around the onset of his first episode of psychosis when he was 22 years old. Since then Peter has experienced two psychotic relapses: he has been diagnosed with schizophrenia and is receiving atypical antipsychotic medication.

Peter lives with his girlfriend, they have been together for more than eight years. At the moment of referral, Peter was not working. Prior to his last relapse, he had been working as an administrator in a college. Peter has an older brother who is a barrister and one younger sister who is an architect. Before becoming unwell, Peter was studying English literature but stopped after his first psychotic episode. Peter's mother is a housewife, and his dad is an engineer. Peter says his childhood was a happy one; however, his father was rarely home due to working abroad.

Treatment context

Peter was referred to a clinic for therapy-resistant positive symptoms for CBT therapy for his persistent voices.

Assessment

The Auditory Hallucination (AH) sub-scale of the psychotic symptom rating scales (PSYRATS, Haddock *et al.*, 1999) was used to assess the severity of the auditory hallucination. The PSYRATS is sensitive to changes over treatment and has two sub-scales: the Auditory Hallucinations sub-scale (AH, 11 items) and the delusions sub-scale (six items). Various dimensions of voices and delusions are assessed over the last week. Each item of the PSYRATS can be scored on a five-point ordinal scale of increasing severity. The PSYRATS-AH assesses frequency (How often the voices occurred last week), duration (How long they lasted), location (inside or outside the head), loudness (How loud the voices sound), beliefs about the origin of voices (internally or externally generated), amount and degree of negative content, amount and intensity of distress, disruption of life caused by voices, and controllability (perceived control on the occurrence of voices). Peter's results are discussed below in outcome.

Case formulation

When we first met, Peter said that all his present difficulties gravitated around the voices he was still hearing. He had recovered well from his most recent relapse, but the voices were still present all the time and annoyed him. He said he believed the voices were a symptom of his illness, but he still could not ignore them and would spend a lot of time listening to them or getting angry at the fact that they were there.

The voice often commented on his future or 'warned him' about things that could happen to his loved ones, e.g., 'you will never find another job', 'your girlfriend is going to be run over by a car', or 'your mum will die soon'. Peter said he did not really believe what the voices were saying, but he recognized that they were tapping in the worries he had about his future and hearing them made him even more anxious. He could not ignore the voices, and he would spend hours ruminating about what they were saying and try to argue with them that they were not right. He would also call his girlfriend and his mother on the phone to check that they were OK.

Rationale for ATT

The way Peter responded to the voices he was hearing could be explained using the cognitive attentional syndrome model: the voices were preservative and he worried and ruminated about them, he spend a lot time and attention appraising and monitoring the possible threat they formed and as a result, he could not concentrate well on other tasks or activities, and finally his reassurance seeking behaviour and arguing with the voices maintained the symptoms and prevented new self-regulation.

Treatment

Based on the rationale, the therapist decided to suggest using ATT, as a technique to change the way Peter was responding to the voices he was hearing. Linking in with the information Peter presented during the assessment the therapist and Peter discussed how the tendency to focus attention on the voices increased the level of anxiety and distress. The therapist also explored how Peter's focus on the voices consumed all his time and prevented him from engaging in more fruitful activities like looking for another job. Finally, they also discussed how his reassurance seeking behaviour was influencing in a negative way the relationship with his girlfriend and his mother, and how it was preventing him from learning new ways of processing and coping with his voices. Together, Peter and the therapist agreed that it would be useful if Peter could change the way he was processing the voices, and how ATT could be a helpful way to modify his attention. Peter said he was very keen to try ATT. Peter was asked to identify, before the next session, sounds he could hear in his living room and this could be used to practice later in the training. The session ended completing a session report worksheet (Beck, 1995), writing down the homework, and a brief summary of the treatment rationale for Peter to take home with him.

Using a session bridging worksheet (Beck, 1995) at the beginning of the next session, the therapist and Peter set an agenda, summarized the rationale for doing ATT, and reviewed the homework. Peter had carried out his homework assignment and had identified the following sounds in his living room, which has an open kitchen: a ticking clock, the noise of the dishwasher, the white noise of an un-tuned radio, and the traffic outside. The therapist compliments Peter for finding so many suitable noises and suggests using similar sounds present in the therapist's office to start the training: a ticking clock, the sound of a pen ticking on the table, the zooming sound of a computer, and the sounds of the traffic outside. Following Wells' protocol (2000), Peter is asked to focus his gaze on a dot on the wall and to keep his eyes open during the practice. He is then asked to start by telling himself 'Focus outward!' and the therapist asks him then to focus on each of the sounds for 15 s and to rest for 5 s between sounds. This sequence is repeated three times. Peter is then asked to score how well he could focus on the sounds on a practice form. The score range between 0 and 10 where 0 means 'I could not focus at all' and 10 means 'I could focus very well'. He gives a score of 2. He found it difficult to focus on the neutral sounds and said that the voices were distracting him; however, he was able to follow the instructions of the therapist, and at times, he could focus his attention on the neutral sounds. Next, Peter is asked to focus on each of the sounds, then to switch between the sounds, and finally to be aware of all the sounds at the same time. The exercise is repeated five more times, and after each time, Peter scores on the form how well he could focus. The scores increase to a 5 for the last sequence. The therapist praised Peter for his achievements during the session and asks Peter to practice ATT each day, once in the morning and once in late afternoon, six sequences each time, and to fill in the form after each sequence. Peter is asked to do his homework at home, in his room.

In the next two sessions, Peter reports that he has been able to practice each day and his scores have risen to a 6 and then to a 8. He stills finds it difficult not to engage with what the voices are saying but says he has started to notice that it is becoming easier to switch his attention away from what the voices are saying. He has looked for vacancies online and is thinking about applying for a job.

Peter and the therapist agree to proceed to the next step of the training, and during the session, the therapist asks Peter to practice to focus on and to switch between the neutral sounds in the office. Next, Peter is asked to focus on the sound of the voices and to switch between the voices and the neutral sounds.

Again, Peter is asked to rate how well he could master his attention. Peter said he found it a bit unsettling to focus on the voices at first but that he was able to switch his attention to other sounds easier than he thought. Peter was pleasantly surprised by this; he said he did not expect to be able to do this so easily. As homework, Peter is asked to practice switching his attention between the voices and other sounds.

At the beginning of the next session, Peter reports things are going much better; he has been able to switch his attention away from the voices. Peter says he feels much more in control of his attention now and that the voices are loosing their grip on him. Peter still hears the voices, but he said they are moved to the background now. The therapist encourages Peter to keep practicing shifting his attention away from the voices.

Next, the therapist and Peter address his reassurance-seeking behaviour of calling his girlfriend and mother to check if they are OK. Peter's reassurance-seeking behaviour is relabelled as a safety behaviour that prevents him from discovering that his thoughts and the voices about his loved ones will come to harm are not leading to the catastrophic outcome he fears. Motivated by his increasing control over his attention and by the effect that this has on the voices, Peter agrees to carry out a behavioural experiment. As homework, the therapist asks Peter to think that she will be run over by a car.

The following session, Peter reports that the voices have decreased in intensity. Peter says he feels much more in control of his attention now and that the voices are loosing their grip on him. Peter still hears the voices, but he said they are only in the background now. Peter also described how having to think the therapist would be run over by a car has made him realize how unlikely it was that the fact that he was thinking it would actually cause the therapist to have an accident. He spontaneously discussed this with his girlfriend and with his mother one evening when they were having dinner together, and with their support and encouragement, he has stopped calling them to check if they were OK. Both his girlfriend and mother have responded very well to this and said how nice it was to have 'the old Peter back'.

Peter has also decided to enrol in a computer course at the local college to update his software knowledge before applying for a new job.

In the final stage of therapy, Peter and the therapist spent time on a 'staying well' plan (Gumley & Schwannauer, 2006), aiming at consolidating the strategies learned during the therapy and at developing an action plan for a possible psychotic relapse.

Outcome

PSYRATS-AH

The PSYRATS-AH was administered at baseline and at the end of therapy. At baseline, Peter reports that has been experiencing voices for the last six years. The voices occur at least once an hour and can last for several minutes and sometimes more than one hour. The voices are about the same loudness as his own voice and sound mostly like they are coming from inside his head. Peter believes the voices are due to his illness. The voices say unpleasant or negative things about him and 'warn' him about bad things happening to his loved ones. Peter's voices are very distressing and cause a moderate amount of disruption to his daily life. Peter feels he has no control over the occurrence of the voices he hears.

After therapy, Peter reports that the voices have decreased in both intensity and duration. They have become less negative and are like a whisper in the background. Peter is no longer distressed by the voices and feels he can choose whether to pay attention to them or not on the majority of occasions (see Table 8.1).

At six months follow-up, Peter is still doing well, the voices have remained in the background, and with the help of his brother, he has found a part-time administrator job, which he enjoys. He no longer needs to use ATT in his daily life.

In summary, Peter has changed the way he processes the voices he hears; he no longer pays attention to them and is no longer preoccupied by them; and he has also dropped the safety behaviours that maintained the problem.

Table 8.1 PSYRATS-AH scores at baseline and after therapy for Peter

	Baseline	End of Treatment
Frequency	3	2
Duration	3	1
Location	1	1
Loudness	2	1
Beliefs regarding origin of voices	1	1
Amount of negative content	4	2
Degree of negative content	4	2
Amount of distress	4	1
Intensity of distress	3	0
Disruption of life	2	0
Controllability	4	1

Acceptance and Commitment Therapy—A case example 'Amanda'

Amanda, a 23-year-old white British woman, had been hearing voices for three years prior to the intervention. She had been diagnosed with schizophrenia and is receiving atypical antipsychotic medication, with positive symptoms considered to be treatment-resistant. Psychological therapy was considered as a treatment option due to the amount of distress and functional disability that Amanda was experiencing, as well as the treatment-resistant nature of her symptoms described below.

Amanda lives with her parents and is an only child. Amanda does volunteer work part-time for an animal shelter for several hours a week; she was in receipt of disability living benefits. She otherwise spends most of her free time at home, listening to music, reading, and watching TV. Amanda reported that she has few friends: she keeps in touch with an old friend from school via emails and text messages, but they rarely meet.

She reported that she had a happy childhood, although when she got to secondary school, she experienced a long period of bullying, which affected her confidence around others. Amanda reported that she did not do particularly well academically at school, leaving when she was 16 years old. She completed GCSEs and went on to secretarial college to achieve national vocational qualifications in administration. Amanda worked for a year as a secretary before her temporary contract was not renewed. She then struggled to find further work, and then started to become unwell, being seen by the early intervention service after a period of six months.

Although she admits to using cannabis in the past, Amanda denied current use of cannabis or other substances.

Treatment context

She was seen by an early intervention service for psychosis and had been prescribed several different antipsychotic medications, with limited impact on reducing voice frequency and intensity. Amanda reports that her current medication regime does reduce the loudness and frequency of the voices; however, she continues to experience daily derogatory and command hallucinations. Amanda was referred for psychological therapy in order to help manage distress and disability with persisting voice hearing.

Assessment and formulation

Voice hearing and mood

Amanda described hearing the voice of an unidentified male, who makes comments about her actions and occasionally gives her commands to harm herself. Amanda reported that the voice tells her to kill herself and to 'give up, why try when you are useless', but also gave other commands, such as telling her to stop talking or to stop certain activities (such as reading). Amanda reported that she hears the voice several times a day, lasting for a minute or two on each occasion. The voice is variable in volume, although mostly it is softer than her voice.

At the time of therapy, Amanda described a depressed mood, with self-critical and pessimistic thoughts, poor appetite, and sleep disturbance. Amanda described having thoughts of suicide, although she denied an urge to act upon them. ACT was considered an appropriate intervention due to the behavioural activation focus of the model: ACT and contemporary behavioural activation approaches share a similar philosophical and theoretical basis in functional contextualism and operant conditioning principles (Martell, Addis, & Jacobsen, 2001).

Beliefs about the identity and intentions of the voice

Amanda reports that she thinks that the voice is a man who tried to assault her when she was 15 years old. This incident occurred while she was waiting for a bus after a music class: she was waiting by herself and a man approached her, asking for money, when Amanda declined his request he hit her with his fist and threatened to hurt her further unless she gave him her money. She gave him the money and he fled the scene. Amanda states that she now thinks that this man had been following her for a long period and that she was at risk of being sexually assaulted by him. She stated that after this incident, she worried about being attacked by this man again, and for a period, would not attend music lessons or go on the bus route.

Amanda stated that she believes that her voice is evil and that it intends to destroy her. She stated that the voice is trying to control her life and to trick her into killing herself. She stated that she believed that the voice was very powerful and knowledgeable, although she did not believe that the voice could control her, instead it was trying to persuade her to give up. She believed that the voice knew of the intentions of others and could read their minds to know what people thought of her.

Coping with the voice

Amanda reported that she typically copes with the voice by distracting herself by listening to music or watching TV. She reported that while this helps, she continues to be troubled by the voice as its comments interfere with her enjoyment of music/TV. She stated that she occasionally argues back with the voice, out-loud when she is by herself, or in her mind if she is around other people.

Amanda also described limiting her contact with things that appear to 'excite' the voice: such as socialising with friends and going out for activities that she enjoys (such as shopping). She stated that she finds it very difficult to tolerate the voice's comments.

She also reported a fear that she might accidentally argue back with the voice out loud when she is out in public—this fear also limits the amount that Amanda goes out.

When asked about how the voice acts as a barrier in her life, Amanda reported that the voice affects her confidence to do new things and plays upon her worries about other people (telling her that others will reject her). She stated that she dismisses plans to take positive risks with her life, as she fears what the voice will say. She also described that she becomes angry and depressed when the voice 'interrupts' activities that she does; she reported that she avoids doing nice things for herself for fear that she will hear the voice making derogatory comments during the activity. Amanda described an example of this of where she would like to be able to meet her friend in a café, but has not mustered the courage to do this because she is worried that the voice may intrude on the conversation. She stated that she worries about being stuck in public, hearing the voice, and that she might respond to it, so that other people might think she was 'mad'.

Case formulation

A case formulation was developed, informed by a functional analysis of the problems that Amanda was describing.

In ACT, the case formulation focuses on the role that experiential avoidance and fusion play in distress and disability, keeping in focus the effects of these upon the client being able to take a psychological flexibility stance to life (Hayes, Luoma, Bond, Masuda, & Lillis, 2006).

Central to the formulation was the role of experiential avoidance and cognitive fusion in Amanda's circumstances, particularly around the problems that she experienced with doing more activities outside of the home and socializing with others. It was hypothesized that Amanda's situation was strongly influenced by negative reinforcement, with her distress and limited social functioning affected by her efforts to control and eliminate the experience of the voice. The functional analysis suggested that Amanda's appraisals and methods of coping with voice hearing were functionally related to avoidance in committing to valued actions of seeking and making new friends and seeking employment.

It was hypothesized similarly that Amanda's mood was a response to the limited positive reinforcement that she received from her current routine, as well as negative reinforcement in the form of avoidance of situations where she may experience increased voice activity and unpleasant emotions, memories, and thoughts (such as seeking friend-ships or committing to work goals).

The ACT approach

Amanda was seen for 12 sessions of ACT in a community clinic. The sessions were up to 45 min in duration, although the earlier sessions were briefer as Amanda engaged with the therapist and approach.

The ACT sessions focused on helping Amanda pursue increased life meaning and vital-ity, through encouragement to do more of the activities that she values and to noticing how struggling with the voice related to increased distress and operated as a barrier to living.

As part of the informed consent procedure to ACT, Amanda was informed that the approach was not about trying to eliminate the voice, that in fact the therapist did not know how to do this, but instead ACT would involve helping to do what is important to her, and to develop a different relationship with her emotions, thoughts, and feelings, including the voice, so that these did not get in the way of her choices and actions.

There were several steps to the sessions:

1. Validating the struggle with auditory hallucinations and suggesting acceptance as an alternative strategy.
2. Clarifying values and identifying directions for action.
3. Through mindfulness, developing present moment focus and de-centring from voice experience as arbiter for action.
4. Making plans and commitments to carry out valued actions; reviewing progress on this from session to session.

The ACT sessions typically involved using several exercises to help Amanda to adopt a stance of mindfulness and acceptance toward the voice and identify and commit to actions that would help her to move forward in life guided by her values. Homework tasks involved practicing mindfulness by using a CD recorded by the therapist, engaging in planned activities and some written exercises to reflect on valued actions.

Mindfulness, cognitive defusion, and present moment focus

Regular use of mindfulness was introduced during the first few sessions: consistent with the suggested procedure by Chadwick *et al.* (2005), mindfulness was introduced by teaching a focus on the breath, with a brief meditation (10 min) and limiting periods of silence by the therapist. Amanda was given a CD of mindfulness exercises to practice in between sessions. She reported that she did listen to the CD and practice some of the brief sitting meditations.

As a component of the mindfulness exercises, Amanda was encouraged to notice her mind and voice hearing as *experiences*, by drawing attention to the non-arbitrary properties of these, such as the tones and rhythm of the voice. For particular phrases that the voice used that were distressing, as well as for self-critical thoughts, Amanda was encouraged to do an exercise that involved putting the content of the phrases/thoughts on cards and then practicing various ways of responding to these, such as carrying them around with her, holding them lightly in her hand, noticing the contrast between pushing them away and 'accepting' them by letting herself be in contact with them without struggle.

Another part of the mindfulness practice involved the therapist encouraging Amanda to notice the difference between being present 'in the moment' and being caught up in memories about the past or worries about the future. This was then linked to valued actions and as a method to step in to the present when she noticed that she was getting caught up in ruminating or worrying.

Self as context

To help Amanda to experience more consistently a sense of self that was transcendent of her voice hearing, the therapist used the *chessboard metaphor* (Hayes, Strosahl, & Wilson, 1999). This metaphor asks the client to imagine that their experience may be akin to a chessboard that extends in all directions, upon which are pieces made up of their psychological experience (thoughts, feelings, urges, memories, etc.) and that these pieces can be at war with each other, that perhaps it even feels like you are one of the pieces on the board, at risk of being harmed by your experience. The client is then encouraged to consider how this would be if instead they were the board, rather than the pieces.

Amanda related to this metaphor, and in subsequent sessions, we were able to encourage this stance by saying 'are you at piece level or board level right now? What would help you to carry all the pieces (including the voice) with you, and do what you care about?'

Acceptance

Acceptance was introduced as an alternative strategy to responding by obeying or struggling with the voice. The therapist engaged Amanda in discussion about the various ways that she had used to cope with the voice, and how these had worked out in the short- and long-term, particularly in light of what she cared about (values).

Amanda was initially reluctant to give up some of the ways that she had attempted to control the voice. A metaphor was then introduced, equating the efforts at controlling the experience of the voice to feeding a baby tiger (Hayes, Barnes-Holmes, & Roche, 2001, p.232), where, in order to make sure it did not attack her, it was being fed various bits of her life. Unfortunately, the cost of this was a life that was getting smaller and smaller and lived on the terms of the voice, rather than Amanda's.

We then worked on experimenting with giving up some control of the voice, in order to be able to have more choices about what she wanted to do with her time. An aspect of this was experiencing the discrimination between control of private experience and control of her body, and how she could act on her values with her hands, feet, and mouth, even if her mind and the voice were telling her not to, or coming up with reasons why this wasn't a good idea.

Values clarification and committed actions

One of the early phases of therapy involved talking about what was important for Amanda in her life. This was difficult initially, as Amanda's conversation tended to focus back on the voice and the personal cost to her of having this experience.

An exercise, involving Amanda imagining that she was an older woman who had won a 'lifetime achievement award', was used to try to clarify for her what was important. In this exercise, Amanda was asked to imagine what her closest friends would say about what she had stood for in her life, and while picturing this to get in touch with what is important to her in terms of values. Discussion from this exercise led to clarifying valued directions in life that Amanda held, validating what she had given up in her struggle with the voice. An analogy was used of a 'Values compass', where the life directions that were important to her were considered as 'north'. This led in later sessions to clarifying valued actions by asking Amanda, 'where is north for you?'.

Finally, a metaphor of Amanda's life like being a bus driver in charge of a bus (The 'Passengers on the Bus' metaphor: Hayes, Strosahl, & Wilson, p.157) was used to link these valued directions with action. It was suggested that some of the problems that she was struggling with, such as the voice, were like passengers that had got onto the bus and were now shouting at her to go in the directions they wanted her to go.

Amanda was able to identify that for her the important directions in life that she wished to pursue were friendships and employment. The therapist then asked her to identify how she would like to act in those two areas of her life and to imagine that the voice and her mood were not barriers for these actions. Amanda was then encouraged to compare her descriptions of how she would optimally like to act with the current situation, and whether, through a stance of acceptance and mindfulness, she could do some of these things while also having the voice.

Outcome

Over the course of therapy, Amanda started to take more 'risks' with the voice, disobeying them by making choices and taking actions in line with her personal values, rather than what the voice told her to do. Although these were not easy choices to make, she progressively practised an alternative stance of mindfulness and acceptance to obedience and resignation to the voice's demands. This involved using these skills *in vivo* while going out of the house, making and meeting friends (through her volunteer work and a social club), and exploring her options for employment (going to the job centre, contacting her former employers, registering at a temp agency). Toward the end of therapy, Amanda described that while she would never enjoy hearing the voice or choose to have it as a life experience, she was more willing to have it 'travel' with her as an 'uninvited guest', rather than spend her time struggling with it.

Values/committed action and social functioning

Amanda completed a measure of consistency in taking valued actions, in the form of a bulls-eye around the life areas of 'love, work, and play' (Dahl & Lundgren, 2007, p.250).

This measure asks the client to rate how consistently they have been acting on their personal values in each of these life domains, by placing a mark on a bull's-eye figure, with ratings close to the bull's-eye representing taking actions 100% in line with values and ratings far away from the bull's-eye representing values-inconsistent actions. Amanda also rated another bull's-eye on how much she persisted in following valued directions despite difficulties and barriers.

At the start of therapy, Amanda rated her actions as being far from the bull's-eye in each of the life domains, suggesting that she was engaging in a number of value-inconsistent actions. She described, for example, that in the area of 'work' that she would like to spend her time engaged in employment where she helped people; however, she could contrast this life direction with her current actions of spending her time at home, avoiding facing the prospect of work by listening to music and watching TV.

At the end of therapy, Amanda was making bull's-eye ratings that suggested greater consistency with acting on her personal values, particularly in the domains of 'work' and 'love/relationships'. In addition, she rated herself as being more persistent in acting on her values when faced with unwanted internal experiences.

On the Social and Occupational Functioning Assessment Scale (SOFAS; DSM-IV, Goldman *et al.*, 1992), Amanda's clinical presentation received a rating of 35 ('Major impairment in several areas') at assessment. At the end of therapy, her social functioning was rated at 60 ('Moderate difficulty') (See Table 8.2).

Symptoms—PSYRATS

Amanda's experience of voice hearing was rated on the PSYRATS-AH (Haddock *et al.*, 1999). On initial assessment, Amanda's description of her voice-hearing produced an overall score of 31, with high scores on frequency, distress, degree of negative content, and life disruption due to the voice.

At the end of therapy, Amanda's report of voice hearing produced an overall score of 23. The main changes in her report were reductions in the level of distress and disruption associated with hearing the voice, with a slight reduction in voice frequency.

General distress—CORE-OM

Amanda completed the Clinical Outcomes in Routine Evaluation–Outcome Measure (*CORE-OM*: Evans *et al.*, 2000), a measure of global distress (subjective well-being, problems or symptoms, and life functioning) and risk items. On initial assessment, her global distress score was 2.09, above the clinical cut-off for females. She endorsed items that she had thought of hurting herself and made plans to end her life. Her responses also suggested that she regarded her ability to function to be strongly affected by her current problems (functioning sub-scale score = 2.58).

At the end of therapy, Amanda's CORE-OM global distress score was 0.70 and the functioning sub-scale score was 0.75. The change in these scores suggests that Amanda experienced a significant change in her levels of distress, as well as her perception that her functioning was less affected by problems. Moreover, she did not rate any items regarding intentions to engage in self-harm or suicide.

Voices Acceptance and Action Scale (VAAS; Shawyer *et al.*, 2007)

Amanda completed the voices acceptance and action scale, a measure of acceptance of voices *as experiences* and personal autonomy from command hallucinations. At assessment, Amanda scored low in both acceptance of the voice and personal autonomy: her responses suggested that she tended to be unwilling to have the voice as part of her life, that she spent time resisting it, and that she did not regard herself as having much personal choice over her own actions. This was in contrast with the end of therapy, where Amanda's VAAS scores suggested that she experienced much greater personal choice over actions and more accepting of having the voice as an experience.

In summary, Amanda appeared to develop greater personal autonomy from her voice hearing over the course of ACT through the practice of mindfulness and acceptance skills that were introduced in the sessions. Moreover, the pattern of Amanda's actions shifted from efforts to avoid or control the voices to activating herself by committing to behaviours based on her personal values. Through a more open, accepting stance, voice hearing appeared to be less of a barrier to sticking to social and employment plans that she had made for herself, opening up the possibilities for Amanda to engage in meaningful activities to improve her quality of life.

Table 8.2 Outcome measures at baseline and after therapy for Amanda

	Baseline	End of Treatment
PSYRATS-AH		
Frequency	2	1
Duration	2	2
Location	4	4
Loudness	1	1
Beliefs regarding origin of voices	3	2
Amount of negative content	4	4
Degree of negative content	4	4
Amount of distress	3	1
Intensity of distress	2	0
Disruption of life	2	0
Controllability	4	4
CORE-OM		
General distress	2.09	0.7
Functioning	2.58	0.75
SOFAS	35 (Major impairment in several areas)	60 (Moderate difficulty)

Discussion

These two case descriptions illustrate how ATT and ACT can be used with auditory hallucinations. There are similarities in the two approaches. A functional analysis of the presenting problems is the cornerstone of both treatments. Equally, they focus on learning how to live with or accepting the voices instead of trying to eliminate them or explain where they come from. Both treatments are process-orientated approaches and target the personal relationship that the person has with their voices. The content or presence of auditory hallucinations are not challenged, rather the patient learns how to separate him/herself from the symptoms. In contrast with traditional cognitive approaches for voices, the meaning of these experiences, such as appraisals of voice power or intention, is not a direct target of change in ATT or ACT. Patients are taught how to detach themselves from the symptoms, rather than engage in experientially avoidant responses (such as safety-seeking behaviours, distraction, or suppression) and to seek other, more functional targets for attention and action.

Both therapies also focus on the *control agenda* rather than attempting to eradicate or modify the voices or the content of what the voices are saying: in ATT, Peter is asked to approach the voices as if they were just another sound he can observe, attend to if he wants, or switch his attention away from; while in ACT Amanda is encouraged to accept the voices instead of struggling with them or try to control them. In both cases, there is an explicit focus on altering the stimulus functions of voices, from experiences that need to be obeyed, controlled, or suppressed to greater response flexibility and choice over actions in response to the voices, including being able to encompass the experience of voice hearing as part of larger patterns of behaviour. Therefore, each approach is functional in focus and has a behavioural component, in which the patients learn how to drop their avoidance/safety behaviours and to develop a more adaptive set of responses to voice hearing and life problems.

The two treatments also differ from each other. The theoretical background, underlying assumptions, and language are different. ATT is a technique that should be embedded in metacognitive therapy or CBT while ACT is a complete therapeutic model. According to ATT, the process of change is driven by enhancing the metacognitive control of attention. By targeting dysfunctional cognitive attentional syndrome, ATT enables new functional self-regulation patterns and new, more functional, metacognitive beliefs to flourish. On the other hand, ACT is based on an operant account of language (relational frame theory) and a functional contextualistic philosophy, with a model of treatment that draws upon principles from behaviour analysis. The processes of change in ACT focus on increasing psychological flexibility, where the person learns to respond more flexibly to internal events by adopting a mindful, accepting stance, in order to more effectively take actions based on personal values. It is theorized that such flexible responding leads to behaviour that is more contingency-shaped rather than rule-governed, allowing the client to better learn from experience, access greater intrinsic reinforcement, and to have more personal influence over their environment. ACT can be thought of as a motivational intervention: by encouraging mindfulness toward internal experiences the client is better able to commit to actions that involve behavioural activation and exposure to previously avoided stimuli. As a result, the ACT model is not exclusive in terms of technique and can be used in conjunction with established behavioural methods. However, the contextual ACT model of working with thoughts and other internal experiences is inconsistent with cognitive therapies that emphasize direct change or control of the content or frequency of these experiences (Hayes & Wilson, 1995; Hayes, Strosahl, & Wilson, 1999).

Finally, a word of caution, both treatment approaches are relatively new and there is very limited evidence for ATT or ACT in the treatment of auditory hallucinations. Research is needed to investigate the effects of each treatment, only then may we be able to draw any conclusions about which treatment should be offered to which patients.

References

Bach, P.A.P., & Moran, D.J. (2008). *ACT in Practice: Case Conceptualization in Acceptance and Commitment Therapy* (1st ed.). Oakland: New Harbinger Publications.

Bach, P., & Hayes, S.C. (2002). The use of acceptance and commitment therapy to prevent the rehospitalization of psychotic patients: A randomized controlled trial. *J Consult Clin Psychol*, **70**(5), 1129–1139.

Beck, J.S. (1995). *Cognitive Therapy: Basics and Beyond*. New York: Guilford Press.

Cavanagh, M., & Franklin, J. (2000). *Attention training and hypochondriasis: Preliminary results of a controlled treatment trial*. Paper presented at the World Congress of Cognitive and Behavioral Therapy. Vancouver, Canada.

Chadwick, P., Barnbrook, E., & Newman-Taylor, K. (2007). Responding mindfully to distressing voices: Links with meaning, affect and relationship with voice. *Tidsskrift for Norsk Psykologforening*, **44**(5), 581–587.

Chadwick, P., Newman-Taylor, K., & Abba, N. (2005). Mindfulness groups for people with psychosis. *Behav Cogn Psychother*, **33**, 351–359.

Dahl, J.C., & Lundgren, T.L. (2007). *Conditioning mechanisms, behavior technology and contextual behavioral therapy*. In S.C. Schachter, G.L. Holmes, & D.G.A. Kasteleijn-Nolst Trenité (Eds). Behavioral Aspects of Epilepsy. New York: Demos Medical Publishing.

Ensum, I., & Morrison, A. P. (2003). The effects of focus of attention on attributional bias in patients experiencing auditory hallucinations. *Behaviour Research & Therapy*, **41**, 895–907.

Evans, C., Mellor-Clark, J., Margison, F., *et al.* (2000). Clinical outcomes in routine evaluation: The CORE-OM. *J Ment Health*, **9**, 247–255.

Gaudiano, B.A., & Herbert, J.D. (2006). Acute treatment of inpatients with psychotic symptoms using acceptance and commitment therapy: Pilot results. *Behaviour Research and Therapy*, **44**, 415–437.

Goldman, H.H., Skodol, A.E., & Lave, T.R. (1992). Revising axis V for DSM-IV: A review of measures of social functioning. *Am J Psychiatry*, **149**, 1148–1156.

Gumley, A., & Schwannauer, M. (2006). *Staying Well After Psychosis: A Cognitive Interpersonal Approach to Recovery and Relapse Prevention*. Chichester: John Wiley & Sons.

Haddock, G., McCarron, J., Tarrier, N., & Faragher, E.B. (1999). Scales to measure dimensions of hallucinations and delusions: The psychotic symptom rating scales (PSYRATS). *Psychol Med*, **29**(4), 879–889.

Hayes, S. C. (1989). *Rule-Governed Behavior: Cognition, Contingencies, and Instructional Control*. New York: Plenum Press.

Hayes, S.C., Barnes-Holmes, D., & Roche, B. (Eds.). (2001). *Relational Frame Theory: A Post-Skinnerian Account of Human Language and Cognition*. New York: Plenum Press.

Hayes, S.C., Luoma, J., Bond, F.W., Masuda, A., & Lillis, J. (2006). Acceptance and commitment therapy: Model, processes and outcomes. *Behaviour Research & Therapy*, **44**, 1–25.

Hayes, S.C., Strosahl, K.D., & Wilson, K.G. (1999). *Acceptance and Commitment Therapy: An Experiential Approach to Behavior Change*. New York: Guilford Press.

Hayes, S.C., & Wilson, K.G. (1995). The role of cognition in complex human behavior: A contextualistic perspective. *J Behav Ther Exp Psychiatry*, **26**, 241–248.

Johns, L.C., Rossell, S., Frith, C., *et al.* (2001). Verbal self-monitoring and auditory verbal hallucinations in patients with schizophrenia. *Psychol Med*, **31**(4), 705–715.

Luoma, J., Hayes, S., & Walser, R. (2008). *Learning ACT: An acceptance and commitment skills training manual for therapists*. Oakland, CA: New Harbinger Press.

Martell, C.R., Addis, M.E., & Jacobson, N.S. (2001). Depression in Context: Strategies for Guided Action. New York: WW Norton.

Morrison, A.P., & Haddock, G. (1997a). *Cognitive factors in source monitoring and auditory hallucinations*. Psychol Med, **27**, 669–679.

Morrison, A.P., & Haddock, G. (1997b). Self-focused attention in schizophrenic patients with and without auditory hallucinations and normal subjects: A comparative study. *Pers Individ Dif*, **23**, 937–941.

Morrison, A.P., Wells, A., & Nothard, S. (2002). Cognitive and emotional predictors of predisposition to hallucinations in non-patients. *Br J Clin Psychol*, **41**, 3–70.

Morrison, A.P., Beck, A.T., Glentworth, D., *et al.* (2002). Imagery and psychotic symptoms: A preliminary investigation. *Behaviour Research & Therapy*, **40**(9), 1053–1062.

Papageorgiou, C., & Wells, A. (1998). Effects of attention training on hypochondriasis: A brief case series. *Psychol Med*, **28**, 193–200.

Shawyer, F., Ratcliff, K., Mackinnon, A., Farhall, J., Hayes, S.C., & Copolov, D. (2007). The voices acceptance and action scale (VAAS): Pilot data. *J Clin Psychol*, **63**(6), 593–606.

Valmaggia, L., Bouman, T.K., & Schuurman, L. (2007). Attention training with auditory hallucinations: A case study. *Cogn Behav Pract*, **14**, 127–133.

Wells, A., & Matthews, G. (1994). *Attention and Emotion: A Clinical Perspective*. Hove: Psychology Press.

Wells, A., & Matthews, G. (1996). Modelling cognition in emotional disorder: The S-REF model. *Behaviour Research and Therapy*, **34**, 881–888.

Wells, A. (1990). Panic disorder in association with relaxation induced anxiety: An attentional training approach to treatment. *Behav Ther*, **21**, 273–280.

Wells, A. (2000). *Emotional Disorders and Metacognition. Innovative Cognitive Therapy*. Chichester: John Wiley & Sons.

Wells, A. (2007). The attention training technique: Theory, effects, and a metacognitive hypothesis on auditory hallucinations. *Cogn Behav Pract*, **14**, 134–138.

Wells, A., White, J., & Carter, K.E.P. (1997). Attention training: Effects on anxiety and beliefs in panic and social phobia. *Clinical Psychology and Psychotherapy*, **4**, 226–232.

Chapter 9

Competitive Memory Training

Mark van der Gaag and Kees Korrelboom

Introduction

Psychotic features are quite common in the population. In the Netherlands, 17.5% of the population reports one psychotic symptom on the Comprehensive International Diagnostic Interview (CIDI) (van Os *et al.*, 2000). In another large survey among 18,000 people, the lifetime prevalence of hearing voices was 10–15% of the population with a yearly incidence of 4–5% (Tien, 1991). Only a part of these voice hearers in the general population will develop a psychiatric disorder. Auditory hallucinations are not always a symptom of a disease or a disabling disorder. For instance, in the past, the hearing of voices was not associated with disease, but with ecstatic religious experiences. The hearing of voices during epileptic seizures was considered divine and epilepsy was called the 'Sacred disease' (Eadie & Bladin, 2001). An example of the different value that was attached to hearing voices is Socrates. He heard voices and when he told his friends about these voices, he was respected even more than before. The general opinion in his time was that only the most noble of men could be in contact with the Gods by the demons. Demons could be evil, but also good, and they were messengers between the world of the Gods and the world of the people (Leudar & Thomas, 2000). In the Christian tradition, demons are fallen angels and are associated with evil and the devil.

The route from harmless extraordinary experiences to disabling psychopathology

Hearing voices is not an isolated symptom in the population. People who hear voices are part of the genetically vulnerable subgroup with psychosis-proneness (Sommer *et al.*, 2008). In most people, voices are a transient phenomenon. However, a psychosis will develop in only some. What processes are involved that in the largest majority of people, the extraordinary experiences wane and disappear but that in some people they become persistent and cross the severity border into frank psychosis? To answer this question, we will address four issues: (1) cognitive appraisal processes, (2) social processes, (3) historical and schema processes, and (4) personal processes such as the loss of self in the battle with voices. All these topics will be discussed extensively in the chapters by Trower *et al.*, and Romme and Escher, both this volume. Therefore, we will not elaborate on these issues, but integrate these concepts into a model of auditory hallucinations that connects to a novel intervention: Competitive Memory Training (COMET).

Appraisal processes

A number of authors have demonstrated that the phenomenology of voices in healthy voice hearers was not different from patients (Langdon *et al.*, 2008) and that voices are well distinguished from inner speech (Hoffman *et al.*, 2008). Studies by Romme and Escher and collaborators and other research groups showed that healthy voice-hearers had more benevolent interpretations of their voices (Romme & Escher, 1989; Honig *et al.*, 1998; Choong *et al.*, 2007). Chadwick and Birchwood (1994) found that 100% of the psychiatric voice hearers had malevolently appraised voices. Close and Garety (1998) also found patients with benevolent voices. Van der Gaag and colleagues (2003) demonstrated that the appraisal of the intentions of the voices and not the content of the voices was associated with anxiety and depression. So the beliefs about voices have been the target of CBT in voices. The main beliefs that are a target for modification are (1) the belief that voices are caused by another person or creature, (2) the belief that the person behind the voice is very powerful and has control over the voice hearer, and (3) the belief that the voice can also do harm.

Social processes

People are constantly ranking their social position in groups (Cummins, 1999). Dependent on their estimated rank in the hierarchy, they will take initiative and the lead or will be submissive and wait for others. Gilbert and Birchwood introduced the Social Rank Theory into the domain of CBT for auditory hallucinations (Birchwood *et al.*, 2000; Gilbert *et al.*, 2001; Birchwood *et al.*, 2004). The psychiatric voice hearers rank themselves most of the time as much less of worth and competence compared to the voices. The voices are dominant and sadistic and the voice hearer is submissive, obedient, and is trying to appease the voices. This means that individual therapy with a voice hearer actually is a group therapy or sometimes a family therapy. A barrier to engagement in CBT is that the relationship with the therapist is less important than the relationship with the voices. The voices are always with the patient and the patient has to deal with them. The therapist is only there every now and then. Gilbert introduced drama techniques in restructuring the relationship to the voice hearers. The main target in these therapies is the development of a caring and compassionate imagined other to outbalance the sadistic voices.

Personal history and schema processes

Voices are often frightening because they threaten to harm the voice hearer. This often evolves into appeasing and obeying of the voices' commands. The goal of obedience and appeasements by the voice hearer is to prevent harm or punishment by the voices in a future event. The association is a sequential one. This means that the message of the voices predicts harmful events. Thus, the obedient behaviour is avoidance behaviour, reinforced by the consequences that the anticipated future harm does not happen and anxious feelings diminish. Several CBT interventions have proven to be successful in these anticipating situations. The omniscience and omnipotence of the voices can be challenged verbally and by behavioural experiments. Once the beliefs about external origin and their appraised capacity to act harmfully are undermined, the patient can stop listening and obeying his voices and he can commit himself to more fulfilling activities.

In some cases, there is also a referential association. For instance, when the patient no longer believes in the external origin and power of the voices, but is reminded by the voices of sad or frightening memories, or when the voices activate negative self-schemata of incompetence, being unloved, being expelled, being worthless, etc. In these situations the voices do not predict negative events, the actual occurrence of which can be challenged. Behavioural experiments cannot be used to contradict opinions or facts that happened in the past. In referential associations, the voices make the patient think of emotion-evoking memories or of negative opinions about the self or the world that the patients live in. In classical conditioning, referential associations are identified with the procedure of evaluative conditioning as opposed to the procedure of signal learning. While in signal learning, the Conditioned Stimulus (CS) predicts the actual occurrence of the Unconditioned Stimulus (UCS), in evaluative learning, the CS acquires the emotional valence of the UCS, often without any specific reference to it (Baeyens *et al.*, 2001). COMET can be used when the therapeutic objective is to re-evaluate the meaning of stimuli that have been acquired by processes of evaluative conditioning. In auditory hallucinations, the target is to associate the voices with benevolent memories, emotions, and thoughts about the self, which are incompatible with the negative content they normally provoke.

Personal processes and the loss of self

Many patients are completely engulfed by the hallucinatory experiences. They pay exclusive attention to their voices and neglect their social relations and participation in society. The voices and the patient interact for many hours each day and they are involved with each other like wrestlers. Sometimes, the voice hearers are angry and shout back to the voices to try to scare them off. Other patients obey all the time and involve themselves in dangerous and harmful behaviours. Reflection on the self and the voices is absent. The voices are real for the voice hearer, and the self is taken hostage by the voices. What the voices say are considered by the patient to be facts. Defusing or decentring is necessary to bring about change. Decentring is the ability to observe one's thoughts and feelings as temporary, objective events in the mind, as opposed to reflections of the self that are necessarily true. Although defusion is presented as a new technique by Hayes and other proponents of Acceptance and Commitment Therapy (ACT) (Hayes, 2004), Beck already mentions in his early work the necessity that the patient 'learns to "distance" himself from his thoughts; that is, that he begins to view his thoughts as psychological events' (Beck *et al.*, 1979). Ingram and Hollon describe the process as distancing or decentring. The patient has to learn to view his thoughts as momentary mental events and not necessary a representation of the truth. It is conceptualized that one of the reasons of the long-term effectiveness of cognitive therapy may lie in implicitly teaching patients to initiate this process in the face of future stress (Ingram & Hollon, 1986).

Developmental psychology also stresses the necessity of decentring in the development towards an adult and balanced personality. Piaget marked the phenomenon of decentring as pivotal to developmental changes in cognitive structures. Decentring involves the combining of perspectives of an object into a unified mental representation, thereby minimizing distortions produced by attending only to isolated or compelling properties of that object. The child is enabled by increasingly more balanced, decentred cognition to transcend his initial egocentricity and develops differentiated and abstract models of conceptualization (Piaget, 1950).

Fresco and colleagues examined whether cognitive therapy would lead to increases in decentring, and further, whether the ability to take a decentred perspective would result in fewer relapses in depressed patients. CBT treatment responders demonstrated significantly higher levels of decentring than did patients treated to remission with medication. Moreover, CBT treatment responders endorsed greater levels of decentring than did CBT non-responders. Importantly, higher levels of decentring were associated with decreased relapse across the 18-month follow-up period, particularly for patients treated with CBT (Fresco *et al.*, 2007).

Despite the successes of the primarily rational–verbal approach of CBT, it is thought that there are other, associative routes to emotion that are much less susceptible to these techniques. Power and Dalgleish have proposed a multi-level processing model of emotion (Power & Dalgleish, 1997; Power & Dalgleish, 1999). In this model, there are four representation modes (Schematic, Propositional, Associative, Analogue Representation Systems: SPAARS) and two routes to emotion. One route to emotion is the well-known route in CBT and appraisal models of therapy: verbal propositions lead to emotions via schemata that integrate propositions and sensory information. The second route is associative and is not mediated by verbal reasoning.

Based on the basic rational assumptions of CBT, the appraisals of external origin and power that psychotic patients attribute to their voices are challenged in a rational process of hypothesis testing and developing alternative explanations for the experience of voices. Thereafter, the induced doubt must be followed by behavioural experiments of exposure.

In some patients, metacognitive change is not sufficient to take away distress. The patient then (rationally) knows that he should not be afraid of the voices, but (on an emotional level) the anxiety still persists. This is an example of change in the schemata and not change in the emotional associations. In some other patients, the therapist cannot apply CBT with positive results, because people are too emotionally involved in their hallucinatory experiences. In both these subgroups of patients, a more direct intervention on the associative emotional level is necessary, as reflection on thoughts and behaviour and a rational–verbal approach is not effective or not even possible. To this end, two other ways of treatment are needed to modify the emotional response to voice content. First, the easily and too often accessed negative experiences from memory that continuously evoke negative emotions must be deactivated. Second, distancing and decentring must be taught as a way to interpret voices and thoughts as mental events that are not necessarily true. Incompatible memories can be used as a tool to modify the strength association of the voices with negative memories and emotions.

The development of COMET and decentring techniques for auditory hallucinations

Competitive Memory Training (COMET) is designed by making use of recent insights and knowledge of the process of change in therapy. A copy of the protocol for COMET for auditory verbal hallucinations has been translated into English and can be requested from the authors. Other translated protocols for COMET for obsessions and for low self-esteem are also available.

The original cognitive model that is endorsed in CBT postulated that memories and schemas are directly modified by taking in new and incompatible information. This is what Barber and De Rubeis (1989) call the accommodation model. Two problems cannot be explained by this model: (1) why do not all people benefit from the modifications by new information? and (2) how can people have a relapse when the dysfunctional memories and schemas have been changed into more neutral ones?

Barber and De Rubeis demonstrated in an extensive review of the experiments in the domain of learning theory literature that it is more probable that the old representations have not been modified, but deactivated by installing and activating incompatible and positive representations. This is what they call the activation–deactivation model of CBT. So in this model, the old learned representations are not unlearned, but are deactivated by new learning.

This view is in line with findings in basic research, pertaining to phenomena as 'renewal', 'reacquisition', 'reinstatement' (Bouton, 1994), and 'UCS-inflation' (Hosoba *et al.*, 2001). In all these instances, seemingly forgotten (or weakened) associations become active (or stronger) again after a change of context or after new experiences with old stimuli have occurred. They were 'forgotten' or 'weakened' because old knowledge had been temporarily overlaid by new knowledge, not because the old knowledge had been 'eradicated'.

Incorporating this view on therapeutic change, Brewin suggests a retrieval competition model to explain how and why different forms of therapy work (Brewin, 2006). According to Brewin, all concepts are represented in memory with different meanings attached to them. These different meanings are in competition with each other to be retrieved, retrieval being a function of the nature of the eliciting stimulus, the context in which this stimulus is embedded, the level to which certain memory processes have already been primed, etc. In psychopathology, dysfunctional meanings are triggered too often in the wrong circumstances. Thus, psychotherapy should influence the retrieval competition in such a way that the chances of functional meanings to be retrieved are increased. This is not achieved by directly changing dysfunctional meanings, but by enhancing access to alternative meanings. Retrieval chances are increased by making the positive and incompatible meanings emotionally more salient, by repeated activation of them (overlearning), and by strengthening associations between different triggers and these positive meanings.

Imagery, exposure, and the Socratic challenging of automatic thoughts all help the patient to install competing representations and strengthen the memory access of these competing representations so as to deactivate the dysfunctional representations.

Retrieval competition is a pivotal process and this opens the opportunity to create new representations without directly disputing the evidence of the dominant negative representations. We can use autobiographical memories of incompatible events. For instance, in patients with voices who tell the patient that he is incompetent and that make the patient remember failures, a competing memory can be one of extreme feelings of competence, e.g., passing an exam, or scoring the winning goal in a final match.

How about distancing and decentring? ACT uses distancing. In a study by Bach and Hayes, 80 in-patients (43 schizophrenia, 19 schizoaffective disorder, 12 mood disorder with psychotic features, 3 delusional disorder, 3 psychosis NOS) were randomized into Treatment As Usual (TAU) versus ACT plus TAU. The ACT group had four sessions. The results after four sessions were that the ACT patients showed significantly higher symptom scores and lower symptom believability scores, and their frequency of rehospitalization was reduced to half the frequency of the TAU group after 4 months. What was done in these four sessions? The first session was 'take the mind for a walk'. It was explained that many people have thoughts, but they do not act on it, e.g., thoughts about food without going to eat. The patient and the therapist went out for a walk. The therapist walks behind the patient and gives a running commentary on things and events they encountered during the walk. The remarks were descriptive and evaluative of nature and predicted events and recommended certain actions. The patient was asked just to listen to this 'mind', without talking back or reacting to the comments and suggestions: 'Just listen and then do what you were doing or would like to do yourself'. This is a cognitive defusion exercise and teaches the patient to observe mental events and not to identify with the events. The second session demonstrated that trying to control discomfort will result in extra discomfort. In the third session, the coping styles were evaluated in the light of a valued goal. For instance, living independently is endangered by taking illicit drugs to cope with voices. The patient is asked only to involve in coping behaviour that does not jeopardize their valued independent living. In the fourth session, just before discharge from hospital, the concepts that were taught in the first three sessions were rehearsed. This study shows that distancing from troublesome voices can be achieved by training to pay attention to mental events without rating them (Bach & Hayes, 2002). It can be argued that the discomforting meanings attributed to these voices had become less accessible in the retrieval hierarchy.

COMET for auditory hallucinations makes use of two different strategies to influence the retrieval competition. First, during the re-evaluation phase, incompatible memories with positive emotions are strengthened to help deactivate the dominant negative memories accompanied by negative emotions. Second, during the decentring phase, COMET will help the patient not to identify with the voices and the voice-victim, but to identify with the observer of these mental events in a detached non-emotional way. Clinical experience in another bi-phasic COMET protocol (COMET for the treatment of obsessions) suggests that some patients need both phases, while others benefit more from either the re-evaluation phase or the decentring phase only (Guijken et al., 2008).

The incompatible memories must be relived to induce the full experience of the positive emotions. How can these self-induced positive mental states be accomplished? Mimicked facial emotions do induce the corresponding emotions (Santibanez & Bloch, 1986). For instance, when the feedback from facial muscles to the amygdala is blocked by botulinum toxin, then the emotion is not experienced (Hennenlotter *et al.*, 2008). So mimicking facial expression of positive emotions can induce the experience of these emotions. Different emotions have both aspects in common and different aspects, and this is reflected in the brain studies as well. Mimicking emotions activate overlapping and different brain regions in different emotions (Lee *et al.*, 2006; Pelletier *et al.*, 2003).

What words and thoughts cannot accomplish on an emotional level might be accomplished by posture, mimicking, and imagining. There is evidence that images are much more effective than self-talk in emotion induction as measured by pulse and blood pressure (Kunzendorf *et al.*, 1996). Mimicked words with implicit laughter activate the reward areas in the brain while non-mimicked words do not have this effect (Osaka & Osaka, 2005). Music can also enhance the experience of positive emotions (Mitterschiffthaler *et al.*, 2007).

Thus, during the re-evaluation phase of COMET, patients learn first to identify positive aspects of them that are incompatible with the meaning they attribute to the messages they receive from their voices. Then they learn to make these incompatible aspects more emotionally salient with the aid of imagery, posture, facial expression, and self-verbalizations and by repeatedly activating memories of them. In some COMET protocols, music and the writing of small self-referent positive stories are also used as means to enhance the emotional salience of the incompatible personal self-aspects. Finally, they have to 'activate' this positive knowledge while deliberately confronting them (*in vivo* or in imagination) with stimuli (i.e., the voices) that used to trigger negative self-knowledge.

In the second phase of COMET, the patient has to decentre and distance himself from the meaning of what the voices say. Again, imagination, posture, facial expression, and self-verbalization are applied to achieve this. The voice hearer has to confront himself once again with the triggers of his negative self-interpretations (the voices). But this time, the patient uses imagery (by looking at or listening to his voices from a distance or through a cloud), posture and facial expression (by looking uninterested or by yawning from sheer boredom) and self-verbalizations (by saying things like 'this is really boring', 'I've seen this hundreds of times and it won't get very interesting'). The combination of re-evaluation and decentring is supposed to help the patient not to be bothered anymore by his voices, by setting back the dysfunctional negative meanings they are associated with lower in the retrieval hierarchy.

The basic COMET protocol is actually a transdiagnostic protocol. Independent of psychopathology, variants of it can be used in all cases with persevering strong emotional responses to evoking stimuli. We will discuss later the first and preliminary results of COMET in treating quite different psychopathologies such as obsessions (Korrelboom *et al.*, 2008b), low self-esteem (Olij *et al.*, 2006), panic disorders (Peeters *et al.*, 2005, Korrelboom *et al.*, 2008a), eating disorders (Korrelboom *et al.*, submitted), rumination and worrying in generalized anxiety disorders and depression (Korrelboom *et al.*, 2004), and a case study with a schizophrenia patient who had auditory hallucinations (de Haan *et al.*, 2008). Some of these protocols are highly pertinent for people with auditory hallucinations, because low self-esteem, obsessions, and depressions are highly prevalent co-morbid disorders in auditory hallucinations. Combining the protocols can be tailored to the psychopathology of the hallucinating patients. There are now randomized clinical trials going on in depression in the elderly, obsessions, and auditory hallucinations. This chapter will present the protocol used in auditory hallucinations. The COMET technique can be administered in about seven sessions to a variety of disorders. Six consecutive steps are done to accomplish the therapy results. In the protocol for auditory hallucinations, the steps are:

1. Interview the patient extensively about the voices,
2. Monitor and register the content of the voices and determine the theme and the counter-theme of the voices,
3. Shift attention to evidence for the counter-theme to be true,
4. Re-experience the counter-theme and make this memory including thoughts and feeling easily accessible by the use of over-learning,
5. Engage the retrieval competition by strengthening the counter-theme memory, emotion, and thoughts in the presence of the (imagined) voices, and
6. Decentring or distancing from the voices.

The first step is to interview the patient extensively about the voices. The interview questions are integrated in the COMET protocol for auditory hallucinations. Three levels of information on the voices are gathered: topographical information, meaning and appraisals, schemas and themes.

Topographical information is gained about the number of voices, whether they are male, female, or both, what their identity is, how loud the voices are, what the frequency and duration of the voices are, whether they are heard inside or outside the head, are the voices commenting, commanding, or criticizing, in what time of the day, and in which situations? Are the voices speaking in the first, second, or third person? Also the emotional response to the voices is determined: which emotions and in what strength. At last, the behavioural reactions are explored. Are these behaviours aggressive, submissive, appeasing, avoiding, and/or obeying?

Meaning of and goals of the voices is gathered in the second part of the structured interview. These are metacognitions about the identity of the voices, the power of the voices, the reason why they have chosen the patient, what goals they pursue, and how it will all end.

Schemas and themes are explored in the third part of the interview. What are the consequences of the voices for the person? Which self-schema is elicited by the voices most often, and what does the theme of the voice content tell about the self of the patient? The theme and counter-theme are chosen with the help of the next pairs of concepts:

◆ Vulnerable versus resilient,
◆ Powerless versus in control,
◆ Unloved versus loved,

◆ Rejected versus accepted,

◆ Bad versus good enough,

◆ Weak versus strong,

◆ Worthless versus useful and worthy, and

◆ Incompetent versus competent.

The information is comprehended in a problem formulation that relates the cognitive behavioural aspects to the personal history and current thoughts, and activated schemas are combined in the formulation. This clarifies for the patient and the therapist what historical events in the patients' life laid the groundwork for the problem, how thoughts and appraisals determine distress and behaviour, and by what mechanisms the problem is perpetuated.

The second step in the transdiagnostic protocol is to monitor and register the content of the voices and to determine the theme of the voices and the counter-theme. A thought record scheme is used to register the voice content.

Mr A hears the voices of three classmates from elementary school. At first, the power of the voices was challenged by not obeying the voices in classical CBT. This was quite successful and although he is now convinced that the boys are not involved in these voices and he no longer obeys the commands, he is still hearing them. Because the voices call him a loser, he thinks about the many failures in his life and the many humiliations by the boys during school, and he feels very depressed and has started to believe that he is incompetent and rejected.

The third step shifts the attention to evidence for the counter-theme to be true and away from the dominant negative memories and self-ratings. This evidence can be found in daily occurrences, but also in actual memories of earlier instances in which the patient experienced moments of competence.

The counter-theme of Mr A was being competent and accepted by others. He registered all events during the week in which he was competent and/or accepted. He found out that he could do many routines very well and that he was especially good at repairing things with friends and his mother's washing machine. He was complemented quite often and felt accepted by friends and by the people in the shops he frequented.

The fourth step is to re-experience the counter-theme and make this memory including thoughts and feeling easily accessible by the use of over-learning. Lang proposed that memories about events are stored in three ways. There is a memory of sensory information with the audiovisual and other perceptual information of the event: a store of procedural knowledge with response representations on how to act in the situation. Lastly, there is a store of declarative knowledge with the personal meaning of the event (Lang, 1979; Lang et al., 1998). We will integrate the three memory stores during recall to enhance a strong and vivid re-experience of the positive emotion. Making positive experiences more emotionally salient, influences the retrieval hierarchy in a beneficial way.

In the case of Mr A, this was his graduation from secondary education. He had a phone call from school that he had passed all his exams with an A and his cry of joy and relief was welcomed by his parents and relatives, who congratulated and hugged him. This memory was elaborately explored: where did it all happen, what time of day was it, what objects were there, what people were at the place, what kind of clothing did they wear, was the sun shining or was it raining, etc. This is done until a very vivid recall of the memory is there in the audio–visual mode of the memory. When this part of the memory is clear, the patient is asked to take on the correct posture and movements: picking up the phone, hearing the message, make a cheerful cry and jump up and being hugged by the others. In other cases, the posture and mimics are used that fit the feeling in general. The patient is asked 'How do you sit or stand when you are proud of yourself? How do you look then?' At last, the semantic memory is added. In his case, it was the thought 'success'.

Re-installing the audio–visual imagery of the memory, the right posture, facial mimic, and movements together with the semantic meaning of the memory also brings back the original emotions of happiness and feelings of competence and acceptance by others. This is carefully checked by asking a percentage score of the vividness of the memory and the reliving of the situation. When the score is under 80% the practice is rehearsed. In most cases, this is accomplished within a session. The homework is to practice the emotional recall five times each day and to report on successfulness of the exercise and the degree of realized relived positive emotion.

The fifth step is to engage the retrieval competition by strengthening the counter-theme memory, emotion, and thoughts in the presence of the (imagined) voices.

Mr A. was asked to recall his counter-theme. When he was cheerfully standing up, he was asked to then imagine his voices telling him he was a loser and at the same time look glad, stand upright and preserve his experience of competence and acceptance. Herewith, he was able to experience that he was a worthwhile person, in spite of anything the voices might say. As in ACT, the patient was encouraged to observe mental events without identifying with these events. In the beginning, the voices still elicited the depressed feeling and as soon as the strong and cheerful posture and mimic waned, Mr A. was asked to stop imagining the voices and concentrate on the counter-theme again to restore the incompatible strong feeling. Once it is restored, this is combined again with the content of the voices. Most patients are capable of feeling competent and accepted while thinking about the voices. Mr A. reported that a strange thing happened to him. He was able to preserve the counter-theme and then the voices were different. Actually a little bit silly. He could not understand why he was so affected before.

This step also has to be over-learned. This over-learning 'deepens' the memory trace and makes the experience more easily accessible. The goal is that it will be more accessible than the depressing memories. Mr A. was asked to practice five times each day the recall of the counter-theme combined with the imagined voices, and preserve the pleasant and positive posture and feeling.

The sixth step is distancing or decentring from the voices. This brings the patient one step further and could also be helpful in the future to prevent relapse. Fresco and colleagues have demonstrated this in depression. CBT responders exhibited significantly greater gains in decentring compared to medication responders. High levels of decentring and low cognitive reactivity were associated with the lowest rates of relapse in an 18-month follow-up period (Fresco et al., 2007). Several decentring techniques can be used dependent on the voice hearing situation.

Mr A. was asked to sit in a chair and say what his voices usually tell him. Then he was asked to change the chair with the chair directly next to the 'voice' chair. He was asked to tell about his general reaction that he uses to give to the voices. The therapist tells Mr A. that he will now be cut in two. One part will stay in the chair and the other part will step back with the therapist and is seated on 'the very last row of the movie theatre'. He is now a witness of himself and his voices sitting next to him on the movie screen. He is asked to imagine that he is looking at the film of his life. Then the therapist starts interviewing. 'What is your favourite movie? How often have you seen it? Why did you get bored after six times? Now the film of your life; how often have you seen it? Why are you still emotionally involved and did you not get bored after the sixth time? Mr A. was then asked to look very bored, sit inattentively, yawn, and make a throw-away gesture with his hand and say, 'And now for something completely different'. The experience was that Mr A. could really distance himself (sitting on the very last row in the theatre) and decentre (be a spectator of himself).

The therapist stressed that this attitude of not identifying with your thoughts and feelings, but to identify with the spectator of the thoughts and the feeling gives room in order to allow thoughts and feelings to emerge and go by. By not engaging and by not fighting, the thoughts and feelings can be better tolerated and they will wane fast to make place for other thoughts and different feelings.

A variant on the theatre technique can be the fading out of the sound of the voices or by zooming out of the visual scene to very small characters that can hardly be seen.

Evidence for the effectiveness of COMET

At the moment, several attempts have been made to evaluate the effectiveness of different COMET protocols in routine psychiatric practice. Until now, five different protocols have been used in pilot studies. Most of these studies pertained to the treatment of low self-esteem. But COMET protocols for the treatment of panic, obsessions, rumination/worrying, and auditory hallucinations have also been tested. In this paragraph, all those studies will be briefly reviewed. Because most (but not all) of them were pilot studies without adequate controls and some other results are only preliminary and not yet properly published, the results can only be regarded as tentative indications for the possible effectiveness of COMET in clinical practice and not as conclusive evidence.

With the exception of the protocols for obsessions and auditory hallucinations, all COMET treatments were delivered in small groups, consisting of 5–8 patients and led by two therapists. Number of sessions varied from 6 to 8, with a frequency of once a week and the duration of sessions varying between 90 to 120 min. While COMET was performed on several sites of two large psychiatric institutions, more than 25 therapists were involved in delivering the treatments.

COMET for treating low self-esteem

Olij *et al.* (2006) assessed the effectiveness of the COMET protocol for low self-esteem in a pilot study with patients with different psychiatric disorders (personality disorders, major depression, eating disorders, post-traumatic stress disorder, and employment-related disorders). While receiving Treatment As Usual (TAU) for their main complaints at different outpatient departments, these patients were treated with seven weekly sessions of COMET for low self-esteem in small groups (5–7 patients). Self-esteem and depression were evaluated (Beck et al., 1961; Rosenberg, 1965). In a pre-post design without controls, mean scores on the Rosenberg Self-Esteem Scale (RSES) of the 75 COMET completers changed from 10.85 (SD = 4.73) to 16.56 (SD = 4.88), while mean scores on the Beck Depression Inventory (BDI) changed from 23.69 (SD = 11.22) to 14.47 (SD = 10.27). These changes were significant (RSES: $t = -9.59$, $p <. 001$; BDI: $t = 10.22$, $p < .001$) and large. The within-group Cohen's d for RSES was 1.19 and for BDI was 0.86 (Olij et al., 2006).

A similar study was performed with 86 patients with different depressive disorders. In an intention-to-treat-analysis the COMET group and improve on the RSES from 20.7 (SD=3.8) to 27.8 (SD=2.9). On the BDI, scores changed from 24.7 (SD=10.4) to 9.7 (SD=5.5). These changes were significant (RSES: $t = -14.5$, $p < .001$; BDI: $t = 15.2$, $p < .001$) and large. The within-group Cohen's d for RSES was 2.1 and for the BDI was 1.8. When the group was split into four diagnostic categories: major depressive disorder ($N = 51$), bipolar disorder ($N = 10$), other depressive disorders ($N = 17$), and depressive disorder in full remission ($N = 8$), there were no significant differences between these groups in their level of self-esteem at the start of COMET. After COMET, there were still no differences on level of self-esteem between groups. However, differences within groups from pre- to post-COMET were significant and large. The within-group Cohen's d varied from 1.3 to 2.3. It seems that COMET for low self-esteem in depressive disorders has comparable results in different subgroups of depressed patients (Maarsingh et al., submitted).

In a cohort of 40 hospitalized and day treatment patients with diagnoses of personality disorder, eating disorder, or a combination of both, 30 patients completed COMET. The patients had been in regular treatment for at least two months and received seven weekly sessions of COMET for low self-esteem in groups in addition to TAU. Measurements were taken at the start of their regular treatment (M1), after at least 2 months of regular treatment (mean = 16.4 (SD = 9.9) weeks) at the start of COMET (M2), 8 weeks later at the end of COMET (M3), and after at least 3 weeks after the end of COMET (mean = 14.8 (SD = 11.6) weeks) at the end of their regular treatment (M4). There were no relevant changes on the RSES between M1 and M2 ($t = 0.46$, n.s.) or between M3 and M4 ($t = -0.15$, n.s.). However, during COMET (M2–M3; duration 8 weeks), changes on the RSES ($t = -5.76$, $p < .001$) as well as on the BDI ($t = 6.89$, $p < .001$) were significant and large. Mean RSES scores rose from 9.2 (SD = 3.8) to 15.5 (SD = 5.9), mean scores on the BDI dropped from 26.9 (SD = 7.3) to 15.3 (SD = 11.2). The within-group Cohen's d on the RSES was 1.27 and was 1.22 on the BDI. Moreover, in a post hoc comparison with similar patients that followed the same regular treatment but not COMET, the COMET patients had higher self-esteem at the end of their total treatment than the comparison group. Results suggest that COMET for low self-esteem + TAU is more effective in changing self-esteem and depression scores than TAU. Moreover, these effects remained stable during follow-up (mean period: 14.8 weeks; SD = 11.6 weeks) (Korrelboom et al., 2009).

In a first Randomized Controlled Trial (RCT) on the COMET for low self-esteem protocol, 52 patients with eating disorders who had been in regular treatment for at least 2 months were randomized over two conditions: 8 weeks of TAU + COMET versus 8 weeks of TAU. Patients in COMET + TAU scored significantly better than that of patients in the control condition. Mean scores on the RSES went up from 20.0 (SD=5.2) to 23.6 (SD=5.5), while those for the BDI went down from 22.1 (SD=11.8) to 15.2 (SD=12.0). The univariate ANCOVA over the post-treatment data with the pre-test data as covariates was statistically significant for the RSES ($F(1,49)=7.58$, $p<.01$), as well as for the BDI $F(1,50)=5.17$, $p<.05$). Between-group effects were large. Cohen's d was 0.80 at the RSES and 0.60 at the BDI. COMET for low self-esteem is effective compared to TAU in improving self-esteem and reducing depression in patients with eating disorders (Korrelboom et al., 2009).

A similar RCT for the treatment of low self-esteem was conducted with patients with personality disorders. After randomization, 91 patients were randomized to either 7 weeks of COMET + TAU or 7 weeks of TAU only. The COMET group improved significantly more than the control group for both the RSES and the BDI. Mean RSES score changed from 20.7 (SD=3.4) to 25.8 (SD=4.6) during COMET. BDI scores in the COMET group changed from 24.3 (SD=10.1) to 16.7 (SD=10.5). The univariate ANCOVA over the post-treatment data with the pre-test data as covariates was statistically significant for the RSES $F(1,88)=16.05$, $p<.001$, as well as for the BDI $F(1,88)=10.02$, $p<.005$. The between group effect size was large for the RSES (Cohen's $d = 1.1$) and for the BDI (Cohen's $d = 0.8$). We conclude that COMET for low self-esteem + TAU compared to TAU is effective in improving self-esteem and reducing depression in patients with personality disorders (Korrelboom et al., submitted).

At this moment, yet another RCT into COMET for low self-esteem is still in progress. Depressed patients with low self-esteem were randomized into two conditions: COMET + TAU versus TAU.

COMET for treating obsessions

Research with the COMET protocol for the treatment of obsessions in patients with obsessive compulsive disorder, suggested that 'treatment resistant' OCD-patients with marked obsessions would benefit from COMET. Seventeen patients who were treated with regular therapy (Exposure and Response Prevention) for at least 7 weeks (mean: 29 weeks; SD = 21 weeks), but who were still symptomatic for obsessions, were individually treated with seven weekly sessions of COMET as an addition to their TAU. At the end of this period, scores on the obsession subscale of the Yale-Brown Obsessive-Compulsive Scale (Y-BOCS: Goodman et al., 1989) changed from 12.80 (SD = 3.41) to 8.33 (SD = 2.16), while scores on the Beck Anxiety Inventory (BAI) dropped from 18.79 (SD = 5.42) to 12.43 (SD = 5.05). These changes were significant and large (Within-group Cohen's d was 1.57 on the Y-BOCS obsessions subscale and 1.21 on the BAI) (Korrelboom et al., 2008b).

Recently, we started an RCT with OCD patients who are being randomized into either Exposure with Response Prevention (ERP) or COMET.

COMET for treating panic disorder

In an uncontrolled pilot study with 41 patients who were treated with the COMET protocol for panic, 29 patients completed COMET for panic as an addition to their regular treatment. Twenty-five patients completed the Agoraphobic Cognition Questionnaire (ACQ) and the Body Sensations Questionnaire (BSQ) at pre- and post-measurements (Chambless et al., 1984). During a 7-week period of COMET for panic training in groups, patients continued with their regular therapy (TAU). Changes between pre- and post-COMET on both ACQ ($t = 6.00$, $p < .001$) and BSQ ($t = 3.69$, $p < .001$) were statistically significant. ACQ scores dropped from 2.69 (SD = 0.81) to 1.98 (SD = 0.75). The within-group effect size is large (Cohen's $d = 0.91$). BSQ scores dropped from 2.60 (SD = 0.85) to 2.11 (SD = 0.66), with a medium effect size (Cohen's $d = 0.64$) (Peeters et al., 2005).

A RCT in which patients with panic disorder (with or without agoraphobia) are randomized between 7 weeks of COMET or 7 weeks of applied relaxation is about to be completed.

COMET for treating worrying and rumination

In a first pilot study, COMET for worrying was tested in small groups of patients with generalized anxiety disorders. At the time of an interim analysis, 35 patients were randomized to 6 weeks of group COMET + TAU or TAU. Measurements were taken at baseline, 3 weeks after the start of COMET and 6 weeks thereafter, when COMET was finished. During baseline until week 3, no significant changes were observed with ANOVA repeated measures for the Penn State Worry Questionnaire (Meyer et al., 1990) ($t = 1.67$, n.s.), and for the Intolerance of Uncertainty Scale (Freeston, 1994) ($t = 0.65$, n.s.). However, 6 weeks later at the end of COMET, changes on both scales compared to baseline were significant (PSWQ: $t = 4.87$, $p < .001$; IUS: $t=4.45$, $p<.001$' with medium within-groups effect-sizes (PSWQ: Cohen's $d = 0.7$; IUS: Cohen's $d = 0.5$). State Anxiety ($t=2.3$, $p<.05$) and Trait Anxiety ($t=4.9$, $p<.001$)(Spielberger, 1983) also changed during COMET. Results suggest that COMET for worrying could be an effective treatment method for patients with generalized anxiety disorder (Martens et al., 2009).

In a RCT, the COMET for rumination protocol + TAU was compared with TAU in 93 elderly depressed patients. Patients after a 7 weekly sessions group treatment of COMET + TAU ruminated less as indicated by the Ruminative Response Scale (RRS: Nolen-Hoeksema & Morrow, 1991) compared to patients in TAU. In the COMET, group scores on the RSS diminished from 47.35 (SD=10.22) to 43.35 (SD=6.53). The univariate ANCOVA over the post-treatment data with the pre-test data and age as covariates show a statistical tendency $F(1,10.33) = 4.29$ $p<.1$. At the same time, depression as measured with the Quick Inventory of Depressive Symptoms (QIDS: (Trivedi et al., 2004)) diminished in the COMET group significantly, in comparison with the control group. In the COMET, group scores for the QIDS went down from 12.67 [SD = 3.84] to 9.46 [SD = 4.59]. This was significant in an univariate ANCOVA over the post treatment scores with the pre-test data and age as covariates $F(1,46,98)=5.03$, $p<.001$). Effect sizes of the differences between COMET and the control group were medium for the RRS (Cohen's $d = 0.45$) and the QIDS (Cohen's $d = 0.49$). COMET for rumination is an effective intervention for elderly depressed patients in diminishing rumination and depression (Ekkers *et al.*, in preparation).

COMET for treating auditory hallucinations

A RCT with 77 schizophrenia-spectrum patients with persistent auditory-verbal hallucinations has just finished. A publication is in preparation by the first author. The target of the treatment was not to diminish the frequency of the voices as these had been unaffected by any therapy for many years in most patients. The target of this COMET protocol was to change the appraisal of the voices and to distance the person of the voice hearer from the voices. Intention-to-treat analysis with a MANOVA found an overall treatment effect ($F(5)=3.2$, $p<.05$) and the step-down showed a decrease in the attributed power to the voices (Beliefs About Voices Questionnaire-Revised, Chadwick & Birchwood, 2000: $F(1,75)=9.7$, $p<.005$); a decrease in submissiveness towards the voices (Social Comparison Rating Scale, Birchwood *et al.*, 2002: $F(1,75)=7.9$, $p<.01$); an increase of acceptance of the voices (Voices Acceptance and Action Scale, Shawyer *et al.*, 2007: $F(1,75)=4.4$, $p<.05$); an increase in internal attribution of the origin of the voices and more control over the voices (Auditory Hallucinations Rating Scale - cognitive subscale, Haddock *et al.*, 1999: $F(1,75)=4.9$, $p<.05$); and an increase in self-esteem (Self-Esteem Rating Scale, Lecomte *et al.*, 2006: $F(1,75)=10.8$, $p<.005$). The Cohen's d effect-sizes were medium to large and ranged from 0.48 to 0.76).

The voices themselves were still ongoing and making the same old negative remarks. The total scores on auditory hallucinations scale improved statistically non-significant ($p=.11$). The depression scores on the Beck Depression Inventory improved $F(1,74)=5,01$, $p<.05$). The protocol accomplishes changes in the appraisal of voices and can easily be made a part of regular CBT. The long-term effects still have to be evaluated. We think that boostering of the accomplishments is necessary to prevent erosion of the treatment results in the process of ongoing voices which might re-activate the negative memory networks again and gain dominance in retrieval over the positive memory networks.

Tentative conclusions about the preliminary evidence

Most studies on COMET are pilot studies without adequate controls. However, all results show that COMET might be able to change psychopathology and attitudes in different psychiatric conditions. Moreover, all referred studies have been performed in routine clinical practice. There were not very strict criteria for inclusion and exclusion for subjects into the study. Actually, all patients with the specific targeted symptom were included. The therapists had only relatively little specific training in and supervision over the application of COMET.

At the moment, most indications for therapeutic effectiveness are found in studies with the protocol for treating low self-esteem. Effect sizes within COMET groups in the several pilot studies pertaining to the treatment of low self-esteem are comparable to those found in both controlled COMET studies on low self-esteem.

The COMET procedures are based on some firmly established findings in experimental psychology. This supports the idea of an effective procedure. It is well known that the activation of action tendencies is a powerful instigator of emotional experience. Posture and facial expression, such as these are applied in COMET, have been shown to influence mood and emotional experience in several studies (Camras *et al.*, 1993; Flack *et al.*, 1999). The same holds true for imagination (Holmes *et al.*, 2008), self-verbalization (Velten, 1968; Lange *et al.*, 1998), and music (Pignatiello *et al.*, 1986; van der Does, 2002). All these procedures are part of the COMET protocol. The triggering of action tendencies associated with alternative emotions during exposure to anxiety provoking situations is a practice in cognitive behavioural therapy with a long and successful history (Barlow *et al.*, 2004).

There are some limitations of the COMET protocol that need to be addressed. Some patients do not have any experiences of success or superiority or that memories of these events have waned. In these patients, it is very difficult to find a proper experience that can be used in countering the negative feelings and thoughts that accompany the voices. In talking therapies, the ability to verbally express oneself can be rate limiting; in COMET, the capacity to visualize images is a necessary prerequisite. Some patients are just not visually oriented. And when they have construed a visual image, the image sometimes is not vivid enough to re-experience the positive feelings that accompanied the original event.

There are several ongoing studies evaluating the COMET protocol, using adequate control groups in randomized controlled clinical trials. In some studies, COMET is compared with other active interventions and in other studies with treatment as usual.

References

Bach, P., & Hayes, S. C. (2002). The use of acceptance and commitment therapy to prevent the rehospitalization of psychotic patients: A randomized controlled trial. *J Consult Clin Psychol*, **70**, 1129–39.

Baeyens, F., Vansteenwegen, D., Hermans, D., & Eelen, P. (2001). Chilled white wine, when all of a sudden the doorbell rings: Mere reference and evaluation versus expectancy and preparation in human Pavlovian learning. In columbus, F. (Ed.) *Advances in psychology research*. Huntington: Nova Science Publishers, Inc.

Barber, J. P., & Derubeis, R. J. (1989). On second thought: Where the action is in cognitive therapy for depression. *Cogn Ther Res*, **13**, 441–57.

Barlow, D. H., Allen, L. B., & Choate, M. L. (2004). Toward a unified treatment for emotional disorders. *Behav Ther*, **35**, 205–30.

Beck, A. T., Ward, C., & Mendelson, M. (1961). Beck depression inventory (BDI). *Arch Gen Psychiatry*, **4**, 561–71.

Beck, A. T., Rush, A. J., Shaw, B. F., & Emery, G. (1979). *Cognitive Therapy for Depression*. New York: Guilford.

Birchwood, M., Meaden, A., Trower, P., Gilbert, P., & Plaistow, J. (2000). The power and omnipotence of voices: Subordination and entrapment by voices and significant others. *Psychol Med*, **30**, 337–44.

Birchwood, M., Meaden, A., Trower, P., & Gilbert, P. (2002). Shame, humiliation, and entrapment in psychosis. A social rank theory approach to cognitive intervention with voices and delusions. In Morrison, A. P. (Ed.) *Casebook of cognitive therapy for psychosis*. Hove, east Sussex: Brunner-Routledge.

Birchwood, M., Gilbert, P., Gilbert, J., *et al.* (2004). Interpersonal and role-related schema influence the relationship with the dominant 'voice' in schizophrenia: A comparison of three models. *Psychol Med*, **34**, 1571–80.

Bouton, M. E. (1994). Conditioning, remembering, and forgetting. *J Exp Psychol: Animal Behav Process*, **20** (3), 219–231.

Brewin, C. R. (2006). Understanding cognitive behaviour therapy: A retrieval competition account. *Behav Res Ther*, **44**, 765–84.

Camras, L. A., Holland, E. A., & Patterson, M. J. (1993). Facial expression. In Lewis, M. & Haviland, J. M. (Eds.) *Handbook of emotions*. New York: Guilford Press, Guilford Press Print.

Chadwick, P., & Birchwood, M. (1994). The omnipotence of voices. A cognitive approach to auditory hallucinations. *Br J Psychiatry*, **164**, 190–201.

Chadwick, P., Lees, S., & Birchwood, M. (2000). The revised beliefs about voices questionnaire (BAVQ-R). *The British Journal of Psychiatry: J Ment Sci*, **177**, 229–32.

Chambless, D. L., Caputo, G. C., Bright, P., & Gallagher, R. (1984). Assessment of fear of fear in agoraphobics: The Body Sensations Questionnaire and the Agoraphobic Cognitions Questionnaire. *J Consult Clin Psychol*, **52**, 1090–7.

Choong, C., Hunter, M. D., & Woodruff, P. W. (2007) Auditory hallucinations in those populations that do not suffer from schizophrenia. *Curr Psychiatry Rep*, **9**, 206–12.

Close, H., & Garety, P. (1998). Cognitive assessment of voices: Further developments in understanding the emotional impact of voices. *Br J Clin Psychol*, **37** (Pt 2), 173–88.

Cummins, D. D. (1999). Cheater detection is modified by social rank: The impact of dominance on the evolution of cognitive functions. *Evol Hum Behav*, **20**, 229–48.

De Haan, G., Van der Gaag, M., & Korrelboom, K. (2008). Competitive memory training (COMET) bij een psychotische vrouw met auditieve hallucinaties. *Directieve Therapie*, **27**, 145–60.

Eadie, M. J., & Bladin, P. F. (2001). *A disease once sacred: A history of the medical understanding of epilepsy*. Eastleigh: John Libbey & Co Ltd.

Ekkers, W., Korrelboom, C. W., Huijbrechts, I., & Van der Gaag, M. (submitted) Competitive memory training for rumination in depressed elderly patients: A randomised controlled trial.

Flack, W. F., Jr., Laird, J. D., & Cavallaro, L. A. (1999). Separate and combined effects of facial expressions and bodily postures on emotional feelings. *Eur J Soc Psychol*, **29**, 203–17.

Freeston, M. H., Rheaume, J., Letarte, H., Dugas, M. J., & Ladouceur, R. (1994). Why do people worry? *Pers Individ Dif*, **17**, 791–802.

Fresco, D. M., Segal, Z. V., Buis, T., & Kennedy, S. (2007). Relationship of posttreatment decentering and cognitive reactivity to relapse in major depression. *J Consult Clin Psychol*, **75**, 447–55.

Gilbert, P., Birchwood, M., Gilbert, J., *et al.* (2001). An exploration of evolved mental mechanisms for dominant and subordinate behaviour in relation to auditory hallucinations in schizophrenia and critical thoughts in depression. *Psychol Med*, **31**, 1117–27.

Guijken, K., Dommanschet, C., & Korrelboom, C. W. (2008) COMET: de behandeling van obsessies met contraconditionering. *Directieve Therapie*, **28**, 251–72.

Haddock, G., Mccarron, J., Tarrier, N., & Faragher, E. B. (1999). Scales to measure dimensions of hallucinations and delusions: The psychotic symptom rating scales (PSYRATS). *Psychol Med*, **29**, 879–89.

Hayes, S. C. (2004). Acceptance and commitment therapy, relational frame theory, and the third wave of behavioral and cognitive therapies. *Behav Ther*, **35**, 639–65.

Hennenlotter, A., Dresel, C., Castrop, F., *et al.* (2008). The link between facial feedback and neural activity within central circuitries of emotion—New insights from botulinum toxin-induced denervation of frown muscles. *Cereb Cortex*, **19**, 537–42.

Hoffman, R. E., Varanko, M., Gilmore, J., & Mishara, A. L. (2008). Experiential features used by patients with schizophrenia to differentiate 'voices' from ordinary verbal thought. *Psychol Med*, **38**, 1167–76.

Holmes, E. A., Mathews, A., Mackintosh, B., & Dalgleish, T. (2008). The causal effect of mental imagery on emotion assessed using picture-word cues. *Emotion*, **8**, 395–409.

Honig, A., Romme, M. A., Ensink, B. J., Escher, S. D., Pennings, M. H., & Devries, M. W. (1998). Auditory hallucinations: A comparison between patients and nonpatients. *J Nerv Ment Dis*, **186**, 646–51.

Hosoba, T., Iwanaga, M., & Seiwa, H. (2001). The effect of UCS inflation and deflation procedures on 'fear' conditioning. *Behav Res Ther*, **39**, 465–75.

Ingram, R. E., & Hollon, S. D. (1986). Cognitive therapy for depression from an information processing perspective. In Ingram, R. E. (Ed.) *Information processing approaches to clinical psychology*. Orlando: Academic Press.

Korrelboom, C. W., Visser, S., & Broeke, E. T. (2004). Gegeneraliseerde angststoornis: Wat is het en wat kun je ertegen doen? *Directieve Therapie*, **24**, 276–95.

Korrelboom, C. W., Peeters, S., Blom, S., & Huijbrechts, I. (2008a). Competitive memory training voor paniekstoornis. *Directieve Therapie*, **28**, 233–50.

Korrelboom, K., Van Der Gaag, M., Hendriks, V., Huijbrechts, I., & Berretty, E. (2008b). Treating obsessions with competitive memory training: A pilot study. *Behav Ther*, **31**, 29–36.

Korrelboom, C. W., Van Der Weele, K., Gjaltema, M., & Hoogstraten, C. (2009). Competitive Memory Training (COMET) for treating low self-esteem: A pilot study in a routine clinical setting. *Behav Ther*, **32**, 3–9.

Korrelboom, C. W., De Jong, M., Huijbrechts, I., & Daansen, P. (2009). Competitive Memory Training (COMET) for treating low self-esteem in patients with eating disorders: A randomised clinical trial. *J Consult Clin Psychol*, **77**, 974-80.

Korrelboom, C. W., Marissen, M., & Van Assendelft, T. (submitted). Competitive Memory Training (COMET) for treating low self-esteem in patients with personality disorders: A randomised clinical trial.

Kunzendorf, R. G., Cohen, R., Francis, L., & Cutler, J. (1996). Effect of negative imaging on heart rate and blood pressure, as a function of image vividness and image 'realness'. *Imagination, Cogn Personality*, **16**, 139–59.

Lang, P. J. (1979). A bio-informational theory of emotional imagery. *Psychophysiology*, **16**, 495–512.

Lang, P. J., Cuthbert, B. N., & Bradley, M. M. (1998). Measuring emotion in therapy: Imagery, activation, and feeling. *Behav Ther*, **29**, 655–74.

Langdon, R., Jones, S. R., Connaughton, E., & Fernyhough, C. (2009). The phenomenology of inner speech: Comparison of schizophrenia patients with auditory verbal hallucinations and healthy controls. *Psychol Med*, **39**, 655-663.

Lange, A., Richard, R., Gest, A., De Vries, M., & Lodder, L. (1998). The effects of positive self-instruction: A controlled trial. *Cogn Ther Res*, **22**, 225–36.

Lecomte, T., Corbière, M., & Laisné, F. (2006). Investigating self-esteem in individuals with schizophrenia: Relevance of the self-esteem rating scale-short form. *Psychiatry Research*, **143**, 99–108.

Lee, T. W., Josephs, O., Dolan, R. J., & Critchley, H. D. (2006). Imitating expressions: Emotion-specific neural substrates in facial mimicry. *Soc Cogn Affect Neurosci*, **1**, 122–35.

Leudar, I., & Thomas, P. (2000). *Voices of reason, voices of insanity: Studies of verbal hallucinations*. London: Routledge.

Maarsingh, M., Huijbrechts, I., & Korrelboom, C. W. (in preparation). Competitive Memory Training (COMET) for low self-esteem in patients with depressive disorders.

Martens, S., Korrelboom, C. W., & Huijbrechts, I. (in preparation). Competitive Memory Training (COMET) for the treatment of worry in patients with generalized anxiety disorder: A pilot study.

Marten, S., Korrelboom, K., & Huijbrechts, I. (2009). Competitive Memory Training (COMET) for worrying. The anti-worrying training. *Directieve Therapie*, **29**, 254–78.

Meyer, T., Miller, M., Metzger, R., & Borcovec, T. (1990). Development and validation of the Penn State Worry Questionnaire. *Behav Res Ther*, **28**, 487–95.

Mitterschiffthaler, M. T., Fu, C. H., Dalton, J. A., Andrew, C. M. & Williams, S. C. (2007). A functional MRI study of happy and sad affective states induced by classical music. *Hum Brain Mapp*, **28**, 1150–62.

Olij, R., Korrelboom, K., Huijbrechts, I., *et al.* (2006). De module zelfbeeld in een groep: werkwijze en eerste bevindingen [Treating low self-esteem in a group: Procedure and first results]. *Directieve Therapie*, **26**, 307–25.

Osaka, N., & Osaka, M. (2005). Striatal reward areas activated by implicit laughter induced by mimic words in humans: A functional magnetic resonance imaging study. *Neuroreport*, **16**, 1621–4.

Peeters, S., Korrelboom, K., Voermans, M., & Huijbrechts, I. (2005). Paniekmanagement revisited: Ervaringen met een nieuwe groepsbehandeling [Training inpanic control revisited: Experiences with a new group therapy]. *Directieve Therapie*, **25**, 396–408.

Pelletier, M., Bouthillier, A., Levesque, J., *et al.* (2003). Separate neural circuits for primary emotions? Brain activity during self-induced sadness and happiness in professional actors. *Neuroreport*, **14**, 1111–6.

Piaget, J. (1950). *The psychology of intelligence*. New York: Harcourt, Brace.

Pignatiello, M. F., Camp, C. J., & Rasar, L. A. (1986). Musical mood induction: An alternative to the Velten technique. *J Abnorm Psychol*, **95**, 295–7.

Power, M., & Dalgleish, T. (1997). *Cognition and emotion: From order to disorder*. Hove: Psychology Press.

Power, M. J., & Dalgleish, T. (1999). Two routes to emotion: Some implications of multi-level theories of emotion for therapeutic practice. *Behav Cogn Psychother*, **27**, 129–41.

Romme, M. A., & Escher, A. D. (1989). Hearing voices. *Schizophr Bull*, **15**, 209–16.

Rosenberg, M. (1965) *Society and the adolescent self-image*. Princeton: Princeton University Press.

Santibanez, G., & Bloch, S. (1986). A qualitative analysis of emotional effector patterns and their feedback. *Pavlovian J Biol Sci*, **21**, 108–16.

Shawyer, F., Ratcliff, K., Mackinnon, A., Farhall, J., Hayes, S. C., & Copolov, D. (2007). The voices acceptance and action scale (VAAS): Pilot data. *J Clin Psychol*, **63**, 593-606.

Sommer, I. E., Daalman, K., Rietkerk, T., *et al.* (2008). Healthy individuals with auditory verbal hallucinations: Who are they? Psychiatric sssessments of a selected sample of 103 subjects. *Schizophr Bull* [Epub ahead of print].

Spielberger, C.D. (1983). *Manual for the State-Trait Anxiety Inventory (STAI-form Y)*. Palo Alto California: Consulting Psychologists Press.

Tien, A. Y. (1991). Distributions of hallucinations in the population. *Soc Psychiatry Psychiatr Epidemiol*, **26**, 287–92.

Trivedi, M. H., Rush, A. J., Ibrahim, H. M., *et al.* (2004). The inventory of depressive symptomatology, clinician rating (IDS-C) and self-report (IDS-SR), and the quick inventory of depressive symptomatology, clinician rating (QIDS-C) and self-report (QIDS-SR) in public sector patients with mood disorders: A psychometric evaluation. *Psychological Medicine*, **34**, 73–82.

Van Der Does, W. (2002). Different types of experimentally induced sad mood? *Behav Ther*, **33**, 551–61.

Van Der Gaag, M., Hageman, M. C., & Birchwood, M. (2003). Evidence for a cognitive model of auditory hallucinations. *J Nerv Ment Dis*, **191**, 542–5.

Van OS, J., Hanssen, M., Bijl, R. V., & Ravelli, A. (2000). Strauss (1969) revisited: A psychosis continuum in the general population? *Schizophr Res*, **45**, 11–20.

Velten, E., JR. (1968). A laboratory task for induction of mood states. *Behav Res Ther*, **6**, 473–82.

Chapter 10

Hallucinations-focused Integrative Therapy (HIT)

Jack A. Jenner

Introduction

Auditory Vocal Hallucinations (AVH), voice hearing, as well as musical hallucinations do not by themselves provide sufficient evidence of an underlying psychiatric illness and are not pathognomonic for any specific disorder. First, population studies show that the incidence of AVH in the general population is far greater than traditional estimates of incidence of psychotic disorders (van Os *et al.*, 2000; Rossler *et al.*, 2007). Second, hypnagogic and hypnopompic voices are normal phenomena according to DSM-IV-TR criteria. Third, more than 60% of American college students report to hear at least once a year a voice calling their name in the absence of an external stimulus. It is unlikely that all of them were psychotic at that time (Barrett & Etheridge, 1992). Fourth, hallucinations may be caused by a wide range of somatic disorders and physiological conditions. Last but not least, many religions such as Pentecostal Christianity, Buddhism, Sufism, and Shamanism label persons who have hallucinatory experiences with the Divine as 'chosen'.

Nevertheless, the combination of AVH and psychological or behavioural complications is highly suspect for the presence of psychiatric disorder. The lifetime prevalence rate of AVH as a symptom in individuals with dissociative disorder (80%), schizophrenia spectre disorders (70%), psychotic depression (30%), and personality disorders (borderline personality disorder about 30%) is much higher than in the general population (Sidgewick *et al.*, 1894; Landmark *et al.*, 1990; Tien 1991; Yee *et al.*, 2005). Although positive and useful voices are fairly common (Jenner *et al.*, 2008), the great majority of voice hearers with a psychiatric disorder suffer from rather persistent AVH with negative content.

Need for psycho-social interventions

Despite the effects of Antipsychotic Medication (AP) and the reduction of side effects following the introduction of atypical AP, AVH are most often refractory to medication. This is mainly due to patient non-compliance with medication treatment plans. Medication non-compliance in schizophrenia patients is about 40% in the first year and rises to 70% over time (Young *et al.*, 1987). In addition, AVH persist in about 30% of AP-compliant patients (Johnstone *et al.*, 1991). Hence, medication refractory AVH may be assumed to exist in about 50% of voice-hearing schizophrenia patients demonstrating a great need for effective treatment. These patients may benefit from newly developed psychosocial interventions, particularly because disabling social handicaps remain in most patients, despite symptom reduction (Bustillo *et al.*, 2001).

In 1994, the Voices Outpatient Clinic was started at the University Medical Centre Groningen with the aim of developing an AVH-tailored therapy. From the very beginning, the foci of therapy have been optimizing compliance, reducing the burden of the disorder and related symptoms, and improving control, quality of life, and social functioning. In 1996, HIT was designed and has been improved upon in the intervening years. In this chapter, the format, content, and cost effectiveness of HIT will be described.

Format of HIT

The HIT format requires psychiatric diagnosis as well as hallucination assessment to be done according to protocol (see under diagnostic AVH protocol). However, the diagnostic and the intervention stages of treatment are not strictly separated. From the very beginning, the therapist intervenes even during his assessment, e.g., through his manner of conducting the diagnostic interview, through the framing of questions and the (positive) reframing of answers and his summarizing. We have even noticed that assessing AVH with the Auditory Vocal Hallucination Rating Scale (AVHRS; Jenner & van de Willige, 2002) may initiate reattribution in many of our patients. Phasing and timing of the various steps in and modules of HIT occur in a flexible manner and are adjusted to the abilities, eagerness for treatment, and personality traits of both patient and relevant others.

The effectiveness of therapeutic programs and interventions depends, to a great extent, on patient compliance. Hence, programmatic aspects of HIT having the aim of improving compliance will be described first. These compliance-enhancing aspects are (1) building and maintaining a therapeutic relationship, (2) integrating interventions with clinical evidence, (3) application of problem-oriented, instead of disease-related psycho-education, (4) family therapy, and (5) a directive and strategic approach applying operant conditioning, embedded in around-the-clock outreach-service.

The HIT program has been empirically developed and has been organized according to current scientific evidence. For example, cognitive handicaps in verbal and visual memory are common among patients with schizophrenia. It may be argued that the greater the number of therapists involved in treatment, the more patient handicaps become noticeable. Pursuing this reasoning, patients may benefit from as few different therapists as possible and, conversely, may suffer from multi-disciplinary teams with shared patient loads. Hence, our rule of thumb is 'less is more', which implies that HIT is preferably administered by one therapist. If consultations are needed, which occurs repeatedly, these are singular and are preferably done in the presence of the primary therapist.

HIT employs multiple modalities to maximize control of persistent AVH. In this approach, a variety of evidence-based treatment strategies have been integrated (e.g., CBT, problem-solving family treatment, supportive counselling, psycho-education, coping training, mobile crisis intervention, and antipsychotic medication). The HIT program consists of one-hour sessions—with a mean of 15—over 9 to 12 months (Jenner, 2002). Patients are advised to involve relevant others in the treatment. If the patient agrees, family members as well as other therapists are invited in sessions as much as they can, preferably in all sessions.

HIT modules are implemented according to flexibly applied protocols that take into account individual needs and preferences, stage of motivation and peoples' personality structure.

Indicators for selecting the most appropriate strategy are patient and voices histories, meaning of and attributions of voices, anxiety levels, and patient explanations regarding voice origins.

Therapeutic alliance

Establishing and maintaining a therapeutic alliance with patients suffering from psychiatric disorders with a high prevalence of AVH is far from easy. To achieve an effective working relationship, it may be helpful to keep the following points in mind: (1) voice hearers tend to share an 'allergy' to psychiatric treatment, (2) accept that voice hearers hear voices (neurons in the Broca and Wernicke brain nuclei fire when patients report AVH), (3) aim at a workable reality that is acceptable for both patient and relatives as well as the therapist rather than at a dogmatic reality (see two-reality principle, motivating strategies, flexibility, and operant conditioning), (4) use a step-wise diagnostic protocol, and (5) Socratic reasoning about AVH is to be the preferred style of communication because it is more productive than confrontation and interpreting AVH and psychotic reasoning as reality disturbances. The Socratic interviewing style seeks to give as little direct advice to the patient as possible and does not focus on proving that the therapist is right and the voice hearer is wrong. Rather it seeks to elicit suggestions for change and solutions from the voice hearer. Preferably, the therapist helps or seduces the patient to draw his own doubt with an indirect style of disputing and testing the patient's inferences about the power of his AVH (Chadwick *et al.*, 1996). Sentences such as could it be possible that …, have you ever considered …, and what do think of … have proved their effectiveness.

Voice hearers' 'allergy' to psychiatry: Disease or relation bound?

Studies report a 40–70% treatment non-compliance rate among voice hearers with psychiatric disorders. Confronting voice hearers with their disturbed reality testing and psycho-education sessions about cognitive deficits, preferably given with conviction, are seemingly logical interventions for therapists who consider non-compliance to be disease related in terms of lacking insight, disturbed reality testing, or resistance. However, voice hearers often feel personally rejected by such a direct and confrontational approach (Cohen & Berk, 1985). Voice hearers want a therapist who is willing to listen to their strange experiences that they themselves do not understand, can neither explain or effectively articulate, and may find scary, certainly in the beginning stage. The more we try to convince voice hearers of being mentally disordered, the more they may feel misunderstood and their experiences to be neglected. From this perspective, patient non-compliance becomes a normal, although disastrous, reaction to an unproductive therapeutic approach. Therapists who interpret non-compliance as (partly) interpersonal will prefer motivational interviewing, re-labelling, and reframing to confrontation. HIT aims to achieve a workable reality that is acceptable for all involved: patient, relatives, and therapist. For this reason, the psychiatric outpatient clinic has been renamed as a 'voice hearer clinic' and the hospital organization has been replaced by a 'customer'-oriented approach guided by the slogan 'the customer is always right'.

Accepting the reality of voice hearing, the two realities approach

In line with the 'customer is always right' slogan, AVHs are accepted as real experiences. This is a sign of both good salesmanship and applied science, as fMRI and PET studies illustrate synchronicity of AVH and neurons firing in the Broca and Wernicke areas of the brain (David, 1999; Weiss & Heckers, 1999; Stephane et al., 2001). The other reality is that *we* do not actually hear voices. This makes voice hearers experts compared to therapists in terms of their subjective experience. When voice hearers accept this 'two-realities' reality, and most of them eventually do, they also indirectly and implicitly take on the role of an 'experience expert' and the responsibilities that go with this title. Then, therapists explicitly call voice hearers to account for their expert role. We have noticed this 'experience expert' role to have great consequences in terms of less negativism and more patient willingness to independently monitor AVH characteristics and their consequences, and their relatives' behaviour too. It has also been our experience that this elevation of the patient to the role of 'expert' improves cooperation and compliance with homework tasks.

Then, patient, relatives, and therapist identify all possible causes and explanations of voice hearing. Explanations are ordered consecutively by all involved in this identification process. We have found that this approach makes patients more willing to accept the therapist's non-psychosis-driven explanations. Each participant is requested to connect his explanations with logical plans of action for which duration, responsibilities for implementation, and parameters of success are determined. For example, trauma may be connected with a period of mourning, witchcraft with rituals, diseases with medication, while patients who are convinced that their voices come from the devil or are God's punishment for sins they have committed may start prayer and psalm-singing. Finally, therapist, patient, and relevant others discuss the feasibility of each plan of action. Some intriguing consequences of this stepped approach have been noticed in our practice. Patients who accept the therapist's explanations also appear to accept relatively easy to try his plans of action, which of course are non-psychosis-driven. This leads to better cooperation and compliance, while resistance and dropout may decrease. Unexpectedly, we have seen patients determine that some of their delusion-driven plans of action are unfeasible and independently withdraw them, something that they seldom did before at the suggestion of therapists or relatives.

Motivational strategies

Motivation for treatment and success rate are significantly and positively correlated. When therapy stagnates, underlying assumptions are that lack of motivation is an inherent part of a patient's personality or is inherent in some psychiatric states. These patient-bound assumptions that neglect the role of communicative and contextual influences easily give rise to a self-fulfilling prophecy that ultimately results in therapeutic stagnation. Treatment implies the creation of conditions that lead to beneficial change. Therapists' attitudes and skills determine this creative process to a great extent. Hence, we prefer Miller and Rollnick's (1991) definition of motivation as a state of readiness or an eagerness to change, which highlights the impact of context-dependent fluctuations that allow for various motivation-focused interventions that are less patient dependent. The illness-awareness model of Prochaska *et al.* (1982) helps to promote this eagerness to change by applying step-by-step stage-dependent strategies.

A variety of motivating strategies are built into the HIT program, both of congruent and paradoxical nature. Labelling patients as 'experience experts' and moving the focus away from a disease/medical model towards one based on consumer needs and demands have already been delineated. For instance, medication non-compliance is viewed as a request for medication adjustment, resistance is regarded as consumer complaints, and symptoms and behaviours are labelled positively.

Prochaska and DiClemente (1982) have developed a stage model of the process of change that allows for assessing a person's readiness for change according to different stages. Each stage requires stage-specific motivational strategies. Patients who have not even considered having a problem are in the pre-contemplation stage. Pre-contemplators may feel coerced by a regular treatment approach. Instead, raising doubt by increasing the pre-contemplator's perception of risks with current behaviour, the cons of hearing voices, and pointing out that treatment might help reduce these cons is the preferred approach. It is not until the action stage that patients are ready to take medication and to carry into effect advices that have been given. Before the action stage, therapeutic 'dos and don'ts may increase resistance and non-compliance.

Positive labelling and reframing are among the most effective motivating strategies. It is change orientation and reattribution that distinguishes positive labelling from compliment. As mentioned earlier, medication non-compliance may be labelled as a request for optimizing medication. Resistance, and hesitation, may be labelled as a request for further information or as a sign of wisdom, suggesting that the patient does not act impulsively but deliberately after having balanced pros and cons. Positive labelling helps to create openness to change, but in itself is seldom sufficient. Two more examples: (a) labelling AVH as a gift may increase self-esteem. This label also allows for drawing the voice hearer into his connected responsibilities. A patient with the delusion of being poisoned repeatedly heard voices commanding him to destroy his parents' kitchen. Because he strongly rejected a congruent approach focusing on insight and due to his severe reality distortion, the therapist switched to a hyper-congruent approach. He compared the patient, who has a protestant denomination, with the Pharaoh's taster and labelled his delusion as a kind of talent. This made him willing and able to replace his delusion-driven destructive behaviour with a more constructive view of protecting his parents. Empathetic Socratic reasoning concerning the risk of civil commitment in reaction to possible aggressive outbursts in shops when confronted with 'poisoned' food made this patient willing to take medication as part of his protecting responsibility. As the reader will notice, the therapist switched from a congruent to hyper-congruent approach because of the patient's absolute rejection of the former approach. By this hyper-congruent approach, the patient is made responsible for the consequences of his psychotic behaviour. This change implies a switch in focus from insight to behaviour and responsibility. This makes sense because enduringly confronting severely deluded patients with their distorted reality testing may fortify their deluded conviction. (b) Labelling AVH as makeshift may be used. For example, monitoring made a sub-assertive female patient aware that her negative voices were connected with specific situations. Labelling her voices as helping makeshifts helped her to apply the appropriate coping behaviour in a more timely way. This not only reduced her fear of the voices, but her self-esteem grew with the successes from her new behaviour. Labelling in a family context helped her husband replace his high-levelled expressed emotions by supporting her instead of questioning her about her psychiatric symptoms. He inquired about the frequency and success of using her voices as makeshifts and complemented her.

Hyper-congruent reactions may be indicated when a congruent approach does not work. This may occur in some psychotic states, especially deluded ones and also in cases of severe ambivalence, as may be encountered in cluster B personality disorders. Severely ambivalent persons demand the therapist to solve both their opposing needs at the same time, which in itself is impossible. Hence, therapist advisements that regard only one pole of their ambivalence often evoke acting-out behaviour from the patient. Advisements should always deal with both poles. Psychotic patients may be held responsible hyper-congruently in line with their psychotic reasoning, not by confrontation, but by Socratic reasoning. Someone with the delusion that God orders him to convert the world may be questioned about the efficacy of his actions and about the likelihood that his smelly clothes keep people away from God. Quite a few of our patients have improved their self-care and hygiene after a debate about how to become an effective advertisement for God.

Flexibility

Thorough psychiatric assessment is mandatory. How to do this is a matter of debate. Regular medical questioning focuses more on symptoms and handicaps than on empowerment and successful coping. Unintentionally, this focus may reinforce the patient's hopelessness, impotence, inability, and passivity. HIT attempts to minimize these side effects by translating symptoms and handicaps into goals to achieve: e.g., the goal of disorganized thinking becomes mastering one's mind, the goal of thought insertion translates into the patients being the 'boss' of their brain, and of AVH controlling one's senses. These examples illustrate that HIT intermingles diagnostic and intervention stages from the very beginning of the program. The various treatment modules are implemented according to protocol. However, the HIT program is very much a tailor-made one, permitting voice hearers to select the timing and sequence of modules. Most voice hearers prefer to start with the coping–training module. Furthermore, interventions are adjusted to match the patient's degree of awareness of the illness. Homework tasks are adjusted to patient capacities. For example, patients and relatives are urgently requested to monitor characteristics of voices, the subjective burden the voices induce, the feelings, thoughts, and actions they generate, and last, but not least, the effectiveness of these associated thoughts and actions. However, the mentally handicapped may monitor their voices by counting them in fives or using a counting machine, while the illiterate may monitor by making use of a tape recorder. According to neurolinguistic programming (Bandler & Grinder, 1979; Knowles, 1983), the therapist also joins both verbally and nonverbally the person's predominant representational system: visual (I *see* what you mean), auditory (that *sounds* clear to me), or kinaesthetic (I have a *sense* that is a *touchy* issue for you). Flexibility also entails the therapist searching for words and explanations that join in with an individual's concept about the origin of voices. For example, one may expect patients who reject the schizophrenia concept also to object to psycho-education about neuro-transmitters, while the schizophrenia concept may help to mitigate guilt feelings of parents. Patients with delusion of thought insertion or withdrawal who deny psychosis may object to psychiatric help anti-psychotics included but may be interested in testing the effectiveness of the 'chemical' cage of Faraday. An exhausted patient may be willing to try restorative (anti-psychotic) tonics. After the principle of the Faraday cage—a metal wire construction that prevents electrical and magnetic waves to enter the inside of the cage—has been explained, the patient is told that some drugs have a similar anti-intrusive effect on thought insertion. Similarly, after an introduction about the effectiveness of restorative tonics and vitamins in physical exhaustion, anti-psychotics are suggested as a kind of restorative to the mind. In neither situation, the term anti-psychotics will be used.

Last but not least, messages should be conveyed according to a person's personality traits. For example, most people with histrionic personality traits appreciate a warm, empathetic therapist, while schizoid persons may feel uncomfortable with such an approach, and paranoid persons may consider such behaviour a reason for self-defence. Similarly, avoidant persons appreciate clear and direct advices more than passive-aggressive persons, and it is advisable to offer narcissistic individuals the choice of more than one option. In summary, careful selection of the packing material improves the chances that your present will be accepted.

Operant conditioning

Success reinforces behaviour and is a strong motivator for continuation and compliance. It is our opinion that cutting a task into many small pieces is to be preferred. The smaller the task, the greater the chance of success, and more pieces means more chances for reinforcement. Also, smaller tasks may reduce the interval between attempts and success, and the sooner success is achieved, the greater its reinforcing power. Therefore, homework tasks and changes are cut into as many small pieces as possible. Another reason for this approach is that the larger and more complex the step, the greater the chance of failure.

HIT also applies operant conditioning in 'dosing' the next appointment. The regular interval between appointments varies from 2 weeks, in the initial stage, to 4–6 weeks during the coping–training stage. The interval is adjusted according to the patient's achievements, which is shorter when tasks have been applied, irrespective of the results. Except for treatment-avoiding patients and for severe danger, suicide, or need for involuntary admission, the interval is extended for patients who repeatedly do not comply with tasks. This approach is fairly different from regular Dutch mental health care practice that shortens the interval in such cases.

There are several points of argument for this approach. First, some patients just need more time to accomplish a task. Prolonging the interval corresponds with their potential, whereas earlier appointments confront them, unintentionally, with being unable to perform adequately. Second, in other patients, non-compliance with tasks is a form of avoidance behaviour. Suspect for this avoidance are patients who complain about being unable to perform but have not yet even tried and those who despite adjustment of their task continue to debate the sense of their task or to complain. Complying with their request to forward the next appointment is a pitfall that reinforces their avoidance because their talking is avoidance behaviour that safeguards them from doing the assigned task. Third, non-compliance may be functional in the therapeutic relation and have no relationship whatsoever with content or difficulty of a task. In these cases, hyper-congruent interventions may be indicated. These hyper-congruent interventions serve the purpose of disconnecting behaviour and functionality, resulting in a loss of the destructive power of the latter. The therapist apologises for having misjudged the time this patient needs for the task and then makes the next appointment dependent on the patient's ability to accomplish the task. The patient is given more time than is actually needed. However, a guarantee is given by the therapist that he or she will get an appointment immediately after having accomplished the assigned task. Hyper-congruent interventions have been shown to be very effective when properly indicated. Most of our patients succeed in accomplishing earlier problematic tasks within 3 weeks. Lastly, in narcissistic patients, a task will often be deliberately described by the therapist as being very difficult, probably beyond the patient's capacities. The patient is told that the next appointment will be postponed for this reason, while also being given a guarantee of an appointment at an earlier time in case the therapist may have underestimated patient's capacities. Personality traits will allow narcissistic patients to 'beat' their therapist.

Diagnostic AVH protocol

As already mentioned, diagnostic steps and interventions are interwoven in HIT. For example, assessing AVH characteristics may be combined with empathy and compassion as well as with seeding doubt.

Step 1: Probing whether the voices are really heard—their physical qualities is needed to differentiate AVH from illusions, delusions, and obsessive-compulsive thoughts.

Step 2: The mortal danger of most AVH is fairly low. In the case of command hallucinations, the danger, in part, depends upon the degree of obedience to the voices and of compliance with treatment. It is mainly the accompanying delusions that make these command hallucinations dangerous.

Hence, assessing both compliance and delusions of being controlled, of paranoid content, and of reference, is mandatory.

Step 3: Somatic and psychiatric disorders, as well as side effects of medication, have to be assessed.

Step 4: Habitual reaction patterns and personality traits of voice hearers and their relatives are indicative of the preferred style of communication. Some examples: while most people appreciate empathy, schizotypal persons prefer more distance; paranoid persons may interpret our compassion as frightening proof that we can read their minds. The grandiose sense of self-importance of narcissistic persons may prevent them from accepting even the best advice. Hence, advisements to narcissistic persons should preferably be presented as a choice with at least two options.

Step 5: Assessing the characteristics of AVH, their possible sense and meaning, and how patient and relatives explain the voices with the Auditory Vocal Hallucination Rating Scale (AVHRS; Jenner & van de Willige, 2002) and the Positive and Useful Voices Inventory (PUVI; Jenner et al., 2008) are the aims of this step. AVHRS is a structured interview used to assess the number, content, frequency, duration, context, organization and location, degree of control, emotional experience, meaning and explanation, and perceived impact of the voice. The reliability coefficient for the AVHRS, based on 92 ratings by four raters, was 0.84 (weighted kappa), for lifetime assessment = .71. Internal consistency was 0.84 (Cronbach's alpha). The AVHRS sum score was substantially associated with the Exchange PANSS total thru $p < 0.005$) through: SCL'90 dimension scores. Pearson's correlation coefficients between AVHRS severity index and SCL'90 dimension scores were with $p < 0.01$: psychoticism $r = 0.66$, depression $r = 0.71$. phobic anxiety $r = 0.54$, somatisation $r = 0.52$, total score $r = 0.62$, and with $p < 0.05$ paranoid ideation $r = 0.40$. Significant ($p < 0.01$ and 0.05) correlations were calculated with PANSS dimensions total score, negative symptoms, emotional distress and hallucinations. According to patients, face validity was very good (Bartels-Velthuis et al., submitted). The majority of voice hearers hear positive voices too, and almost half of them have useful voices (Jenner et al., 2008). Assessment of positive and useful voices is mandatory because some patients' treatment non-compliance may result from their fear that these voices will disappear as an undesirable side effect of treatment. The PUVI is a 53-item self-report AVH inventory that assesses prevalence, course and characteristics of positive and useful AVH, and emotional attribution, and two subscales exploring reasons for attributions. These subscales have good internal consistency (Cronbach's alpha: positive voices subscale = 0.92, useful voices subscale = 0.89).

Step 6: To what extent are the voices functional for the patient in terms of secondary gain?

Step 7: Do reactions from relatives selectively reinforce the existence of voice hearing?

Step 8: Probing the habitual coping repertoire with the GLOS (Groningen Inventory Coping with Voices: Jenner & Geelhoed-Jenner, 1998).

Step 9: Estimating the balance of unwillingness and incapacity.

HIT treatment modules

Medication

The medication regime adopted for HIT is in accordance with the Dutch Psychiatric Association guidelines for schizophrenia spectrum disorders, delirium, and bipolar disorders; these guidelines closely mirror those of the American Psychiatric Association. Prescription of medication is related to diagnosis, i.e., anti-psychotics for patients with schizophrenia spectrum disorder and mood stabilizers for patients with affective disorders with anti-psychotic addition when indicated. Patients are strongly advised not to take benzodiazepines for more than 10 consecutive days. Motivation strategies are an essential part of successfully offering medication. Specific strategies are selected according to the patient's stage of readiness to change, his usual behaviour pattern and personality traits, and the presence and content of psychotic reasoning. In general medication advises will not be given before an extensive discussion about the cons of hearing voices and the mentioning of successes of HIT in other patients. It is only when patients have entered the action stage that medication directives are given. As outlined earlier, we may offer anti-psychotics as restoratives to patients who feel exhausted and as a chemical alternative of Faraday's cage in order to protect against insertion of thought.

Coping training

The results from studies of coping-behaviour interventions are equivocal, which may be partly due to lack of a uniform coping classification system. Another complication in measuring effectiveness of coping-behaviour interventions is that voice hearers apply similar coping-behaviour with different intentions and attributions. Patients of the Groningen Voices Outpatient Clinic have given positive reports about following our coping training. The training involves teaching patients and relatives a repertoire of skills for anxiety management, distracting attention from the voices, and focusing attention on the voices when necessary. Focusing may take the form of just asking questions, negotiating, scolding, or evoking. The voice hearer's habitual coping pattern is assessed by daily monitoring of the characteristics of the voices, contextual aspects, and coping-behaviour and its effects. This has been found to be fairly crucial for developing an appropriate set of coping strategies. Relatives are requested to monitor which signs of AVH they notice, contextual aspects of the AVH, their reaction toward the voice hearer, and their impact of the voices and voice hearer. As a next step, the voice hearer draws up an inventory of which GLOS coping behaviour items (50) he has applied (Jenner & Geelhoed-Jenner, 1998). The items have been subdivided into the following domains: vocal (speaking, singing), motor (walking, cycling), cognitive (reattribution, thought stop), physical (ear plug, auto-mutilation), social (withdrawal, contacting), physiological (sleeping, relaxation), spiritual (meditation, prayer), and chemical (alcohol, medication, eating). The items encompass actions as well as talking to and with the voices. The frequency of application, whether this has been done consequently, and degree of beneficial and/or ineffective effects, are monitored for each GLOS item reported. GLOS-items endorsed by the patient are then categorized as anxiety reducing, distractive, or focusing-on-voices, according the divisions made by Bentall *et al.* (1994).

Finally, the trial and error period starts with testing the effects of packages of coping behaviours for at least six consecutive weeks per coping package. A combination of vocal, cognitive, and another class of coping behaviour is advised. It is safe to start with simple and congruent items such as singing, distraction, and physical activities. Evoking voices, a hyper-congruent focusing action, may be advised when congruent strategies give insufficient relief. Hyper-congruent focusing actions have also been shown to be indicated in severe psychotic states. Evoking may induce strong emotions and anxiety, not the least in relatives. Hence, the first focusing session should always to be conducted in the therapist's office or the patient's home, preferably in the presence of relatives. In the end, the patient's preferences and monitoring data help in effectively tailoring the coping-package. A final coping-strategy is composed on the principle of keeping what works and replacing ineffective behaviours. After psycho-education on learning theory principles has been given, relatives are trained in selectively reinforcing the voice hearers' attempts at implementing these coping behaviours. The relatives' monitoring provides the therapist data for support, coaching, and selective reinforcement. *In vivo* trials of coping behaviour need time. Therefore, the interval between coping-oriented sessions is increased from 2–4 weeks to 4–6 weeks in length.

Cognitive Behaviour Therapy (CBT)

Learning theory postulates that expectations, assumptions, and misinterpretations of voice hearers are important in the continuation of AVH. Most voice hearers presume that their assumptions and negative expectations are becoming realized; they strikingly test this in an insufficient and inconsistent manner, or may even lack any testing. The aim of CBT, among other things, is changing the voice hearer's interpretation of voices as powerful and malevolent (Chadwick & Birchwood, 1994). Focuses of CBT are (a) attribution of external causes to internally generated ones and labelling them as just annoying symptoms, (b) contesting the power of the voices by examining their predictive power and disobedience to command hallucinations, and (c) removing the supposed meaning of voices and reducing them to annoying noise.

CBT interventions adopted for HIT focus on making sense of the AVH, on precipitating events, on emotional, cognitive, and behavioural actions, and on the reactions of relevant others. When voice hearing is related to past traumatic events, AVH may cause the recall of negative memories that may be selectively increased through operant conditioning. If this is the case, counter-conditioning may be indicated. For patients whose voices have become a link in a sequence of fear and avoidance, *in vivo* behaviour experiments that challenge incorrect assumptions may be indicated. Whatever the intervention, Socratic reasoning remains the preferred style of communication. It is probably the most effective approach for inserting doubt about beliefs and misinterpretations, and, in our experience, has been found to be effective in patients who are uncertain of being in the right.

Psycho-education

The current state of evidence about the effects of psycho-education is also equivocal. It certainly increases the knowledge of patients and relatives, and influences relatives' restrictive social attitudes, especially in families where patient and relatives have few contacts (Holmes *et al.*, 1999). Reduction of the level of expressed emotions has also been reported, which may help reduce the relapse rate. Psycho-education increases knowledge and some insight; however, Trauer and Sachs (2000) found patient insight to be positively correlated with depression and negatively correlated with personal functioning, suggesting that psycho-education might result in depression and reduced personal functioning in at least some patients. Other negative consequences have also been reported. Amador *et al.* (1996) found increased suicidal ideation after psycho-education.

HIT psycho-education focuses on voices and other symptoms, and on the feelings, thoughts, and reactions they induce. Much attention is given to origins of voices, with the aim of reaching a causality model that is acceptable for all. We lecture on and have extensive discussions about the vulnerability concept, selective perception, reality testing, and the impact of life events and stress. The mechanisms of operant conditioning and selective reinforcement are extensively elaborated on. Contrarily, psycho-education specifically about disorders is limited and given only on indication.

We attach much value to timing, i.e., connecting the psycho-education topics to the issue under discussion. For example, discussing possible origins of voices is part of the two-realities approach as described above. When the voice hearer speaks about the origins he has in mind, we give psycho-education about internal speech and lecture on the stress-vulnerability model. When incest is mentioned during biographical assessment, we lecture on research that has found an association between traumatic events and hallucinations. We bring the mechanisms of selective perception up at the time that voices are assessed with the AVHRS. However, lecturing on selective reinforcement and supportive reactions of relatives is postponed till the phase that patient and relatives monitor the effects of their coping behaviour.

Family treatment

HIT has integrated elements of the problem solving, psycho-education, social constructivism, and strategic and narrative family treatment schools. Fifteen years of working with voice hearers has taught us that each patient-system requires its own mixture. Joint sessions with the patient and relatives are favoured, although separate individual sessions are held when indicated. Additional sessions are held with important others such as additional therapists, the family doctor, and the patient's case-manager.

Relatives monitor the patient's behaviour, their own feelings, cognitions, and behaviour toward the patient, and patients in turn monitor their relatives' reactions. These data help both the patient and the relatives to gain insight and deliver material for changing behaviour and for selecting optimal ways of reducing the level of expressed emotions. We have noticed that self-monitoring data are more convincing than therapist's convictions that change is needed. Monitoring has been found to be an effective motivating intervention. Relatives are trained in positive labelling and in selectively reinforcing the patient's coping behaviour, self-care, and daily activities.

Rehabilitation

Social isolation, self-neglect, and insufficient self-care are quite common among voice hearers with schizophrenia. HIT applies the rehabilitation methods that are known for self-care, structuring daily activities, social contact, and so on. In keeping with the method, they are offered as coping behaviours that are weapons against the voices instead of rehabilitative interventions aimed at reducing handicaps. The reason behind this approach is to increase the attraction of the interventions, to enlarge feelings of mastery, and to minimize connections between handicaps and disorders. Our patients appreciate viewing rehabilitation as a strategy that shows the voices that it is they, the patients, who are in command. Most of them enjoy nagging their voices, e.g., some voice hearers who alarmingly neglected their self-care accepted to take showers daily in order to surprise and hence spite their voices.

The art of integration

It will be clear by this point that HIT cannot be anything but tailor-made. It requires the tailor to be experienced in various diagnostic systems, styles of communication, and methods of intervention. These systems, styles, and methods refer to different causal models of care and illness (Siegler & Osmond, 1966; Jenner & Tromp, 1998). For example, medical and psychodynamic models attribute no causal role to patients in becoming ill. In contrast, cognitive behaviour therapy being based on a moral model postulates that illness results from behaviour applied at the wrong time or in the wrong situations, which implies that disorders are causally related to the patient's behaviour. Both psychiatric and psychological treatments aim at recovery, which certainly is not the primary goal of rehabilitation.

The HIT interventions that emanate from these models cannot be simply added up; without proper adjustments, integration will not be possible. Adjustments must consider individual therapists, as well as the management of therapeutic processes and the collaboration within teams. For example, regular practice that labels voice hearing as psychotic signs and voices as hallucinations might interfere with positive labelling applied in HIT. Similarly, extending the interval between sessions, as has been described in the operant conditioning section, may come up against a wall of resistance because common practice is reducing the interval. Even when extending has been done carefully and on indication, resistance may be great in the beginning. Now to speak about labelling voices as a gift. Considering whether such a label has an ethical ground, we vote yes in specific circumstances. For example, the patient we described in the motivational section had been unsuccessfully treated with a congruent approach based upon the orthodox psychopathology view. Neither psycho-education nor convincing and confrontation had been effective, they had even resulted in a request for civil commitment. In such cases, labelling symptoms as gifts may be the only alternative for joining in, for allowing entrance in the patient's delusional system. As our case illustrates, this label opened the way for cooperation and helped preventing civil commitment. Initially, interventions, even monitoring, frequently lead to an exacerbation of voices. Problems may arise when one therapist labels the exacerbation as relapse and another therapist suggests the possibility that this may be the start of the voices' death struggle. The former therapist will decide to stop the monitoring, while the latter will suggest the contrary.

Few therapists have been sufficiently trained in all HIT modules. Hence, proper training in the various modules is required, as is sufficient supervision that includes supervision-on-the-spot sessions (with one-way screen) at regular intervals. It has been our experience that it takes trainees about 6 months to get adequately acquainted with timing and phasing and selecting the style of communication that best fits the situation.

Long-term effects of HIT

Studies suggest that HIT is effective for treating AVH in patients with chronic schizophrenia spectrum disorders, patients with dissociative disorders, and in patients with borderline personality disorders (Jenner *et al.*, 1998, 2004, 2006 ; Wiersma *et al.*, 2001, 2004), as well as for first episode psychotic adolescents (Jenner & van de Willige, 2001). In particular, positive effects of HIT have been reported on subjective burden, control of voices, quality of life, and social functioning. Additionally, these positive effects have been shown to last at least up to 9 months after stopping treatment in one study (Jenner *et al.*, 2004, 2006; Wiersma *et al.*, 2004) and up to 24 months in another (Jenner *et al.*, 1998; Wiersma *et al.*, 2001).

In a naturalistic retrospective study, Jenner *et al.* (1998) examined the effectiveness of HIT in 40 chronic patients with treatment refractory AVH and diagnoses of schizophrenia, dissociative disorder, or borderline personality disorder. Their mean duration of voice hearing was 8 years, and 6.5 years for treatment. Treatment results were (1) A dropout rate of less than 10%; (2) Over 80% of patients were satisfied with HIT (mean score 4.3 on a 5-point score); (3) AVH remitted completely in 20% of participants, in another 50% frequency, and duration of AVH decreased, while intensity was reduced in 30%; and (4) 40% experienced additional improvement in social functioning. At 4-years follow-up, i.e., 2 years post-treatment, 60% had maintained improvements, another 30% reported further improvements, and 8% had relapsed, but were functioning better than before treatment (Wiersma *et al.*, 2001).

In an open prospective study, Jenner and Van de Willige (2001) examined the effectiveness of HIT in a group of 14 adolescents with first-episode AVH. Results showed that nine patients became free of voices, while anxiety, thought process, control of voices, and social functioning improved substantially in 80% of participants.

In a Randomized Controlled Trial (RCT), Jenner *et al.* (2004) compared routine treatment with HIT in a group of 76 treatment refractory patients with chronic schizophrenia (mean duration of voice hearing was 10 years). After 9 months of treatment, improvements were significantly greater ($p < 0.05$) in the HIT group in the domains of subjective burden, psychopathology, quality of life, and social functioning. Improvements in subjective burden reached significance in distress and total burden. Both the frequency and duration and the control indices almost reached significance by a conservative 2-tailed *t*-test, but would have reached statistical significance with a justified 1-tailed test. Significant improvements in psychopathology of HIT patients were found on PANSS-scores for hallucinations, disorganization, depression, general psychopathology, and total score. Effect Sizes (ES) were calculated as Cohen's *d* (subtracting mean differential scores (controls–experimentals), divided by pooled within-group SD of controls post-treatment; Cohen, 1977), and Number-Needed-to-Treat (NNT) with Walter's (2000) computation (1/event rate controls—event rate experimentals). NNT is the number of patients that have to be treated with HIT during a certain period of time in order to prevent a symptom, compared to the control treatment. Effective treatments need NNT < 10 with lower NNT, indicating treatment to be more effective. ES and NNT of HIT varied from 0.71/2 (hallucinations) to 0.47/4 (depression), 0.63/4 to 5 (disorganization), and 0.65/3–4 (total PANSS-score). The NNT for the various social functions was 6 and 7 in favour of HIT subjects. While no improvements in social functions were found among controls, 51% of HIT-patients showed more than 20% improvement from their initial status at baseline (Wiersma *et al.*, 2004). The dropout rate was 9% after 9 months and 16% after 18 months. At 18-month follow-up, i.e., 9 months post-treatment, the HIT group had maintained improvements in all of the above-mentioned domains. Improvements remained significant in favour of HIT for the hallucination characteristics, amount and threat of negative content, distress, amount of interference with daily functioning, and the total burden of the voices. However, significant differences between the two groups had disappeared for frequency and duration of voices and for differences in the level of control over voices. Controls had improved during the follow-up period, probably due to the fact that controls were given some HIT modules (Jenner *et al.*, 2006).

In addition to high patient satisfaction with the program and low drop-out rates in all of the above mentioned studies, findings also suggest that the interventions were helpful in motivating formerly medication-refusing (non-compliant) patients to accept medication in later instances. Despite significant and clinically relevant improvements in social functioning, social handicaps remained, however, and warranted follow-up treatment. Hence, a Multi-Family HIT version has been developed (Jenner *et al.*, 2001). In a pilot study, patients showed significant improvements for control of voices, subjective burden, and social functioning, while relatives reported a significant reduction of burden and improvements in their interactions with patients (Jenner *et al.*, 2006).

Cost-effectiveness of HIT

Stant *et al.* (2003) examined the cost-effectiveness of HIT in the 76 treatment refractory patients with chronic schizophrenia who participated in the RCT. In this study, costs (in and outside of the health care sector) and outcomes were registered prospectively during a period of 18 months for patients. Mean costs for the whole study period per patient in the HIT group ($18,237) were lower than the mean costs per patient in the Treatment as Usual group ($21,436), although this difference did not reach statistical significance. Supplementary analyses (which took into account skewed distributions of cost variables) indicated that future cost differences will, in most cases, be in favour of the HIT program. In terms of symptoms (measured with the PANSS), results were in favour of the HIT group, although differences did not reach a statistically significant level.

Indications and contra-indications for HIT

HIT is indicated for AVH irrespective of their origin and duration. Severe disorganization and incoherence, inadequate mastery of language, and primary addiction are contra-indications for HIT. Subnormal intelligence and psycho-organic disorders are relative contra-indications, as there is clear evidence that some adjustments to the program can make HIT suitable for these patients (de Boer, 2006). Examples of adjustments are a strong focus on operant conditioning, mediation through relevant others, flash cards, and communication-related adjustments, especially in speech.

So far, clear disadvantages have not appeared. However, both patients and relatives report that homework and monitoring represents a heavy load for them. Relatives report that attending sessions takes upon their time. Also, not all employers react positively, some object to attending treatment session during working hours. Till now, our fear that deluded patients may include the therapist in their delusional system has not come true. The small number of trained therapists is a serious problem that limits access to HIT.

Discussion

Cost-effectiveness of HIT has been demonstrated, as has the feasibility of program application in community treatment settings. Direct comparison of HIT with other therapies is fairly difficult because most therapies (family treatment, and rehabilitation studies) are disorder and syndrome orientated. Only a few therapies other than HIT focus specifically on symptoms. Comparison is also problematic because few therapies have been examined in RCTs for their effectiveness in the reduction of AVH. CBT has been thoroughly studied in many RCTs, but mainly for efficacy, not effectiveness.

Although CBT is an essential module in HIT, family treatment, flexibility of program, psycho-education, and form of treatment differentiate CBT in the context of HIT from

Table 10.1 Comparison of the effectiveness of CBT and HIT in psychotic patients

Effectiveness	CBT	HIT
Sum of positive symptoms*	(effect size = .44)	(effect size = .64)
Duration of effect upon follow-up	+	+ (+)
Hallucinations **	E.S. = .44, ± (NNT[†] = 7)	E.S. = .71, ++ (NNT = 2)
Duration of effect upon follow-up	−	++
Depression	NNT = unknown	NNT = 4
Social functioning***	Some (NNT = equivocal results)	Good (NNT = 6-7)
Duration of effect upon follow-up	±	++
Drop out rate****	Medium-high up to 40%	Low 9–16%
Quality of Life***	+	++
Generalization of effect	Limited	Substantial

*Nice 2008. Jenner *et al*. 2004. Wykes *et al*. 2008.

**Valmaggia *et al*. Jenner *et al*. 2004, 2006b.

***Wiersma *et al*. 2004.

****Jenner *et al*. 1999, 2004, 2006b.

[†]NNT refers to the number needed to treat, that is, the number of patients that are needed to make the difference with the control treatment. NNTs smaller than 10 refer to a fairly effective treatment; thus, the smaller the number, the more effective the treatment.

CBT-only programs. When one compares HIT with CBT, dropout percentage, patient satisfaction (HIT population scores: 80% good/very good), effect-size, NNT, and generalization of effect to social functioning seem to favour HIT. Durability of effect on AVH is another advantage of HIT. Luteijn (2009) compared several treatment modalities of CBT and HIT (Table 10.1).

Implementation of HIT requires proper training of competent therapists. HIT shares this obstacle with other psycho-social interventions. It is regrettable that the politics of health care management have not been able, or perhaps willing, to solve this problem. To know that voices in psychiatric patients are persistent and represent a severe burden for them, their relatives, and the community, and to realize that these voices improve insufficiently with medication alone makes it difficult to accept that these patients have inadequate access to psycho-social treatments that may alleviate their burden and may improve their social functioning.

References

Amador, X.F., Friedman, J.H., Kasapis, C., Yale, S.A., Flaum, M., & Gorman, J.M. (1996). Suicidal behaviour in schizophrenia and its relationship in awareness of illness. *Am J Psychiatry*, **153**, 1185–88.

Bandler, R., & Grinder, J. (1979). *Frogs into princes*. Moab, Utah: Real People Press.

Barrett, T.R., & Etheridge, J.B. (1992). Verbal hallucinations in normals. I. People who hear voices. *Appl Cogn Psychol*, **6**, 379–87.

Bartels-Velthuis, A.A., van de Willige, G., Jenner, J.A., & Wiersma, D. (2010). Assessing AVH: the psychometric evaluation of the auditory vocal hallucination rating scale (AVHRS). *Br J Psychiatry Suppl*, **196**, 41–46.

Bentall, R.P., Haddock, G., & Slade, P.D. (1994). Cognitive behaviour therapy for persistent auditory hallucinations: from theory to therapy. *Behav Ther*, **25**, 51–66.

de Boer, R. (2006). HIT in minder begaafden, in J.A. Jenner (ed.) *Hallucinaties: kenmerken, verklaringen en behandeling* [HIT in the mentally handicapped. In *Hallucinations: characteristics, causality models and therapies*]. Assen: Van Gorcum and Comp, pp. 141–43.

Bustillo, J.R., Lauriello, J., Horan, W.P., & Keith, S.J. (2001). The psychosocial treatment of schizophrenia: an update. *Am J Psychiatry*, **158**, 163–75.

Chadwick, P., & Birchwood, M. (1994). The omnipotence of voices. A cognitive approach to auditory hallucinations. *Br J Psychiatry*, **164**, 190–201.

Chadwick, P., Birchwood, M., & Trower, P. (1996). *Cognitive therapy for delusions, voices and paranoia*. Chicester: John Wiley and Sons.

Cohen, J. (1977). *Statistical power analysis for the behavioural sciences*. New York: Academic Press.

Cohen, C.I., & Berk, L.A. (1985). Personal coping styles of schizophrenic outpatients. *Hosp Community Psychiatry*, **36**, 407–10.

David, A.S. (1999). Auditory hallucinations: phenomenology, neuropsychology and neuroimaging update. *Acta Psychiatr Scand*, **99** (suppl. 395): 77–9.

Holmes, E.P., Corrigan, P.W., Williams, P., Canar, J., & Kubiak, M.A. (1999). Changing attitudes about schizophrenia. *Schizophr Bull*, **25**, 447–56.

Jenner, J.A., & Geelhoed-Jenner, B.N.W.J. (1998). *GLOS: De Groningse Lijst Omgaan met Stemmenhoren* (The Groningen Coping with Voices Inventory). Internal Publication. Groningen: University Medical Centre Groningen, UCP.

Jenner, J.A., & Tromp, C. (1998). Modellen van zorg. In J.A. Jenner, E.L.M. Maeckelberghe, J.J. Rebel, J. Vermeij (eds.). *Wel bezorgd, geestelijke verzorging en gezondheidszorg*. Kampen: Kok.

Jenner, J.A., van de Willige, G., & Wiersma, D. (1998). Effectiveness of cognitive therapy with coping training for persistent auditory hallucinations: a retrospective study of attenders of a psychiatric out-patient department. *Acta Psychiatr Scand*, **98**, 384–9.

Jenner, J.A., Wiersma, D., van de Willige, G., & Nienhuis, F.J. (1999). Effectiveness of CBT for positive psychotic symptoms: discrepancies between British and Dutch programmes. *Schizophr Res*, **36**(1–3), 326–7.

Jenner, J.A., Mulder, H., & de Boer, R. (2001). MFT *cursiv-HIT: patiënten cursusboek and trainershandleiding*. (Multi Family HIT textbook for voice hearers and their relatives and trainer manual). Internal Publication. Groningen: University Medical Centre Groningen, UCP.

Jenner J.A., & van de Willige G. (2001). HIT, Hallucination focused Integrative Treatment as early intervention in psychotic adolescents with auditory hallucinations: A pilot study. *Acta Psychiatr Scand*, **103**, 148–52.

Jenner, J.A. (2002). An integrative treatment for patients with persistent auditory Hallucinations. *Psychiatr Serv*, **53**, 897–8.

Jenner, J.A., & van de Willige, G. (2002). *The auditory vocal hallucination rating scale.* Internal Publication. Groningen: University Medical Centre Groningen, UCP.

Jenner, J.A., Nienhuis, F.J., Wiersma, D., & van de Willige, G. (2004). Hallucination-focused integrative treatment improves burden, control, and symptoms in schizophrenia patients with drug-resistant hallucinations. *Schizophr Bull*, **30**, 127–39.

Jenner, J.A., van de Willige, G., & Wiersma, D. (2006a). Multi-family treatment for patients with persistent auditory hallucinations and their relatives: A pilot study. *Acta Psychiatr Scand*, **113**, 154–8.

Jenner, J.A., Nienhuis, F.J., van de Willige, G., & Wiersma, D. (2006b). 'Hitting' voices of schizophrenia patients may lastingly reduce persistent auditory hallucinations and their burden: 18-month outcome of a randomized controlled trial. *Can J Psychiatry*, **51**, 169–77.

Jenner, J.A., Rutten, S., Beuckens, J., Boonstra, N., & Sytema, S. (2008). Positive and useful vocal hallucinations: prevalence, characteristics, attributions, and implications for treatment. *Acta Psychiatr Scand*, **118**, 238–45.

Johnstone, E.C., Owens, D.G., & Leary, J. (1991). Disabilities and circumstances of schizophrenic patients: a follow-up study. Comparison of the 1975–85 cohort with the 1970–75 cohort. *Br J Psychiatry Suppl*, **13**, 34–6.

Knowles, R.D. (1983). Building rapport through neurolinguistic programming. *Am J Nurs*, **82**, 1011–4.

Landmark, J., Merskey, H., Cernovsky, Z.Z., & Helmes, E. (1990). The positive triad of schizophrenic symptoms: its statistical properties and its relationship to 13 traditional diagnostic systems. *Br J Psychiatry*, **156**, 388–94.

Luteijn, B. (2009). *Psychosocial interventions in schizophrenia patients: a special role for HIT* (in Dutch). Presentation Symposium: Caring for crumpled souls.

Miller, W.R., & Rollnick, S. (1991). *Motivational interviewing: Preparing people to change addictive behaviour.* New York: Guilford Press.

NICE. (2008). *Core interventions in the treatment and management of schizophrenia adults in primary and secondary care.* (www.nice.org.uk/guidance/index.jsp?action).

Prochaska, J.O., & DiClemente, C.C. (1982). Transtheoretical therapy: towards a more integrative model of change. *Psychotherapy: Theory, Research and Practice*, **19**, 276–88.

Rossler, W., Riecher-Rossler, A., Angst, J., *et al.* (2007). Psychotic experiences in the general population: a twenty-year prospective community study. *Schizophr Res*, **92**, 1–14.

Sidgewick, H., Johnson, A., Myers, F.W.H., *et al.* (1984). Report on the census of hallucinations. *Proceedings of the Society for psychological Research*, **26**, 259–393.

Siegler, M., & Osmond, H. (1966). Models of madness. *Br J Psychiatry*, **112**, 1193–1203.

Stant, A.D., TenVergert, E.M., Groen, H., *et al.* (2003). Cost-effectiveness of the HIT programme in patients with schizophrenia and persistent auditory hallucinations. *Acta Psychiatr Scand*, **107**, 361–8.

Stephane, M., Barton, S., & Boutros, N.N. (2001). Auditory verbal hallucinations and dysfunction of the neural substrates of speech. *Schizophr Res*, **50**, 61–78.

Tien, A.Y. (1991). Distributions of hallucination in the population. *Soc Psychiatry Psychiatr Epidemiol*, **26**, 287–92.

Trauer, T., & Sacks, T. (2000). The relationship between insight and medication adherence in severely mentally ill clients treated in the community. *Acta Psychiatr Scand*, **102**, 211–6.

van Os, J., Hanssen, M., Bijl, R.V., & Ravelli, A. (2000). Strauss (1969) revisited: a psychosis continuum in the general population? *Schizophr Res*, **45**, 11–20.

Walter, S.D. (2000). Choice of effect measures for epidemiological data. *J Clin Epidemiol*, **53**, 931–9.

Weiss, A.P., & Heckers, S. (1999) Neuroimaging of hallucinations: a review of the literature. *Psychiatry Res*, **92**, 61–74.

Wiersma, D., Jenner, J.A., van de Willige, G., Spakman, M., & Nienhuis, F.J. (2001). Cognitive behaviour therapy with coping training for persistent auditory hallucinations in schizophrenia: a naturalistic follow-up study of the durability of effects. *Acta Psychiatr Scand*, **103**, 393–9.

Wiersma, D., Jenner, J.A., Nienhuis, F.J., & van de Willige, G. (2004). Hallucinations-focused integrative treatment improves quality of life in schizophrenia patients. *Acta Psychiatr Scand*, **109**, 194–201.

Wykes, T., Steel, C., Tarrier, N., *et al.* (2008). Conitive behavior therapy for schizophrenia: clinical models and methodological rigor. *Schizophr Bull*, **34**, 523-37.

Yee, L., Korner, A.J., McSwiggan, S., Meares, R.A., & Stevenson, J. (2005) Persistent hallucinosis in borderline personality disorder. *Compr Psychiatry*, **46**, 147–54.

Young, H.F., Bentall, R.P., Slade, P.D., & Dewey, M.E. (1987). The role of brief instructions and suggestibility in the elicitation of auditory and visual hallucinations in normal and psychiatric subjects. *J Nerv Ment Dis*, **175**, 41–8.

Chapter 11

'Normalizing' the voice hearing experience

The continuum between auditory hallucinations and ordinary mental life

Michael Garrett

Unlike mental states such as dreams, feelings of anxiety, or slips of the tongue, which are familiar to all, most people find few analogies between psychotic symptoms such as auditory hallucinations and their own mental life. Clinicians and family members of the mentally ill may find it difficult to empathize with these experiences. In fact, Karl Jaspers, one of the most influential phenomenologists in psychiatry in the last century, believed that the mental states that define psychosis are so alien to ordinary experience as to defy empathic understanding (Jaspers, 1972). Contrary to this view, recent decades have seen mounting evidence that a continuum exists between psychosis and ordinary mental life (Johns & van Os, 2001). The Cognitive Behavioral Therapy (CBT; see Smith *et al.*, and Johns & Wykes, both this volume) of psychosis requires the therapist to appreciate this continuum.

In keeping with the continuum model, Kingdon and Turkington introduced the concept of 'normalizing' as a specific clinical technique in CBT of psychosis (Kingdon *et al.*, 1994, Kingdon & Turkington, 2005). They identified a number of analogies to psychosis that occur in everyday life, such as hypnogogic and hypnopompic hallucinations, and used these analogies to 'normalize' the seemingly alien hallucinations of psychotic patients in treatment sessions. 'Normalizing' psychotic experiences dramatically changes the doctor–patient relationship. The traditional categorical disease model of schizophrenia accentuates the differences between the patient and 'normals', including the doctor. The doctor is an outside expert on the patient's disease. 'Normalizing' within the continuum model emphasizes the similarities between psychotic symptoms and everyday experience, and therefore the similarities between doctor and patient. This shifts the power relationship toward a more equal footing. The doctor is less the all-knowing expert, more a collaborator who can join in an evidence-based exploration of the patient's distressing experiences. The CBT therapist conveys a willingness to see the patient's experiences as connected to the mental life of people in general, and even to himself. Instead of getting the message 'You have a brain disease that sets you apart from the human community', the patient receives the message 'The voice hearing experience is a special variant of a biological and psychological process that occurs to varying degrees in many people, including me, your therapist. I hope to learn more about your voice hearing experiences, particularly any aspects of the experience you find distressing'.

The continuum between psychosis and ordinary mental life

Strauss proposed the idea that beliefs lie along a continuum from odd and idiosyncratic convictions in normals to floridly pathological delusions in psychosis (Strauss, 1969).

> 'This view stresses the notion that schizophrenia and the symptoms that characterize it are understandable exaggerations of normal function and not exotic symptoms superimposed on the personality. When the distortion and exaggeration reach a certain level of eccentricity or begin to impair social function they are called symptoms'. (P. 585.)

Community samples lend support to the continuum model. For example, a random community sample of 7076 men and women aged 18–64 years was studied with the Composite International Diagnostic Interview (Van Os *et al.*, 2000). Of the 7076 individuals in the study, 1237 (17.5%) scored positive on at least one psychosis item. The authors conclude, 'the psychosis phenotype as it exists in nature may be nearly 50 times (17.5% divided by the schizophrenia prevalence of 0.4%) more prevalent than the more narrow medical concept'. (p. 16.) Individuals not otherwise considered mentally ill report delusions and aberrant perceptual experiences. These experiences appear to be one extreme of a complex, multidimensional continuum, which at times overlaps the ordinary mind, rather than a categorically distinct disease state that is discontinuous with ordinary mental processes (Johns & van Os, 2001). While there is continuity between ordinary mental life and psychosis, there are also important differences that distinguish the 'hallucinations of everyday life' from hallucinations in a psychotic illness. The 'voices' of chronic psychosis tend to be more frequent, more persistently critical, distressing, and disruptive of ordinary social functioning. They are also very often entwined with delusional beliefs, which in turn have an adverse impact on the patient's life.

Continuum of beliefs and cognitive processes

Beliefs held by the general public lie along a continuum with psychosis. For example, a 1989 Gallup poll of 60,000 British adults revealed that a substantial percentage of the population holds a variety of parapsychological and magical beliefs (Cox & Cowling, 1989). Fifty percent of this poll believed in thought transference, a mental process reminiscent of 'thought insertion', a Schneiderian first-rank symptom of schizophrenia (Schneider, 1959). In a comparison of a group of normal controls with a group at high risk for psychosis, psychotic and psychosis-prone individuals alike entertained a continuum of aberrant beliefs (Chapman & Chapman, 1988). In many cases, core delusional beliefs could be identified in the pre-morbid concerns of individuals who later became psychotic, suggesting continuity between pre-psychotic and psychotic mental life.

A variety of cognitive biases have been found to characterize psychosis, including attributional biases, attentional biases, a tendency to jump to conclusions, dichotomous thinking, and belief inflexibility (Bentall *et al.*, 2001, Blackwood *et al.*, 2001, Garety *et al.*, 2001, 2005, 2007, Van Der Gaag, 2006). In keeping with a continuum, these processes occur in non-psychotic individuals as well, though to a lesser degree, i.e., psychosis entails an exaggeration of the biases of ordinary mental life. Cognitive research has yet to study a cognitive process that occurs in psychosis alone with no analogue in ordinary thinking.

Most people tend to regard psychotic individuals as irrational and themselves as logical. However, there is considerable evidence that delusional subjects can think logically and that 'normal' people think irrationally (Sutherland, 1994). Delusional individuals are as capable of syllogistic reasoning as normal controls (Kemp *et al.*, 1997). Maher hypothesized that delusions arise when individuals employ logical reasoning to explain anomalous experiences, such as 'voices' (Maher, 1988). Far from being fully rational, ordinary mental life is replete with illogical thinking, at times exhibiting the same cognitive biases that maintain delusions. For example, delusions are typically regarded as fixed beliefs that remain certain in the face of evidence to the contrary. Certainty of belief was studied in a group of normal subjects, who were asked a question, then asked to rate the probability of their answer being correct. Beliefs rated at a 1,000,000:1 confidence level were correct only 90% of the time (Fischhoff *et al.*, 1977). Normal people are irrationally certain of their beliefs, as are delusional patients. Lord (1979) studied the impact of new information on beliefs by examining beliefs about capital punishment as a deterrent to murder in a non-clinical population. In the face of additional information, some of which contradicted their initial beliefs, 23% felt even *more* strongly convinced of the truth of their initial beliefs after reviewing data to the contrary. Just like deluded patients, normal people tend to ignore data that is not in keeping with their prior beliefs.

Continuum of perceptions

Just as beliefs and cognitive processes occur along a continuum, perceptual experiences do as well. Hallucinations occur in a wide variety of disease states including toxic delirium, epilepsy, stroke, brain tumor, syphilis, nutritional deficiency, and hearing loss (Assad, 1990), which suggests that hallucinations most likely arise from a capacity latent in the normal brain, widely distributed throughout the general population. This latent capacity is brought to the fore by a variety of disease processes resulting in hallucinations.

Auditory hallucinations also occur in a significant number of individuals who do not meet criteria for schizophrenia or any Axis I psychotic disorder (Posey, 1986, Romme & Escher, 1989). Posey & Losch studied 375 'normal' college students not known to be mentally ill (Posey & Losch, 1983, Posey, 1986). They administered a questionnaire with 14 types of auditory hallucinations. For example, one question read, 'Almost every morning while I do my housework, I have a pleasant conversation with my dead grandmother. I talk to her, and quite regularly hear her voice actually aloud…Anything similar happen to you?' Five percent of students responded that they had had experiences of a similar sort. This study has been replicated, with very similar findings (Barrett & Etheridge, 1992). A number of studies over the last century substantiate the existence of a continuum of perceptual experiences, including auditory hallucinations, in the general population (West, 1948, McKellar, 1968, Bentall & Slade, 1985, Young *et al.*, 1986, Tien, 1991, Sidgewick *et al.*, 1894, Johns *et al.*, 2002). Healthy volunteers hallucinate and manifest circumscribed delusions in sensory deprivation experiments. It is not uncommon for a grieving widow not otherwise considered mentally ill to hallucinate the voice of her deceased spouse (Grimby, 1988). Individuals in the community who experience auditory verbal hallucinations in the absence of a diagnosable Axis I psychotic disorder appear to have a higher incidence of schizotypal personality disorder and a tendency toward delusional thinking, suggesting that these individuals, while not manifestly psychotic, may share a general vulnerability to schizophrenia (Sommer *et al.*, 2008). Hallucinations also occur in a wide variety of clinical conditions, post-traumatic states, and drug-induced intoxications (Assad, 1990). The above studies indicate that 'voices' occur in a variety of settings in individuals not otherwise considered to be mentally ill.

Hallucinations of everyday life

Most people can find cognitive analogies to the voice hearing experience in the brief 'hallucinations of everyday life'. Many people experience brief sequences of hallucinated images and/or voices when falling asleep (hypnogogic hallucinations) or when awakening (hypnopompic hallucinations). Sounds with a high alert significance are particularly prone to be hallucinated, as when a person 'hears' someone calling his name when no one is speaking, an event reported by 64% of a non-clinical sample (Barrett & Etheridge, 1992). Parents of young children may 'hallucinate' the cry of their baby, only to find the infant sleeping soundly when they arrive at the crib. One may be uncertain whether a phone rang, or one imagined it (hallucinated it), an event which serves as the basis of an experiential exercise to be described below.

Inner speech and the 'dialogic' structure of the mind

Moving from surveys of community samples to an introspective examination of hallucinations of everyday life, one soon encounters the phenomenon of 'inner speech'. Inner speech might be defined as the subjective experience of 'hearing' ones thoughts in mind without an external expression of these thoughts by the vocal musculature in articulated speech. It is a normal mental capacity in which one part of the mind appears to 'speak' while another part of the mind 'listens'. Anyone can locate this capacity in himself by silently counting from one to ten while observing the experience. For most people, this counting in the mind is akin to, but not identical with, hearing numbers spoken aloud. It is closely related to the auditory sensory mode, but has a somewhat flattened, two-dimensional quality compared with external speech. People use inner speech for a variety of mundane functions, like dialing an unfamiliar phone number. As the dialer repeats the number to himself in inner speech, the memory trace of this auditory-like input enters a short-term memory buffer, which then rapidly decays (Baddeley & Logie, 1992). The number slips from consciousness unless the dialer repeats the 'speaker–listener' loop by saying the numbers over again until the dialing task is completed. A similar use of inner speech occurs when transferring information to a form, as when filling in an unfamiliar address, or entering a bank deposit. Inner speech can assume a dialogic quality and may be employed to direct an individual's actions, as when a runner nearing the finish line says to himself, 'Just fifty yards more!' A person on a diet tempted by cheese cake may say to himself, 'Discipline. Discipline'. Or we may talk to ourselves and issue self-evaluations, as in 'You idiot!' or 'Not bad, if I say so myself'. A substantial literature suggests that the normal faculty of inner speech is linked in some way to auditory hallucinations (Gould, 1948, 1949, 1950, Bick & Kinsbourne, 1987; Leudar *et al.*, 1997). Jamming the inner speech mechanism with distracting cognitive tasks like counting can temporarily silence voices, which suggests that 'voices' and inner speech may share an overlapping neurophysiologic mechanism.

The voice hearing experience is an extraordinary example of an ordinary human capacity. Normal and naturally occurring inner speech provides a way for clinicians to 'normalize' the voice hearing experience, for themselves and for patients in treatment sessions. In effect, we all have the capacity to talk to ourselves. How does the ordinary mind come to be structured as a speaker–listener dyad? Vygotsky answers that all higher order internal cognitive functions like inner speech develop from an earlier external, interpersonal, and social form of the same process (Wertsch, 1985; Vygotsky, 1987). In his theory, external speech between parent and child evolves into private speech, where the child talks out loud to himself, which next becomes internalized as thought in expanded inner speech, which eventually edits down to condensed inner speech. Aspects of the mind are structured like a dialogue because inner speech and related thought arise from an internalization of the child's social interaction with parents. The speaker–listener dyad in the ordinary mind is the legacy of the speaker–listener dyad between parent and child.

Psychoanalysis and object relations theory provide another view of the dyadic structure of the ordinary mind. In the process of social interaction over the course of development, people construct internal mental representations of themselves and others. Object relations theory examines the origin of these mental representations and the relationships between them (Klein, 1935, 1946, Greenberg & Mitchell, 1983, Kernberg, 2005). A psychological 'object' is not a physical thing, but rather a mental representation of a thing, a real or imagined person, an entity, or even an abstraction, which is invested with psychological properties and imagined or experienced as having a discrete bounded presence in the mind. All psychological objects, even when they correspond to actual people, are 'internal objects', in that they exist in the internal representational world of the psyche rather than physical reality. From an object relations perspective, 'voices' are a particular type of internal object.

The familiar voice of conscience (the 'superego') is an internal object. The punitive superego may 'say' to the self, 'It is all your fault!' The part of the mind that 'speaks' the internal criticism is not the same aspect of the mind that 'hears' it and feels its sting. They are separate internal objects. The self and the superego are linked in an internal object relationship that regulates self-esteem. Fifty percent of psychotic patients who experienced hallucinations reported that their 'voices' had replaced their 'voice of conscience'

(Nayani & David, 1996). This observation provides a clue as to the psychological origin of critical 'voices'. From a psychoanalytic perspective, the familiar critical 'voices' of psychosis are internal objects derived from a punitive superego, which are experienced as auditory perceptions. Viewing critical 'voices' in this way 'normalizes' the voice hearing experience by linking it to the moral dialogue between internal objects, which occurs routinely in most people.

For example, a man with a history of paranoid schizophrenia reported he first heard a 'voice' say 'Don't!' the first time he masturbated as an adolescent. He heard a second 'voice' say, 'Your brother does it. No big deal'. At first he did not know where the 'voices' came from, or their identity, but over time he came to believe that he was hearing the voice of God laying down rules about what he could and could not do, and the voice of Satan, tempting him to defy God. From a psychoanalytic point of view, the first 'voice' the patient heard was a perceptual experience of his critical superego, which appeared to be originating outside the self. The second voice is also a part of the patient's mind, the part that wants to engage in sexual activity.

Experiential exercises to 'normalize' psychosis

Few techniques exist aimed specifically at increasing the clinician's ability to 'normalize' psychosis by finding analogies to psychotic experiences in his own mental life. In recent years, mental health consumers have taken matters into their own hands to provide better training for mental health professionals. Deegan, a psychologist and 'voice hearer', developed a training exercise to acquaint clinicians with the experience of 'hearing voices' (Deegan, 1996). In this exercise, students wear ear phones and listen to an audiotape, which simulates auditory hallucinations, while at the same time trying to perform a number of routine tasks. It is quickly apparent how difficult it would be to negotiate even the most basic social situations while suffering the constant intrusion of 'voices'. Autobiographical accounts by patients help the clinician to view the world through the patient's eyes (Sommer & Osmond, 1983, Schreber, 1988, Schiller & Bennett, 1995). More recently, multiple internet sites and online groups have emerged for voice hearers, including the Voice Hearing Network in the UK at hearing-voices.org,uk; rethink.org; and health.groups.yahoo.com/group/voice-hearers, to mention a few.

Garrett *et al.*, developed a series of five experiential teaching exercises designed for groups of 10–30 people, which illustrate transient disruptions of mental function, which serve as analogies to psychotic experiences (Garrett *et al.*, 2006). Just as the experience of not being able to remember something on the 'tip-of-the-tongue' can provide clues about how memories are processed (Brown, 1991), other transient disturbances of ordinary mental life may provide clues to the cognitive processes underlying psychosis. The exercises are intended to help clinicians locate in their own minds the latent cognitive and perceptual fault lines along which the ordinary mind fractures in mental illness. For example, many people have 'heard' a phone ring once, or at a distance, and wondered if the ring was real or they imagined it. This 'hallucination of everyday life' is the basis of the exercise described below, *The Phone Rings Once*. The exercise compares the meta-cognitive processes that occur in ordinary people when they are confronted with the single ring (a slightly anomalous perception of uncertain origin), with the meta-cognitive processes in people who hear 'voices'. In both cases, the question, 'Did the experience arise from inside me or from the outside world?' is the central issue.

Garety *et al.*, propose a four-step cognitive model of psychosis in which a triggering event in a predisposed person leads to an anomalous experience, such as hearing a 'voice' (Fig. 11.1) (Garety *et al.*, 2001). The person then makes a meta-cognitive judgment as to whether the experience is believed to originate within the mind or outside the self. In this model, it is not the anomalous experience *per se*, but the belief that the experience originates in the outside world that constitutes the psychosis. In the authors' words, 'The externalizing appraisal is thus a defining decision. Psychosis is recognized as occurring when the individual appraises experiences as externally caused and personally significant'.

The exercises to be described have been used by the author for over ten years as part of the training curriculum for groups of medical students on assignment to psychiatry as part of their general medical school education, and for psychiatric residents engaged in a four-year program of postgraduate training in psychiatry. The purpose of the exercises is to help foster empathy in trainees for psychotic patients who manifest seemingly incomprehensible hallucinations and delusions. In the exercise *The Phone Rings Once*, a person hears a phone ring once while in the shower, but is uncertain whether the phone actually rang. In Garety's model, the masking noise of the shower and the expectation of the call is the predisposing circumstance, the anomalous experience is the single ring of the phone, and the meta-cognitive question is 'Did the phone ring or did I hallucinate it?'

The phone rings once exercise

The group is asked to imagine, [1] 'You have just come back from jogging. You are planning to meet a friend for dinner but do not know the address of the restaurant. Your friend said she would call and tell you the address. You jump into the shower, leaving the door to the bathroom open slightly in case the phone rings. The rush of the water masks outside noise to a degree. You hear the phone ring once. You turn off the shower and listen intently. It does not ring again. What are you thinking now?' The group leader then elicits comments from the group. The group immediately understands that the question is whether they imagined the phone ringing or actually heard it. Perception ordinarily

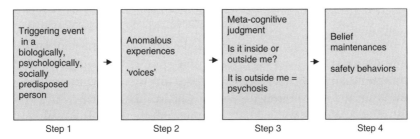

Fig. 11.1 Cognitive model of psychosis.

defines reality (Johnson *et al.*, 1981, 1993, Johnson, 1988). Under normal conditions rich, redundant sensory inputs generate an unambiguous picture of the world. In the shower, the 'white noise' of the water degrades the auditory signal-to-noise ratio. Anticipation of the call further sets the stage to possibly hallucinate the ringing of the phone. The ringing of the phone has an emotional valence. People are more likely to hallucinate sensory elements of emotional significance and survival value than sensory inputs that are indifferent to the organism. In evolution, better a few false positive alerts than a single false negative, e.g., better to be mistaken that you heard a lion three times than miss the real lion once. Just as 'voices' have the subjective quality of perception (Garrett & Silva, 2003), the single ring has the quality of a perception. The person having the anomalous experience cannot determine its origin based on the subjective quality of the experience alone. Meta-cognitive processes, prior beliefs, and judgment must be brought to bear.

Whether in psychosis or ordinary life, people interpret anomalous perceptions in light of their prior beliefs about the world. Divergent attitudes toward the single ring immediately emerge in the group reflecting the individual psychology of each group member. Some in the group say they would conclude they imagined the ring because the shower noise made it difficult to hear and they were expecting a call. They have a meta-cognitive model of their own mind, which includes the possibility of hallucinations in certain set conditions. Others say they would think they imagined the ring because a real caller would have allowed the phone to ring more than once. Others say they would be inclined to believe the ring had been real. Though by no means inevitable in any explanation, many report a belief that immediately imagines a caller on the other end of the single ring. This personifies the situation and makes it interpersonal. Perhaps someone called the number by mistake and hung up after one ring when he realized his error. Perhaps the expected friend was calling, and got interrupted, in which case she will call back.

One clinician reported she heard the phone ring when in the shower so frequently she had come to expect it. She automatically considered any ring in the shower to be a hallucination. Because this experience was predictable, familiar, brief, and contained, it caused no distress. She had over time constructed a meta-cognitive model of her own mind that included this particular type of hallucination. One clinician said he was so confident in his hearing he would have no doubt about the reality of the ring, and certainly would have felt frustrated to have missed the call. Unlike the clinician above, this member of the group claimed to have absolute confidence in the fidelity of his perceptual system, a very different meta-cognitive assessment of his own mind. Different people have different meta-cognitive models of their own minds, models that accept varying degrees of anomalous perceptual experiences and quirky ideas, with varying degrees of confidence in their perceptions, memories, and other cognitive functions. One of the reasons people who hear 'voices' fail to identify the 'voice' as a product of their own mind is that Western culture does not prepare its citizens with a meta-cognitive model of mind that normalizes the voice hearing experience. Children learn about dreams from their parents, from books, and in school, and incorporate the dream state into their meta-cognitive model of their mind. There is no comparable recognition of the dialogic structure of the mind in secondary education. When people hear 'voices', they encounter a new and powerful phenomenon about which their culture has little to say, except to apply the stigmatizing label of mental illness. Cognitive-Behavioural Therapy for psychosis fills in this gap.

Back to the exercise. Occasionally, someone speculates the single ring might indicate a malfunction of the phone. In effect, the phone might be 'ill'. Whether judged to be of internal or external origin, no one at this point is particularly concerned about the ambiguity of the experience because it is infrequent, short lived, and not of pressing personal relevance. From the beginning of the exercise, students begin to invest in divergent 'realities' despite the fact they have no objective evidence in favour of one view or another. The percept-like experience itself remains entirely silent as to its origin. Like beliefs about the single ring, patients who hear 'voices' build alternate realities based upon percept-like experiences that cannot be traced to their internal origin.

The exercise continues. [2] 'You step back into the shower, waiting briefly before you turn the water on. All is quiet. You proceed with your shower, and minutes later, the same thing happens. You again hear the phone ring once. What are you thinking now?' A few in the group would at this point become more interested in the ring because it has happened twice in rapid succession, but most remain unconcerned, and most continue to locate the problem outside themselves. Some students say they would be uncertain whether they heard the ring or hallucinated it, but they would be content to remain uncertain. They hold a meta-cognitive belief in the basic integrity of their own minds, even if there are occasional illusory stretches. An occasional student suggests that there may be no anomalous experience at all, that the phone rang several times as would be expected, and only the last ring was heard. In this version of events, there is nothing amiss. For some, the rapid repetition of the single ring phone calls suggests there is a human intention behind it. They say they might now conclude their friend was trying to call, but there is something wrong with the phone. Some students would submit the question about whether the ring was real or imagined to the authority of an inanimate machine. If there was no record of a call on their answering machine or caller identification, then they would conclude they imagined the ring. These students have a prior belief about the world that their own minds occasionally play tricks, but that answering machines generally do not. Some suggest they would keep the phone next to them to reduce any uncertainty about future rings.

As with the meta-cognitive deliberations of the group about the ring, patients think through their experience of their 'voices'. As in the exercise, the persistence of the 'voice' contributes to its salience. Just as trainees may conclude there must be a person making the repeated phone calls, the 'voice' is experienced as a person engaged in a dialogue with the voice hearer. Like the trainees who suggest strategies to clarify the origin of the ring, patients at times attempt to clarify the origin of the 'voice'. For example, one man noted that his 'voices' seemed particularly intense in the neighborhood where his parents lived. He conducted an experiment in which he approached their apartment on foot, noting the intensity of the 'voices' as he neared their apartment. The 'voices' got louder. He concluded the 'voices' were physically located nearby. Even when the voice hearer employs a tried and true strategy to locate the origin of a sound, by approaching to see if it gets louder, delusional conclusions may prevail. The usual strategies people use to clarify the origin of sounds are of little avail to the voice hearer because the 'voice' does not conform to the patient's prior beliefs about the properties of sound.

The exercise continues. [3] 'You finish your shower and begin getting dressed. Once more, you hear a single ring. Where are you now?' At this point, it is becoming harder to ignore the experience. Depending on one's prior meta-cognitive beliefs about one's own mind, there is more or less tolerance to the mind playing tricks before the situation elicits concern. However, most students say at this point they would be paying attention to the ring and trying to figure out what was going on. The persistence of the ring outside the shower eliminates the shower water white noise theory. Like psychotic patients, most students would continue to believe the problem lies outside their own minds, though an occasional student makes a joke at this point, 'I would start thinking about calling my shrink!' Theories that locate the problem outside the mind fall into two groups, those involving an unseen caller, and those favoring a broken machine explanation. Maybe someone keeps dialing the wrong number by mistake and hanging up. A few students may suggest the possibility of a persistent telemarketer, or even a prank caller. An unfriendly agent may be behind the calls, a watered down version of the full-blown persecutor who will appear later, in the minds of some. The persistent repetition of events is taken to suggest that some intention is directed toward the self. The phone is ordinarily used to communicate, just as the voice hearer believes the 'voices' are attempting to communicate. With repetition, the anomalous experience begins to feel increasingly self-referential and interpersonal, as happens with anomalous experiences judged to have significance for the self in delusion formation. Other students stick to their belief that the problem lies in the phone, not in people behind the phone. The phone is broken, or there is something wrong with the phone lines.

The exercise continues. [4] 'Your friend calls shortly there after to give you the address of the restaurant. You write it down, then pause for a moment, and ask 'Did you just call me?' Your friend says no. Do you believe her answer?' If someone is behind the calls, we would prefer to think it is a friend playing a trick than an unknown person intending some harm. Better a pretend tormentor than a real one. Most students say they would take the friend at her word, but a few admit they would have a moment of doubt, depending on the friend's past history as a joker. Prior beliefs about the world come into play. In most cases, when the friend in the exercise says she hasn't been calling, this would be accepted as true. One can trust a friend to discriminate between what is and is not real. Not so with psychotic patients. Patients often feel betrayed by their families when family members do not corroborate what the patient believes to be self-evidently true. For example, a man 'saw' several secret agents following him. He asked his girlfriend if she too had noticed these men, and when she said no, he concluded that the secret agents had 'turned her' and she had joined the plot against him. The patient felt betrayed by those he most loved and needed. Here the group leader can point out to trainees the enormous leap of faith demanded of psychotic individuals when the therapist asks the patient to surrender their reliance on their own perceptual system to determine what is real in favour of the therapist's version of reality. At this point, the range of beliefs and emotional attitudes toward the anomalous single ring are apparent in the group.

The exercise continues. [5] 'The next day the same thing happens, this time unrelated to the shower. You hear the phone ring once. You call the phone company. They investigate, but they find nothing wrong with the phone'. The group leader asks if they would believe the report of the phone company. Most people would because of prior beliefs about the phone company not being involved in conspiracies, although a moment's reflection opens up a different possibility, often entertained in psychosis, that the phone is bugged and that someone at the phone company is involved. The exercise continues. 'As the week goes on, you hear a single ring once every several hours when you are at home. You are trying to figure out what is going on. It occurs to you that you hear the ring most often when you are standing near your kitchen window. What are you thinking now?'

As with persistent 'voices', at this point, it is extremely difficult to ignore the repeated single ring. The persistent singleness of the ring is odd, which contributes a vague salience to the experience. Just as a succession of anomalous percepts in psychosis requires an explanation, so do the successive single rings. As is the case with ideas of reference, connections begin to form between events. The kitchen window seems a meaningful contingency. Many students say at this point they would believe someone who could see into their apartment through the kitchen window was playing a malicious trick. They would be frightened and angry. The persecutor who inhabits paranoid delusions has arrived in the room. Interestingly, some students would interpret the contingency of the window very differently. Maybe there is a phone in a neighboring apartment that is most easily heard from their kitchen window, and all the concern about the phone has been much ado about nothing. The majority of students inevitably places the problem outside themselves, in a prankster, broken phone, or neighbor's phone, rather than lose faith in the reliability of their perceptual system. Like people who hear 'voices', most students hold fast to their belief that the ring is a real perception. The exercise posits exactly the same percept-like experience in each group member. As with psychotic patients, the amount of distress each group member feels varies considerably depending upon each person's beliefs about the origin and meaning of the perception.

Students readily see the similarity between these ideas and paranoid delusions. Like the students in the class, psychotic patients faced with repeated anomalous percepts of ambiguous origin typically conclude that the world has changed rather than believe their perceptual system cannot be trusted to define reality. Like the rare psychotic patient with insight, only a minority of students in the exercise would wonder if there was something the matter with them. Unlike the student who was certain the ring was real, this minority is able to entertain the idea they might be ill. Whatever their belief, it is important to underscore for students that their belief about the origin of the ring was constructed without the slightest bit of hard evidence one way or the other as to whether it was real or imagined. The exercise concludes with the question, [6] 'What would it take for you to abandon faith in the ability of your perceptual system to determine reality and to surrender this function to another person?' Most students readily grasp in a personal way the near impossibility of doing this and see how often we expect some version of this surrender from patients. Because the perceiver cannot use the subjective quality of his experience to retrace his steps backward from conscious percept to source of origin, he has no definitive field test of what is real. When reality cannot be unambiguously defined, the brain fills in our picture of the world with predisposed fantasies and prior beliefs about the world. And so, in the end, patient and clinician sit across from each other, each confidently asserting a belief in the integrity of their own mind. In one class, toward the end of this exercise, a student began to cry. When she regained her composure, she explained she had just understood for the first time how terrifying it would be to not be able to distinguish reality from imagination. When confronted with a perceptual anomaly, whether a hallucinated 'voice' or a single ring of the phone, most people conclude it is the world that has changed rather than their own minds.

A second brief exercise examines the experience of hearing the voice of God or some other figure with supernatural authority. The instructor announces to the group of students that he has just fallen into a remarkable good fortune! The instructor says he is able to arrange a one-hour conversation between any student and God in which the student can ask God any questions he or she might want to ask, about any subject, from the practical aspects of every day life to the spiritual dimensions of human existence. If the instructor is playfully insistent, students can be easily cajoled into accepting the hypothetical premise. Students are then asked, 'How much would you pay for such an opportunity? Would you pay a week's income? Would you pay a month's income? A year's? Any amount?' As discussion ensues as to what each student would be willing to pay, two points of view typically emerge. One group of more philosophically minded students charges ahead, offering of course they would give a week's salary, of course a month's salary, of course any amount to really be able to speak with God! Generally, a second group of students hangs back, reluctant to commit themselves to the exercise. They are wary of the conversation proposed. They wonder what it would be like to live a life without mystery, in which the future was known, and conclude this would not be altogether a blessing. In short order, what began in the spirit of an auction with rapidly escalating bids gives way to a sobering realization that having a conversation with God would not only cost whatever money was offered, but would forever and irrevocably change ones relationship with every family member and friend. Such an experience would be the most significant of ones life, but one that would create an unbridgeable social divide between the voice hearer and other people. Patients who hear the voice of God believe they stand alone in possession of divine knowledge and remain true to their relationship with God, which costs them their connection to the human community at large.

In addition to two exercises described above, Garrett *et al.* (2006) describe in detail four additional exercises intended to highlight other transient disturbances in ordinary mental function, which provide analogies to psychotic symptoms. Briefly, these exercises include:

1. *The Elevator.* This exercise examines several aspects of attention and disturbances of facial recognition that can be linked to ideas of reference and paranoid delusions.

2. *What a coincidence?* Delusional individuals often believe that behind the mundane appearance of everyday events, some person, entity, deity, or agency is controlling them. This exercise examines occasions of remarkable coincidence in everyday life, which suggest that hidden forces may be operating behind the scenes.

3. *The police car is coming up behind you.* This exercise simulates a transient paranoid delusion in the experience of a motorist who is speeding and who has just passed a police car parked by the side of the road. The police car pulls out in apparent pursuit.

4. *The disappearing cloth.* In this exercise, the group leader performs a simple magic trick easily learned by anyone. Without announcing that he is going to perform the trick, he takes out a small white cloth out of his pocket and makes it disappear. When the trick is properly done, some in the group notice the cloth, while others do not. Two different 'realities' emerge in the group, a minority who have had the anomalous experience of seeing a cloth disappear, and a majority who have not had this experience. This creates an opportunity for the group to examine the role of perception and social consensus in defining reality.

'Normalizing' as clinical technique

'Normalizing' psychotic experiences is a specific clinical intervention to be employed with other techniques in the CBT toolbox (see Smith *et al.*, & Johns & Wykes, both this volume), including peripheral questioning, inference chaining, rating the likelihood and value of evidence, reality testing experiments, and so on. When done with tact and timing, normalizing can foster trust between patient and therapist, and open up an earnest, good faith exploration of the patient's experiences. A central goal of CBT for psychosis is to help the patient reassess his beliefs, substituting alternative beliefs that result in less distress. Recall the cognitive model of psychosis in Fig. 11.1, in which internal mental events receive an external attribution. 'Normalizing' begins the process of reversing this external attribution. When the therapist tells the patient that the patient's experiences are part of a continuum of mental states the therapist shares, the therapist grounds the conversation in the interior of mental life rather than the exterior of the physical world. Consider two clinical examples of the use of 'normalizing' in the CBT of 'voices'.

Patient A

The patient is a 46-year-old man with a diagnosis of paranoid schizophrenia, hospitalized for 10 years after assaulting a stranger he felt had been sent to do him harm. In the sixth treatment session, the patient complained that he had 'heard' one of the nurses making derogatory remarks about his mother, who had recently died. He believed this had occurred on three separate occasions. He was convinced that the nurse was attempting to provoke him into a violent outburst, so as to undermine his efforts to obtain discharge from the hospital. It was apparent the patient had hallucinated the nurse's remarks. The therapist asked if the patient might have misheard what she said. This made the patient angry, as though the therapist were taking sides with his abuser. Feeling misunderstood and betrayed by the therapist, he debated whether to continue in treatment. At this point, the therapist began 'normalizing' the hallucinatory experience. The therapist offered that he sometimes mistakenly heard his name being called, and wondered if anything like that had ever happened to the patient. The patient acknowledged that he sometimes heard his name being called to come to the phone, only to find out someone else was being summoned. The patient granted that he sometimes misheard things, but he remained confident he was not mistaken about the nurse.

Later in the session, the patient spoke of how close he was to his mother, and how much he missed her. At this point, the therapist underscored how powerful feelings are set in motion when a loved one dies, which can be quite stressful. He also shared a personal experience with the patient regarding his own grandmother's death some years prior. The funeral home had been arrayed with flowers with a distinct fragrance. The therapist recalled that when he returned to his apartment, he 'smelled' the same fragrance in his home, though no flowers were actually present. The therapist said the emotions of the day had no doubt contributed to his having that experience. The patient took an interest in the therapist's story and said, unprompted, 'That would be a hallucination, right!' The therapist agreed.

In the next session, the patient's adversarial attitude toward the nurse had softened. He recalled that she had once actually shown him a kindness and given him a soda. He was now willing to explore his experiences with the nurse. When asked to be as precise and specific about what he had heard as he could be, the patient acknowledged that two of the three times the nurse had spoken, her words were indistinct. Perhaps he had mis-interpreted what she said. By relating hallucinations to his own personal hallucinatory experience in the context of loss, the clinician 'normalized' the patient's hallucinations, which allowed the therapist to talk about the nurse without seeming to take sides with someone the patient considered a persecutor. Normalizing salvaged the therapeutic alli-ance. The patient continued in treatment and went on to achieve good insight that the fears that prompted him to attack strangers in the past were 'false fears'.

Patient B

Patient B was an intelligent 58-year-old woman with two psychiatric admissions at age 46 and 48 for schizoaffective psychosis, manic type. Her psychotic illness was precipitated by her divorce and her mother's death, which occurred within the same year. Prior to being hospitalized, she believed that the government was sending her messages through a secret code embedded in automobile license plates. She began to hear 'voices', which appeared to offer cryptic clues regarding the license plate code. The 'voices' persisted after the ideas of reference subsided. At the time she began treatment, she had for many years been hearing 'voices' daily in runs lasting hours at a time. She heard several different 'voices', some with distinct accents and male or female gender, and other 'voices' with less distinct identities. The patient had consistently refused treatment because of previous negative experiences when attempts were made to 'medicate' her. At her family's urging, she agreed to enter treatment if medication was not part of the treatment plan.

The CBT began with the therapist constructing a timeline of the patient's illness. When asked what was the most distressing aspect of her current situation, the patient said the 'voices' made frightening predictions that various individuals were going to die, some named and some unnamed. She believed the predictions were credible. The 'voices' offered what she thought were confusing clues as to who was going to die, and she would spend hours in circular conversations with the 'voices' trying to find out who was in peril. The 'voices' frequently referred to a woman named 'Nancy'. 'Nancy' never spoke to her directly, but played an important role in the death predictions. The patient described a typical sequence with the 'voices'.

> Voices: There will be death.
> Patient: Who is going to die?
> Voices: Nancy knows. She's in town.
> Patient: Where in town?
> Voices: She is at the bridge.
> Patient: Which bridge?
> Voices: You know which bridge. It's bad.

And so on, in loops of circular innuendo that went nowhere. She believed that the 'voices' knew as much as they did because they had access to a government computer. Her conviction that the 'voices' could predict death crystallized when a 'voice' predicted that Frank Sinatra was going to die, and he did. Patient and therapist agreed on the goal of exploring the voice hearing experience with the aim of possibly diminishing the stress associated with the death predictions.

In the second session, the therapist began 'normalizing' the patient's voices, relating them to the continuum of ordinary mental life. Hallucinations of everyday life were discussed, as well as hallucinations in grief and sensory deprivation. The therapist provided a brief overview of the typical phenomenology of the voice hearing experience, adding that there were many individuals who heard 'voices' much like she did. It had never occurred to her that she was not alone in this experience, and learning that others also heard 'voices' increased her comfort in talking about her experience, and heightened her curiosity.

The therapist reinforced the 'normalizing' of the 'voices' with a metaphor and a paper drawing (Fig. 11.2). 'Ordinarily thoughts rise up into our awareness as though we are 'hearing' them through an inner ear in our mind. Everyone's mind has a window in it between this inside world of thoughts, and the outside world of sounds. In most people, that window is open just a narrow crack. An occasional thought, like hearing our name called out loud, can drift through this narrow opening into the outside world. Then we 'hear' our own thought as though it was coming from the outside world. When a person is under stress, that window in the mind can open wide. Thoughts pour out through the

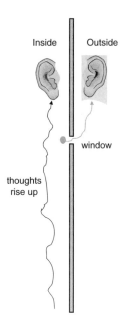

Inside   Outside

window

thoughts
rise up

Fig. 11.2 Ordinary mental life.

open window, and are heard as though they are sounds originating outside ourselves'. The patient followed the metaphor with interest, but did not at this point relate it to her 'voices'.

The next several sessions were devoted to reviewing the stress/vulnerability model of psychological disorders, and the ABC assessment of life events, where 'A' is the activating event, 'B' the belief about the significance of this event, and 'C' the emotional or behavioral consequence of the belief. Patient and therapist sketched out an A-B-C model of her voice hearing experience. 'A' was the 'voice' predicting that someone was going to die; 'B' was her belief that this was a credible prediction; 'C' was the emotional consequence of anxiety and fear, and the behavioral consequence of hours of attention paid to the 'voices' in an effort to figure out who was at risk.

Evidence for her belief that the predictions of the voices would come true was examined. The patient's belief hinged on the fact that the 'voices' had predicted Frank Sinatra would die, and he did. She acknowledged that the 'voices' had also predicted that her children's' pediatrician would die, and he had not. Prompted by the normalizing window metaphor, she offered that she may have had her own expectation, apart from the 'voices', that Frank Sinatra would die because he had appeared on television obviously ailing, and there had been discussion of his ill health. 'Maybe that was something I knew anyway?'

The therapist expressed an interest in how she coped with the 'voices'. She said she had noticed that if she involved herself in meaningful activity that required concentration, the 'voices' were less. The therapist went over a list of 30 possible coping techniques, and suggested a homework assignment of reviewing the list to see what might be of use to her that she wasn't already doing. In the next session, she noted that she was already using several techniques on the list and would be interested to try others. The therapist suggested the analogy of sitting in the back row of a movie theater. 'The 'voices' are at a distance, up on the screen. You are sitting in the back row, far away from the screen. You pay some attention to the voices on the screen, but you can let your attention go elsewhere, and you need not talk back to the voices on the screen' (personal communication, M. van der Gaag). The patient said she would try using this idea when the 'voices' were bothering her.

By the fourth session, the patient was quite curious about her voice hearing experience and was an active collaborator in the therapeutic investigation. She described a manic episode that led to her hospitalization in which she travelled to Europe with no money and no change of clothing. She recalled having racing thoughts and hearing 'voices'. The phenomenology of manic thought disorder was discussed, including the concept of circumstantial thinking, which the patient said she had at that time. The therapist remarked that another hypomanic patient he had worked with, a computer programmer, would address programming problems he was working on to his 'voices' and the 'voices' would suggest possible programming solutions. The patient then offered, 'I think when I was manic I was watching my 'voices' engage in circumstantial thinking'. Like circumstantial thinking, her 'voices' tended to follow a theme, but meandered in an unfocused way, which gave her the impression the 'voices' were dropping hints about some hidden truth. She also recognized that the 'voices' occasionally said phrases her parents used to say when she was a child.

At the beginning of the sixth session, the patient offered, 'I have started to deal with the 'voices' differently. Now when I get the 'voices' I say to myself, 'I am not hearing this. I am thinking this'. She estimated that this meta-cognitive shift had reduced the frequency of the 'voices' by 50%. Her understanding that the 'voices' represented her own thoughts undercut her belief that the 'voices' could accurately predict deaths, and she was no longer afraid of these dire predictions. Though less frequent and less distressing, the 'voices' continued to bother her, in part because they interrupted her thinking, and there were aspects of the voice hearing experience she could not make sense of. While no single explanation of the content of the 'voices' emerged, little by little the patient was able to identify the origin of many aspects of the voice hearing experience as originating within her own mind. For example, one week she had heard a 'voice' say over and over again, 'Throw the five!' She traced this back to a card game she had played the week before in which she had said to herself at a decisive moment in the game, 'Throw the five'. Employing a computer analogy to her mind, she said, 'Some of the stuff the 'voices' say are memories, like there is a hard disk in my brain de-fragging '.

Patient and therapist turned their attention to 'Nancy'. Patient and therapist listed 'Nancy's' traits. The 'voices' often said, 'Nancy, you are not in this'. She was an outsider, like the patient. She was Italian, as was the patient. 'Nancy' hates housework, and would prefer to work in business, as the patient had before she became ill. Her brother, who had a substance abuse problem, had moved in with her and did not do his share of housework. She recalled thinking to herself 'He does nothing', then hearing the 'voices' say, 'He didn't put the Italian bread away!' The patient then suggested, 'Maybe 'Nancy' is like me?'

Lastly, patient and therapist turned their attention to why the 'voices' might have been so concerned with predicting deaths. The patient had by now become familiar with looking for relationships between the 'voices' and her mental life. She offered, 'Maybe the 'voices' are talking about my death anxiety. I was very close to my mother. I miss her terribly'. In the next two sessions, patient and therapist further explored a number of separations and losses that had been deeply upsetting to the patient. The patient took the lead. Her father's death had also been a blow, though less so than her mother. The divorce had been a traumatic ending and separation. Anticipating another painful loss, she frequently worried that her aging dog would become ill and die. And lastly, she thought the 'voices' preoccupation with death reflected her own growing awareness of her mortality. Her psychiatric illness had not gone away, as she had once imagined it would. It had remained, a harbinger of her own aging, human vulnerability, and mortality. The therapist summarized her ideas, saying, 'The 'voices' predicting deaths give voice to your grief and fear of more painful losses in the future.

The therapist consolidated the work of these two sessions by returning to the normalizing 'window in the mind' diagram. He drew in the network of memories and thoughts that had crossed over through the open window in her mind and flowed together to emerge in the 'voices' preoccupation with deaths (Fig. 11.3). The patient was by now familiar with the 'window' schematic. The therapist mentioned that medication was sometimes helpful in closing the biological window in the mind between thoughts and perceptions. The patient had been categorically opposed to medication at the beginning of the treatment, but now expressed an interest. The therapist reviewed the options available, mechanisms of action, and possible side effects of medication. The patient elected to begin aripiprazole, which was slowly titrated upward to 10mg QAM and 5mg QHS, with

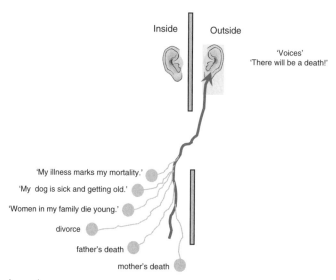

Fig. 11.3 Hearing voices.

complete cessation of 'voices'. The patient began thinking about going back to work. She experienced occasional recurrences of 'voices' when she was 'alone and bored'. After two months taking the medication, she reported that while she was not troubled by 'voices' predicting deaths anymore, but that she occasionally became excessively worried that someone close to her might become ill or die. She recognized this worry as her own thoughts, and knew her fears could not be attached to any realistic concern. Her family was in good health. She found these thoughts distressing, but much less distressing than her literal belief in the predictive power of the 'voices' prior to treatment. At one year follow up the patient was working part-time in a flower shop, and not hearing 'voices'.

Next steps

In summary, an appreciation of the continuum between psychosis and ordinary mental life becomes a practical clinical tool in the form of 'normalizing' interventions in the psychotherapy of psychosis. Relating psychotic mental states to ordinary mental life reduces the stigma of these experiences, which places the doctor–patient relationship on a more equal footing. This encourages open and trusting communication between patient and clinician. Suggesting to patients that analogies to psychotic symptoms can be found in the mental life of most people, including the clinician, begins to reverse the meta-psychological judgment the patient has made to locate psychotic experiences in the out-side world. Normalizing psychotic symptoms places these experiences within the mental life of the clinician and others, which begins the therapeutic process of locating these experiences within the mental life of the patient, as treatment proceeds.

A convincing appreciation of the continuum between psychosis and ordinary mental life should be an important goal in the psychosis curriculum of graduate psychology and psychiatry programs. General training should include lectures, reading material, and experiential exercises relating to the continuum. More advanced training in CBT for psychosis should include the use of 'normalizing' as a clinical intervention. In coming years, the renewed interest in the individual psychotherapy of psychosis will pose two challenges of integration. As a community of psychotherapists, we must ask how to best integrate CBT techniques with psychodynamic perspectives. The ability to listen to clinical material in a psychodynamic frame can help the CBT clinician better recognize and work through resistances to treatment, engage the psychotic patient in a therapeutic alliance, formulate the psychosis in the stress/vulnerability model, understand the personal meaning of hallucinations and delusions, characterize 'negative self-schema', and understand how individual patients regulate self-esteem. The case of voices predicting deaths outlined above illustrates the combined use of CBT and psychodynamic interventions at different points within a single treatment.

Consider another example of how a psychodynamic listening ear can facilitate CBT technique. A 35-year-old woman with chronic paranoid schizophrenia believed that the Dean of the college where she had gone to school had planted a computer chip in her body to observe her thoughts and actions. Over the course of 16 sessions of CBT, she came to understand that her belief about the chip was a delusion. Two years after achieving this insight, during a period she had been doing quite well, she had occasion to contact the school for the first time in many years. She needed to apply to have her college loans forgiven in order to have her college transcript released to a local secretarial school. The woman at the college spoke briefly to a second person while she was talking to the patient on the phone. It occurred to the patient that the other person in the room was likely someone from the Dean's office, which revived the patient's concern that the Dean might be tracking her again. In the several days between the phone call and the patient's next appointment, the patient could not shake her belief she was under surveillance by the Dean. She was sleeping poorly, and had begun to slip into the early stages of a paranoid relapse.

Psychodynamically oriented therapists are trained to help patients put thoughts and feelings that are just out of awareness into words. Sensing the patient's predominant affect was anger, the therapist quickly observed, 'It sounds like it was infuriating to think that after all these years, the school could start tracking you again. Just when you got up the courage to contact them, and you were hoping they would help you move forward, you felt like they were starting to drag you back'. The therapist's psychodynamic training allowed him to quickly articulate the patient's thoughts and feelings with clarity and accuracy. The patient readily agreed that she had felt this way. Helping the patient to express her thoughts and feelings allowed her to dissipate her anger sufficiently to engage in a 'booster' CBT session. Patient and therapist examined alternate explanations for why the woman on the phone might have spoken to someone else in the room while talking with the patient. Together, patient and therapist were able to abate the impending paranoid episode. In the author's opinion, the optimal approach to the psychotherapy of psychotic patients is a cognitive behavioral treatment guided by a psychodynamic frame. As a broad clinical community, we must ask how to increase the availability of CBT for psychosis, and how to combine psychotherapy with psychopharmacology and social interventions.

References

Assad, G. (1990). *Hallucinations in Clinical Psychiatry*, New York: Brunner/Mazel.

Baddeley, A., & Logie, R. (1992). Auditory imagery and working memory. *In Auditory Imagery*, Hillsdale: Lawrence Erlbaum Associates.

Barrett, T. R., & Etheridge, J. B. (1992). Verbal hallucinations in normals, I: People who hear 'voices'. *Appl Cogn Psychol*, **6**, 379–87.

Bentall, R. P., & Slade, P. D. (1985). Reality testing and auditory hallucinations: a signal detection analysis. *Br J Clin Psychol*, **24** (Pt 3), 159–69.

Bentall, R. P., Corcoran, R., Howard, R., Blackwood, N., & Kinderman, P. (2001). Persecutory delusions: a review and theoretical integration. *Clin Psychol Rev*, **21**, 1143–92.

Bick, P. A., & Kinsbourne, M. (1987). Auditory hallucinations and subvocal speech in schizophrenic patients. *Am J Psychiatry*, **144**, 222–5.

Blackwood, N. J., Howard, R. J., Bentall, R. P., & Murray, R. M. (2001). Cognitive neuropsychiatric models of persecutory delusions. *Am J Psychiatry*, **158**, 527–39.

Brown, A. S. (1991). A review of the tip-of-the-tongue experience. *Psychol Bull*, **109**, 204–23.

Chapman, L. J., & Chapman, J. P. (1988). *The Genesis of Delusions*, New York: John Wiley & Sons.

Cox, D., & Cowling, P. (1989). *Are you normal?* London: Tower Press.

Deegan, P. E. (1996). *Hearing Voices That Are Distressing: A Training and Simulation Experience.* Lawrence: The National Empowerment Center.

Fischhoff, B., Slovic, P., & Lichtenstein, S. (1977). Knowing with certainty: the appopriateness of extreme confidence. *Journal of Experimental Psychology: Human Perception and Performan*, **3**, 552–64.

Garety, P. A., Kuipers, E., Fowler, D., Freeman, D., & Bebbington, P. E. (2001). A cognitive model of the positive symptoms of psychosis. *Psychol Med*, **31**, 189–95.

Garrett, M., & Silva, R. (2003). Auditory hallucinations, source monitoring, and the belief that 'voices' are real. *Schizophr Bull*, **29**, 445–57.

Garety, P. A., Freeman, D., Jolley, S., *et al.* (2005). Reasoning, emotions, and delusional conviction in psychosis. *J Abnorm Psychol*, **114**, 373–84.

Garrett, M., Stone, D., & Turkington, D. (2006). Normalizing psychotic symptoms. *Psychol Psychother*, **79**, 595–610.

Garety, P. A., Bebbington, P., Fowler, D., Freeman, D., & Kuipers, E. (2007). Implications for neurobiological research of cognitive models of psychosis: a theoretical paper. *Psychol Med*, **37**, 1377–91.

Gould, L. N. (1948). Verbal hallucinations and activity of vocal musculature. *Am J Psychiatry*, **105**, 367–72.

Gould, L. N. (1949). Auditory hallucinations and subvocal speech; objective study in a case of schizophrenia. *J Nerv Ment Dis*, **109**, 418–27.

Gould, L. N. (1950). Verbal hallucinations as automatic speech; the reactivation of dormant speech habit. *Am J Psychiatry*, **107**, 110–9.

Greenberg, J., & Mitchell, S. (1983). *Object Relations in Psychoanalytic Theory.* Cambridge, London, England: Harvard University Press.

Grimby, A. (1988). Hallucinations following the loss of a spouse: common and normal events among the elderly. *J Clin Geropsychol*, **4**, 65–74.

Jaspers, K. (1972). *General Psychopathology.* Manchester/Chicago: Manchester University Press/ The University of Chicago Press.

Johns, L. C., & Van Os, J. (2001). The continuity of psychotic experiences in the general population. *Clin Psychol Rev*, **21**, 1125–41.

Johns, L. C., Nazroo, J. Y., Bebbington, P., & Kuipers, E. (2002). Occurrence of hallucinatory experiences in a community sample and ethnic variations. *Br J Psychiatry*, **180**, 174–8.

Johnson, M. K., Raye, C. L., Foley, M. A., & Foley, J. H. (1981). Cognitive operations and decisions bias in reality monitoring. *Am J Psychol*, **94**, 37–64.

Johnson, M. K. (1988). Reality monitoring: an experimental phenomenological approach. *J Exp Psychol: Gen*, **117**, 390–4.

Johnson, M., Shahin, H., & Stephen, L. (1993). Source monitoring. *Psychol Bull*, **114**, 3–28.

Kemp, R., Chua, S., Mckenna, P., & David, A. (1997). Reasoning and delusions. *Br J Psychiatry*, **170**, 398–405.

Kernberg, O. (2005). Object relations theories and technique. In person, E., Cooper, A. & Gabbard, G. (Eds.) *Textbook of Psychoanalysis*. Washington DC: American Psychiatric Publishing.

Kingdon, D., Turkington, D., & John, C. (1994). Cognitive behaviour therapy of schizophrenia. The amenability of delusions and hallucinations to reasoning. *Br J Psychiatry*, **164**, 581–7.

Kingdon, D., & Turkington, D. (2005). *Cognitive Therapy of Schizophrenia.* New York: Guilford.

Klein, M. (1935). A contribution to the psychogenesis of manic-depressive states. *Int J Psycho-Anal*, **16**, 145–74.

Klein, M. (1946). Notes on some schizoid mechanisms1. *Int J Psycho-anal*, **27**, 99–110.

Leudar, I., Thomas, P., Mcnally, D., & Glinski, A. (1997). What voices can do with words: pragmatics of verbal hallucinations. *Cambridge University Press*, **27**(4), 885–98.

Lord, C. G. (1979). Biased assimilation and attitude polarization: the effects of prior theories on subsequently considered evidence. *J Pers Soc Psychol*, **37**, 2098–109.

Maher, B. A. (1988). *Anomalous Experience and Delusional Thinking: The Logic of Explanations*. New York: John Wiley & Sons.

Mckellar, P. (1968). *Experience and Behavior*. Harmondsworth: Penguin Press.

Nayani, T. H., & David, A. S. (1996). The auditory hallucination: a phenomenological survey. *Psychol Med*, **26**, 177–89.

Posey, T. B., & Losch, M. E. (1983). Auditory Hallucinations of Hearing Voices in 375 Normal Subjects. *Imagination, Cogn Pers*, **3**, 99–113.

Posey, T. B. (1986). Verbal hallucinations also occur in normals. *Behav Brain Sci*, **9**(3), 530.

Romme, M., & Escher, A. (1989). Hearing voices. *Schizophr Bull*, **15**, 209–16.

Schiller, L., & Bennett, A. (1995). *The Quiet Room*. New York: Warner Books.

Schneider, K. (1959). *Clinical Psychopathology*. New York: Grune & Stratton.

Schreber, D. P. (1988). *Memoirs of My Nervous Illness*. Cambridge: Harvard University Press.

Sidgewick, H., Johnson, A., & Myers, F. W. H. (1894). Report of the census of hallucinations. *Proc Soc Psych Res*, **26**, 259–394.

Sommer, R., & Osmond, H. (1983). A bibliography of mental patients' autobiographies, 1960–1982. *Am J Psychiatry*, **140**, 1051–4.

Sommer, I. E. C., Daalman, K., Rietkerk, T., *et al*. (2008). Healthy individuals with auditory verbal hallucinations; Who are they? Psychiatric assessments of a selected sample of 103 subjects. *Schizophr Bull Advance Access*. E-pub ahead of print.

Strauss, J. S. (1969). Hallucinations and delusions as points on continua function. Rating scale evidence. *Arch Gen Psychiatry*, **21**, 581–6.

Sutherland, S. (1994). *Irrationality. Why We Don't Think Straight!* New Brunswick: Rutgers University Press.

Tien, A. Y. (1991). Distributions of hallucinations in the population. *Soc Psychiatry Psychiatr Epidemiol*, **26**, 287–92.

Van der Gaag, M. (2006). A neuropsychiatric model of biological processes in the remission of delusion and auditory hallucinations. *Schizophr Bull*, **1**, S113–22.

Van Os, J., Hanssen, M., Bijl, R. V., & Ravelli, A. (2000). Strauss (1969) revisited; a psychosis continuum in the general population? *Schizophr Res*, **45**, 11–20.

Vygotsky, L. S. (1987). *The Collected Works of L.S. Vygotsky*. New York: Plenum Press.

Wertsch, J. V. (1985). *Vygotsky and the Social Formation of Mind*, Cambridge: Harvard University Press.

West, D. J. (1948). A mass-observation on hallucinations. *J Soc Psych Res*, **34**, 187–96.

Young, H. F., Bentall, R. P., Slade, P. D., & Dewey, M. E. (1986). Disposition towards hallucination, gender and EPQ scores: a brief report. *Pers Individ Dif*, **7**, 247–9.

Chapter 12

Understanding and shaping adaptive coping with voices

John Farhall

Lisa, who has struggled with voices for almost 10 years, is on the couch in her room, her coat pulled tightly around her, quietly saying, 'No! No!' Arriving for a home visit, Paul, her mental health worker, asks if she is speaking to one of her 'voices', and comments to Lisa that she sounds a bit stressed. Although Lisa says little other than acknowledging hearing voices, the worker gently persists:

> *Is it the sun-god, or the old man that you're hearing now?*
> *—The old man.*
> *Is the voice as loud as yesterday?*
> *—He's gone away now because you came.*
> *How long were you caught up with the voice before I arrived?*
> *—I don't know—half an hour maybe.*
> *I see, so you had noticed the voice for about half an hour, but it stopped when I spoke to you, or when you spoke to me just now?*
> *—Yes. I think so.*
> *Ah, now that's interesting—it reminds me of an idea from your coping list—wasn't there something about the voice stopping when you're listening or talking?*
> *—Yes, I know, and singing and humming too, but I think it just went away anyway this time.*
> *Yes, well, it might be co-incidence, but it did seem to stop when we started talking…What do you think might have happened if you had hummed your favourite tune when you were hearing the voice just now?*
> *—It probably would have got bored and gone away.*

This scenario illustrates some elements of a coping approach for assisting voice hearers that we will take up in this chapter. Paul assists Lisa to *disengage* from the voice and reflect on the experience, seeing it as a phenomenon about which she can deliberately take coping actions. He utilizes in-the-moment work and *learning from experience* to *extend her repertoire of effective coping*, even though insight is relatively low. The suggested strategies involve *vocalization*—an element of coping that has empirical and theoretical support. Finally, although implementing an evidence-based intervention, this home visit gives Paul an *opportunity to work informally*, illustrating how enhancement of coping can be applied by family caregivers, residential care staff, and voice-hearers themselves.

Background and theory

The evidence about coping strategies for voices

Coping is, at heart, a simple and widely applicable idea. When humans are faced with situations that threaten well-being, they feel stressed and will typically do something to either ameliorate the stressor (problem-focused coping) or manage the stressful emotions (emotion-focused coping). It does not matter whether the stressor is an external event, such as running late for an appointment or a bereavement; or whether the stressor is a symptom of a disorder, such as pain or tinnitus or depressed mood—wherever a stimulus is stressful, we are likely to see some coping responses on the part of the person concerned. In psychotic disorders, persisting symptoms including anxiety, depression, retardation, thought disturbance, hallucinations, and delusions are common in patients living in the community, and most patients report self-initiated, or 'natural', coping strategies (Carr & Katsikitis, 1987).

Self-initiated or natural coping with voices

If voices can indeed be defined as a stressor, then we would expect most hallucinators to show automatic or deliberate efforts to try to cope. A recent review (Farhall, Greenwood, & Jackson, 2007) identified studies of natural coping with voices in people with a diagnosis of schizophrenia. Across the 12 studies, more than 90% of the 703 participants reported one or more coping strategies, at least when prompted with a list of examples. Even when no prompting was used (e.g., Farhall & Voudouris, 1996) at least half of the participant group was able to readily describe a coping strategy. The mean number of coping strategies reported by each hallucinator in these studies ranged from 2.2 strategies per person (Frederick & Cotanch, 1995) to 18.3 strategies (O'Sullivan, 1994). It is reasonable to conclude that some degree of 'natural' coping is common, if not universal, amongst hallucinators, and that most have a repertoire of a few strategies they can report.

What are these 'natural' coping strategies adopted by people who hear voices? At least 14 published studies (see, Farhall et al., 2007) have investigated this question, studying hospitalized and community-residing samples and Western and non-Western cultures. Although different methodologies and instruments make summaries and comparisons difficult, some important themes have emerged from this literature.

Although the phenomenon of voices is conceptualized as a single 'symptom', it is clear that it leads to a great diversity of coping strategies. These range from yelling back at voices to ignoring them, from taking substances to talking with a friend, and from searching for the speaker to seeking change via prayer (Carter, Mackinnon, & Copolov, 1996; Tsai & Ku, 2005). This wide range of ways of coping seems to be more similar than different across cultures—coping reported by samples from India (Singh, Sharan, & Kulhara, 2003), Japan (Hayashi et al., 2007), and Taiwan (Tsai & Ku, 2005) are similar to those from Western countries, though some culturally consistent emphases have been observed, including a greater emphasis on religious strategies such as prayer in Saudi Arabia compared with the UK (Wahass & Kent, 1997). Although some strategies, such as using ear plugs or turning up the volume of music to 'drown out' voices, seem tailored to hallucinations, most strategies are not unique to voices: A large proportion of reported strategies are also ways of coping with life stressors that are reported by people without any disorder at all (Farhall & Gehrke, 1997).

The diversity of coping encompasses cognitive, behavioural, and physiological domains (Falloon & Talbot, 1981; Frederick & Cotanch, 1995). Three studies (O'Sullivan, 1994;

Farhall & Gehrke, 1997; Hayashi *et al.*, 2007) have used principal components analysis to identify how strategies may reflect possible styles of coping, highlighting that hallucinators vary in the extent to which they use active *vs.* passive coping strategies, and accept *vs.* resist the voice. A multidimensional scaling analysis (Carter, Mackinnon, & Copolov, 1996) identified groups of strategies that seemed to reflect mechanisms of action: competing auditory stimuli, vocalization, and distraction. The Hayashi study found relationships between coping factors and symptoms and appraisal, for example, fewer distraction strategies where delusions or negative symptoms were more prominent.

The fact that most hallucinators naturally try to cope with hearing voices, and can report their strategies for coping, has led researchers to seek to identify whether some natural ways of coping are better than others. Typically, hallucinators claim moderate benefit from the strategies they report, but no strategies stand out from this literature as being routinely effective for most people (O'Sullivan, 1994; Carter *et al.*, 1996; Farhall & Voudouris, 1996; Nayani & David, 1996; Tsai & Ku, 2005; Hayashi *et al.*, 2007). Nonetheless, a few strategies have been reported by a majority of these studies as relatively effective compared with others: shifting or focusing attention, listening to music, prayer, and talking to others. It is interesting that these could be plausibly assigned to the mechanisms of action suggested by Carter *et al.* (1996), an observation that is given weight by the experimental work reported in the next section. Other strategies (such as yelling back at the voices) have been reported as typically unhelpful (Farhall & Voudouris, 1996), however, not universally so (Nayani & David, 1996), and some strategies, such as self-harm, misuse of prescription or street drugs or smoking have health risks, regardless of any immediate emotion coping or distraction benefit.

Experimental studies of strategy efficacy

Clearer evidence about the effectiveness of verbal and auditory strategies for coping comes from experimental studies. The effectiveness of 'talking to someone' was noted earlier from self-reports. Experimental studies have also demonstrated that actions involving vocalization, such as speaking out loud, counting, and singing can interrupt hallucinated voices. In addition, actions involving *sub*-vocalization, such as reading silently or talking under your breath, can also interrupt voices and serve as a way of coping (Bick & Kinsbourne, 1987; Gallagher, Dinan, & Baker, 1995). The effectiveness of these techniques can be understood from source monitoring theories of voices. If hallucinated voices comprise internal speech that is erroneously attributed to an external source (Slade, 1994), the use of cortical speech pathways to speak or sing should minimize inner speech, making it less likely that any material would be available to be misattributed (Green & Kinsbourne, 1990).

Auditory techniques have also been used to interrupt or inhibit hallucinations, and there is indirect evidence from brain imaging research of auditory competition between hallucinations and external stimuli (David *et al.*, 1996). The reasoning here is similar to that for vocalization techniques—humans have a limited capacity for processing auditory perceptual material and so if these pathways are fully utilized processing real-world stimuli, there is little chance of experiencing an auditory hallucination. This rationale is consistent with patient reports of attempting to 'drown out' voices and clinical observations that hallucinations are more likely to occur in situations of low external auditory stimulation or monotonous noise. Consistent with the relative effectiveness of the natural strategy of 'listening to music', experimental studies have demonstrated efficacy for 'auditory competition' methods. The more meaningful, and the more familiar the stimuli, the more effective they are in 'competing' for attention with voices (Margo, Hemsley, & Slade, 1981). Nelson *et al.*'s study (Nelson, Thrasher, & Barnes, 1991) compared a variety of auditory manipulation methods on practical as well as efficacy grounds, finding that a personal music player was not only effective, but also had the best uptake and continued use over time.

Other techniques have been experimentally investigated, but with less clear results. For example, manipulation of auditory input through use of an ear plug in the non-dominant ear was initially driven by the inter-hemispheric communication theory of Paul Green (Green, 1978) and supported by case studies (e.g., Birchwood, 1986), and Nelson *et al.*'s (1991) uncontrolled trial (8 of 13 who used it reported some benefit). However, both an experimental study (Done *et al.*, 1986) and a successful single-case treatment (Morley, 1987) provided evidence at odds with the theoretical mechanism. Like most coping strategies, its efficacy and mechanism are still unclear; however, it merits being on lists of possible strategies as some patients report benefit.

Implications for clinical practice

The literature reviewed has established that hallucinators typically find voices stressful and automatically attempt to cope, as they would with any other stressor. These 'natural' coping strategies cover a wide range of behaviours and overlap with ways of coping for everyday stressors; few are tailored to the specific stressor of voices. Their reported effectiveness for persisting hallucinations is modest. Both experimental studies and reports of natural coping suggest that strategies involving auditory competition, vocalization and distraction can interrupt or inhibit voices and thereby bring some relief. There may also be benefit in active *vs.* passive coping styles and in a relationship with the voice characterized by acceptance, distance, or insight.

The universality of coping as a human response to stress, combined with the limitations of effectiveness of many natural attempts at coping, suggests that enhancement of coping is a meaningful and potentially useful intervention. As coping is a fundamental survival mechanism of humans, it is arguably a natural and potentially powerful point of engagement as well as an understandable model for assisting clients. It also has the potential to be relevant and understandable across cultures. Logically, programs to assist hallucinators might include one or more of the following elements (Farhall *et al.*, 2007):

1. Encouraging growth in coping repertoires, where patients have few strategies,

2. Helping patients prioritize more efficacious strategies from their existing repertoire,

3. Teaching patients additional strategies that have known efficacy, and

4. Providing information to patients about natural strategies used by other hallucinators, and their reported efficacy, to encourage further self-discovery of personally effective strategies.

Studies using coping strategies in clinical practice

We now turn to programs and therapies that have utilized a coping approach, to consider the approaches taken, and their effectiveness.

Hallucination-specific coping therapies

Two studies have reported a systematic approach to teaching coping strategies, where the stressor has been voices. The 'distraction therapy' of Haddock, Bentall, and Slade (1996) introduced new strategies each session to build a repertoire of suppression and distraction techniques. Distraction therapy was compared with 'focusing therapy' in which a hierarchy of increasing attention to voices is utilized with the aim of reducing or reversing the misattribution of internally generated mental activity assumed to underlie the phenomenon. Both groups improved to a similar extent over the treatment period and to 2-year follow-up (Haddock, Slade, Bentall, Reid, & Faragher, 1998), although there was some evidence that self-esteem was better protected for focusers.

Buccheri *et al.* (1996) reported a group program in which 11 empirically supported behavioural strategies for managing persisting hallucinations were systematically introduced. All participants reported benefit from one or more strategies, with different strategies useful for different people. Narrative reports from participants supported the systematic introduction of coping strategies in a group treatment context, but the small numbers precluded meaningful analysis of treatment *vs.* control conditions. In a second study with 60 participants but no control condition (Buccheri *et al.*, 2004), reductions from baseline levels of hallucination were sustained for up to 1 year post-treatment. A group intervention pilot has also been reported (Perlman & Hubbard, 2000).

Hallucination-specific therapies for voices that include coping

Hallucinations-focused Integrated Therapy (HIT; see Jenner, this volume) is a multi-modal family therapy developed in the Netherlands for patients with persisting hallucinations (Wiersma, Jenner, van de Willige, Spakman, & Nienhuis, 2001). The manualized, 20-session treatment is implemented flexibly and largely replaces routine care. It encompasses six main components: psychoeducation, medication, CBT, coping training, family treatment, and rehabilitation. The coping training, delivered to patients and their relatives, includes anxiety management, distraction, and focusing elements, with exercises and daily monitoring. A randomized trial of HIT versus routine care (Jenner, Nienhuis, Wiersma, & van de Willige, 2004) demonstrated reductions in distress about hallucinations, and in symptom scores. Jenner *et al.*, were unable to say what contribution, if any, the coping component made to the overall benefit.

A novel group program was piloted by Maxwell (2008), in which coping enhancement, psychoeducation and belief modification were taught to family caregivers of hallucinators, who were encouraged and supported by the group to try applicable interventions with their ill relatives. Time series analyses showed a clinically significant reduction in voice frequency in one of the eight hallucinators, though the onset of the improvement was associated with the psychoeducation component.

In contrast to the Buccheri program, the voices groups developed by Wykes and colleagues (Wykes, Parr, & Landau, 1999; Wykes *et al.*, 2005) include psychoeducation and cognitive restructuring in addition to behavioural coping strategies. Where groups were conducted by more experienced therapists, the program improved social functioning and reduced hallucination severity (Wykes *et al.*, 2005). The increase in number of coping strategies employed following treatment was not significant, suggesting that this may not have been the primary route to change.

Coping enhancement therapies for problems including hallucinations

Coping Strategy Enhancement (CSE) introduced the core therapeutic approach of assessing and building upon natural coping (Tarrier, Harwood, Yusopoff, Beckett, & Baker, 1990; Tarrier *et al.*, 1993), although it was not confined to working with hallucinations. Further development led to the addition of problem solving and relapse prevention in a broader CBT for psychosis approach (Tarrier *et al.*, 1998). CSE originally consisted of 10 bi-weekly sessions in which a behavioural analysis of distressing symptoms was made, a priority symptom chosen, natural coping assessed as helpful or not, and enhancements to natural coping made using a variety of behavioural techniques (Tarrier, 1992). On balance, the evidence suggests the approach has merit (Tarrier *et al.*, 1993), but there are little data specifically about the outcome for the symptom of hallucinations, and the contribution of the coping work (*vs.* additional components) to improvements in hallucinations has not been demonstrated directly (Tarrier *et al.*, 2001). Nonetheless, the use of adaptive coping strategies was associated with reduction in the number and severity of symptoms (Tarrier *et al.*, 1993).

Coping enhancement was the most frequently used component in a pilot implementation of a CBT intervention for psychotic symptoms (Farhall & Cotton, 2002). Ratings of positive symptom frequency, distress, and preoccupation improved significantly, but numbers were too small to report hallucinations results separately.

Cognitive behaviour therapies that include a coping component

Coping techniques for positive symptoms have become increasingly known through their inclusion in several variants of CBT for psychosis (Liberman, 1988; Kingdon & Turkington, 1994; Fowler, Garety, & Kuipers, 1995; Hogarty *et al.*, 1995; Tarrier *et al.*, 1998; Pinto, La Pia, Mennella, Georgio, & DeSimone, 1999; Herrmann-Doig, Maude, & Edwards, 2003). A common application of coping enhancement is in the early stages of CBT for psychosis, to provide practical help, especially with distressing symptoms (Fowler, Garety, & Kuipers, 1998). However, coping is not a significant element of some therapies, particularly those based on cognitive therapy (Chadwick, Birchwood, & Trower, 1996; Drury, Birchwood, Cochrane, & Macmillan, 1996; Rector & Beck, 2002). Unfortunately, no CBT for psychosis studies report on the efficacy of coping strategies for hallucinations.

Disengagement and mindfulness

The notion that disengagement from, and acceptance of, voices may be adaptive, is suggested by studies of coping in which shifting attention away from voices was a relatively effective short-term strategy (e.g., Ramanathan, 1984; Nayani & David, 1996; Johns, Hemsley, & Kuipers, 2002) and active acceptance rather than resistance of voices associated with better coping (Romme & Escher, 1989; Farhall & Gehrke, 1997). These themes comprise two of the three emerging theoretical constructs arising from a recent grounded theory analysis of mindfulness for psychosis groups (Chadwick, 2005). Clinical treatments incorporating mindfulness and acceptance include group programs (Chadwick, 2005) and two limited trials of Acceptance and Commitment Therapy (Bach & Hayes, 2002; Gaudiano & Herbert, 2006). Although these themes are not introduced in the form of coping strategies, the studies strengthen the argument that disengagement and acceptance strategies may be beneficial.

A coping model

The literature on natural coping with voices makes few references to theories of coping, although the language, and the concept of natural coping, implies a vulnerability–stress–coping model (Zubin & Spring, 1977) or stress–appraisal–coping model (Lazarus & Folkman, 1984). Some coping-based interventions (e.g., Tarrier, 1992; Liberman, Kopelowicz, & Young, 1994) use a behavioural framework, in which the hallucination is considered a stimulus that is appraised as stressful, prompting selection of strategies from a repertoire of coping in order to ameliorate the experienced stress. Inadequate coping is assumed to relate to having few (Tarrier, 1987) or ineffective (Carter et al., 1996) strategies for coping.

However, a simple behavioural model does not easily explain the phenomenology of coping with voices: hallucinators neither necessarily use more frequently the strategies they rate as being more effective (Carter et al., 1996; Farhall & Voudouris, 1996) nor do they necessarily implement effective strategies they have learned (Allen, Halperin, & Friend, 1985; Bick & Kinsbourne, 1987). These findings imply that we need to understand how the person appraises their hallucinatory experience and what factors influence their choice of coping action. The process of appraisal of voices has been investigated and addressed mainly through cognitive therapy paradigms (see elsewhere in this book). However, appraisal is also a central component of the best-known general model of coping, the stress–appraisal–coping model of Richard Lazarus, and it is a version of this coping model that is outlined here.

A Stress–Appraisal–Coping Model of Voices (the SACMOV model)

In a study of patients' responses during specific 'episodes' or occasions of hearing a voice, Farhall (2005) investigated the applicability of the general stress–appraisal–coping model of Lazarus and Folkman (1984), developing a hallucination-specific version. This Stress–Appraisal–Coping Model of Voices (the SACMOV model) incorporates salient aspects of the phenomenology of voices, and findings from the coping literature within an explicit model that can guide assessment of the process of coping and choice of interventions that may enhance it. Consistent with stress–appraisal–coping theory, the model is situational, that is, it describes the processes that are hypothesized to occur during specific episodes or occasions of hearing a voice.

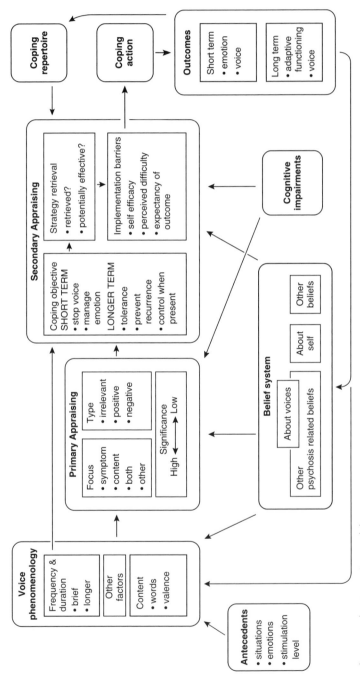

Fig. 12.1 The SACMOV model.

The five main components of the SACMOV model are depicted in Figure 12.1.

1. *Phenomenology.* The duration and the content of the voice each influence how a voice is appraised and what may be a relevant coping strategy. For example, if the voice is typically of a short duration and infrequent—for example, a few words of abuse—strategies aimed at interrupting or inhibiting voices, such as vocalization or listening to music through earphones, make no sense. In addition, voice content, particularly its positive or negative valence, is a significant determinant of appraisal and associated emotions. Other features of the voice such as loudness, who is speaking, and familiarity of the experience can also shape how it is appraised.

2. *Primary appraising.* Primary appraisal refers to a person's evaluation of whether, and in what way, an event is important for their well-being (Lazarus & Folkman, 1984). Applied to voices, the experience may be appraised as negative, for example, ('They drive me mad!') or positive ('They're my friends') or irrelevant for well-being ('I really don't care—I hardly notice them now'). These different *appraisal types* have very different implications for coping therapies. A further distinction is the *focus of appraisal,* that is, whether the person sees their voice as an unusual experience such as a symptom (as implied by the comment, 'I'm so sick of hearing these voices'), or whether their focus of appraisal is on the content of what is heard (as illustrated by 'They have no right to tell me to go and wash my hair'). Encounters with voices also differ in how important or significant for well-being the hearer judges them to be. For example, some voice hearers habituate to their voices, to the extent that they are rarely a source of stress.

3. *Secondary appraising.* Where primary appraisal identifies a threat to well-being, secondary appraisal processes are activated to consider what, if anything, can be done to cope with the situation. Detailed interviewing of hallucinators in the Farhall (2005) study suggested that it may be difficult to assess what is going on in response to voices without an understanding of the hallucinator's *objective* in this coping encounter. Not all coping is directed at stopping voices—sometimes the aim of a coping is to survive the highly stressful moment, which may lead to use of an emotion management strategy or a method of inhibiting the voice. In addition, some coping actions have a long-term aim, such as prevention (e.g., socializing because 'They don't come when I'm with my friends'), and some are forms of tolerance or mindful distancing. Once an aim is emerging, the secondary appraisal process identifies or retrieves strategies from the *coping repertoire* and considers any *implementation barriers* (e.g., I can't use the listening to music strategy if I'm in the classroom).

4. *Coping.* The *coping action* taken is thus dependent on the secondary appraisal process. Deliberately chosen strategies of coping may be easy to identify when talking to patients, but automatic responses (both helpful and unhelpful) may also be usefully conceptualized as a coping response. For example, habitually seeking out a family member to talk with when harassed by voices may be an effective form of 'automatic' coping.

5. *Outcomes.* It follows from the discussion of short- and long-term objectives of coping in (3) above that it is useful to consider both short- and longer-term outcomes of coping. This can be critical in devising a course of coping enhancement, because a strategy that is effective in the short-term (e.g., avoidance of going to the shops for fear of persecutory voices) may be maladaptive in the long-term.

The SACMOV model also includes the influence of the belief system on the content of the voice and on primary and secondary appraisal and acknowledges that cognitive impairments associated with psychosis can play a role in shaping coping. For example, difficulty in concentration, abstract thinking, and memory may make it more difficult to adaptively appraise the experience and implement an effective coping response.

Assessment and treatment

Assessment and formulation for coping enhancement

The SACMOV model prompts assessment in six domains—antecedents, phenomenology, primary appraisal, coping repertoire, secondary appraisal, and coping outcome. The guide to assessment in Table 12.1 gives sample questions for clinical assessment of each domain. The most important questions to consider in developing a formulation of what is happening when voices occur, and then considering priority coping interventions, are discussed below.

Is the voice an acute or persisting symptom?

Where voices have recently arisen or returned, assessment should identify any precipitants. These may be addressed directly, for example, via support and problem-solving for stressors. The use of short-term coping strategies (see below) can bring relief and improve self-efficacy.

Is the person's natural coping oriented to voice content or the phenomenon of hearing a voice?

For some voice-hearers, their natural coping responds to the literal voice content, such as an instruction to do something, or to the relationship with the voice, such as telling it to stop its harassment. Other voice hearers, to varying degrees, can stand back from the experience, recognizing it is a phenomenon that has recurring patterns, and realizing that they sometimes get drawn into its world. The more that voice-hearers can disengage, the more they can choose to take problem-focused coping actions, rather than brief emotion-coping responses. Interventions directed at distancing and mindfulness can be useful to help separate self from the symptom.

What is experienced as the problem by the client and others?

Natural coping is directed at whatever is appraised as stressful—it may be the annoying persistence of the voice, the fear generated by being told to overdose, the shame at being reminded of past humiliations, and it may even be a fear that voices may disappear if medication is taken as prescribed. From the point of view of others, the problem may be seen as poor engagement with the real world, or risky behaviour in response to voices or distress.

Table 12.1 A guide to coping assessment: domains, key variables, and sample questions

Antecedents—the situations and triggers that are associated with voices

Situations: Where are you when you hear a voice?

Stimulation level: What are you doing when you hear a voice?

Emotions: Do you tend to hear voices more when you are relaxed or when you are stressed?

Other: When are you free of voices?

Phenomenology—the nature of the voices experienced

Frequency and Duration: How often has the voice been present over the past few weeks? For how long does each experience of a voice last?

Identity of the voice: Whose voice do you hear?

Description of typical content: What do the voices say?

Verbatim example of content: Tell me about the last time you heard a voice—what did the voice actually say?

Primary Appraisal—the extent to which voices are perceived as helpful or a problem

Type of appraisal: Are your voices good or helpful to you? ...bad or a problem for you? ...irrelevant to you—neither good nor bad?

Appraisal significance: How important to you are the voices you hear?

Focus of appraisal: When appraising the voice, is the person referring to voices as a symptom or experience, or is the appraisal referring to the content of what is heard?

Coping Repertoire—automatic and deliberate actions in response to voices

Unprompted retrieval of repertoire: When you hear a voice that you do not like, is there anything you do to make the voice stop, or to make yourself feel better?

Cued retrieval of repertoire: (Show a list of coping strategies—see Fig. 12.2 for an example) This is a list of ways of coping with voices that that other people have used. Have you done any of these in the past few months when you have heard a voice? Which ones have been helpful?

Secondary Appraisal—the process of constructing a coping action

Coping objective: (Referring to one or more coping strategies) What are you trying to achieve when you do this? What effect do you hope it will have? (i.e., Try to clarify objective.)

Strategy retrieval: When you start to hear voices, can you remember these ways of coping?

Implementation barriers: Do you always do things like this (coping strategies) when you hear a voice? What gets in the way of using one of these ways of coping? (e.g., poor self-efficacy, perceived difficulty, pessimism about outcome.)

Coping outcome—*Emotion-focused and problem-focused outcomes*: When you hear a voice and use one of your coping strategies, do you feel better? ...does the voice stop or change?

Longer-term outcome: Are you coping better with your voice these days compared with a few months ago? Have your ways of coping helped you to prevent or live with your voice better?

What is the person's current objective of coping?

Knowing the client's appraisal of the problem helps clinicians to understand the coping objective and strategy choice. Much research has assumed that the goal of coping strategies is to make the voice disappear; however, other objectives, such as emotion management, may be dominant currently for the client. The problem formulation can prompt ideas for interventions that go beyond immediate coping, including longer-term objectives such as preventing recurrence, increasing tolerance, or gaining better control.

Eliciting coping strategies first, and then exploring the person's objective in using the strategies, and the extent to which the person is aware of impediments to coping (such as retrieval failures or implementation barriers), is a pragmatic way of assessing secondary appraisals.

How collaborative is the relationship?

Some voice hearers are so engulfed in the phenomenon that the notion of joining with the worker to enhance coping makes little sense. Other barriers to collaboration arise where voices instruct non-cooperation or where they are positively appraised as guides or companions, whilst contributing to serious disability. Where voice hearers have little interest in, or capacity for, collaborative enhancement of coping, working with triggers and the environment may help limit engulfment and distress (see below).

What are the points of intervention that may make a difference?

Tying the assessment information together into a problem-focused formulation can help identify where the most important or promising points of intervention might be.

Julia *For assessment, Julia agreed to record her voices for at least 3 days noting the time, voice content, and her response. Both she and her therapist were surprised at the frequency— voices were recorded up to 80 times in one day! Discussion revealed that the recording task had sensitized her to noticing voices, and she agreed that in general, voice activity increased the more she tuned into what they were saying. This was particularly so when she had responded to a voice and was awaiting its reaction. Although agreeing with her diagnosis of schizophrenia, she saw voices as disembodied beings and she felt compelled to listen, frequently carrying out everyday commands such as 'Phone your mother', or 'Leave the queue', even when she didn't want to do this.*

The formulation proposed that Julia had developed an engaged, but anxious relationship with her voices, in which her frequent responding to voices and anxious listening to see what they might say next augmented their frequency. Her coping objective was solely emotion control, usually through compliance with commands or avoidance of going out. Compliance acted as a form of safety behaviour that reinforced the perceived power of her voices—fears of retribution for non-compliance could never be tested. Because collaboration with the therapist was good, and engagement with voices so frequent, distancing strategies were chosen as the initial focus.

Interventions: Coping with and diminishing hallucinations

Coping interventions can be divided into three main groups: disengagement, coping with emotions, and directly influencing the voice. These core interventions may be supported by the management of environments and triggers, and minimization of maladaptive strategies. An outline of these interventions is followed by a presentation of the steps that can be taken to implement a coping interventions approach.

Disengagement

Voice hearers frequently get drawn into responding to the *content* of the voice. The SACMOV model suggests that coping can be improved by helping the person disengage from the symptom, preferably learning to appraise the *presence of the voice* as being the problem to be coped with, rather than the content of the voice. Disengagement may have short-term emotion-coping benefits: standing back from the experience can defuse emotion, and noticing the voice as a recurring experience can feed into growing self-efficacy. It also prepares for problem-focused coping: In the moment, it may allow space to decide what to do about the problem; and in the longer term, thinking about voices as an experience can hasten psychoeducation and foster more adaptive coping styles.

Strategies

1. *Describing the experience of voices.* Disengagement can start by encouraging the person to become an interested observer of their voices and to share their observations with another. 'Focussing Therapy' (Haddock *et al.*, 1996) illustrates how to take an observer stance whilst building confidence in sharing the detail of voice experiences. Conceptualized as a form of 'desensitization', the process starts by asking clients to describe the physical characteristics of voices, such as loudness or tone (which may be less anxiety provoking to disclose), before encouraging sharing of the content of what is heard.

2. *Systematic monitoring of voices.* Monitoring, too, can take a graded approach, starting with recording voice frequency and distress between sessions, and adding elements as required to further assess phenomenology or coping implementation. Monitoring itself can lead to a reduction in voice frequency (Sims, 1998). Where hallucinators decline monitoring homework, retrospectively completing the monitoring during a session can give experience in the desired observing stance.

3. *Practicing mindfulness.* Mindfulness is an attitude of non-judgemental acceptance of inner experiences (Shawyer, Farhall, Sims, & Copolov, 2005). It means noticing and accepting the presence of the voice without necessarily trying to change or suppress it, hopefully coming to see that such disengagement frees one to choose actions that are more compatible with valued goals. Clinicians familiar with mindfulness therapies can apply simple techniques to help the hallucinator develop an attitude of non-judgemental acceptance. This can start with mindfulness of the breath, and then incorporate mindfulness of sounds, of thoughts, and of voices.

4. *Practicing tolerance.* Where therapists are not familiar with mindfulness, and the client is willing, an exposure paradigm can be an alternative (Herrmann-Doig *et al.*, 2003). Relaxation is learned and practiced in the absence of voices, and then the hallucinator is encouraged to bring voices on in the session whilst practicing relaxation, in order to build tolerance of an experience that is difficult to prevent.

5. *Self-instruction.* Disengagement from voices can also be supported by self-instructions, such as, 'It's my voice again. That's OK. I'll let it be and get on with what I want to do'. These work best where the person *wants* to stop being caught up by the voice or doing what it says. If the voice is very attention-getting, successful disengagement may be difficult; however, some degree of distancing via continuous self-talk may still be possible: 'It's becoming insistent now, so I'll just talk out loud and describe it...It's very

loud now, and it is saying the same stuff as yesterday'. Collaboratively devising a cue card, with helpful information and self-talk, may assist.

Coping with distress arising from hallucinations ('Emotion-focused coping')

Emotion management is a natural starting point for collaborative assistance, especially where people are distressed or annoyed by voices. It leads naturally to a coping enhancement approach because natural emotion-focused coping strategies are easy to identify, but usually insufficient. Where the person is ambivalent about, or intimidated by voices, emotion-coping strategies may be more acceptable than strategies aimed at reducing voices. However, the aim of therapy should be to rely more on distancing and problem strategies for their adaptive advantages over time.

Strategies

1. *Reducing tension.* Some natural coping strategies are aimed at tension reduction or self-soothing. These include relaxing, taking a bath, or listening to calming music, as well as release of tension through physical exercise. Hallucinators' use of risky strategies such as alcohol or other substances may also be directed at tension reduction. Identifying the objective of these attempts to cope and their level of success, and then discussing together their disadvantages and possible alternatives may build motivation towards replacement with more adaptive actions.

2. *Changing thinking.* Cognitive coping also plays a role in management of emotion. This ranges from simple self-talk, such as, 'You'll be OK', 'Keep calm'; to self instruction 'I'll leave them alone and listen to the music—then I'll feel better'; to recall of psychoeducation 'It's just my mind playing tricks again'; 'I'm not a freak—Lots of people hear voices' or de-catastrophizing self-talk 'They always go away', 'They are just bully voices—words can't harm me'.

Interrupting, reducing, and stopping hallucinations

The evidence reviewed earlier that certain techniques can interrupt or inhibit the experience of a hallucinated voice provides a powerful base for crafting possible coping strategies, as well as an explanation for the apparent effectiveness of some natural strategies.

Strategies

1. *Distraction.* Regularly listening to voices makes the experience more likely to recur through sensitization or via associative connections. Distraction strategies can break this cycle and bring relief by deliberately redirecting attention away from voices. Attention can be redirected via thinking ('I'm going to see if I can remember every track of my favourite music CD' or 'I'll count backwards from 100') or by doing activities likely to draw attention away from internal preoccupations (e.g., playing ball with the dog). If voices are particularly persistent, thought-stopping techniques (Lamontagne, Audet, & Elie, 1983) may be used to interrupt the flow of the voice and enable engagement in an alternative distracting activity. Note that interrupting or redirecting attention should not be confused with *suppression*. Directly trying to stop

listening to or thinking about a voice paradoxically focuses attention on it (to see if it is being suppressed!), thus defeating the intention of the action.

2. *Auditory competition.* A rationale along the lines of 'Our brains can't concentrate on too many things at once, so they automatically tune into what seems most important', can be followed by discussion of strategies that include highly salient auditory input. Try working together on strategies that include louder volumes, enjoyable sounds, personal meaning, familiarity, and where possible, social reinforcers (e.g., conversations, listening to music together).

3. *Subvocalization.* The model of voices as misattributed subvocal speech suggests a range of strategies aimed at interrupting and replacing such subvocalization. These can involve subvocalizing (e.g., talking to oneself or reading silently) or vocalizing (e.g., talking to someone, singing, humming, reading out loud).

Julia *Capitalizing on Julia's monitoring, distancing work proceeded through conversations about the voices as a phenomenon, identifying that the more she responded to a voice, the more it seemed to be there, and that, conversely, when she didn't respond, it often 'gave up' and 'went away'. She was able to 'name' some recurring patterns, such as 'It's the telling-me-what-to-do voice'. Although she gained some distance on the phenomenon when voices were not present, it was still difficult for her to deliberately disengage. This led to the introduction of some mindfulness skills. Julia practiced mindfulness of the breath in sessions and at home, focusing on just noticing sounds and thoughts without responding to them, gently returning attention to the breath each time. She enjoyed these exercises and progressed to role play practice through a version of the acceptance and commitment therapy exercise, 'Taking your mind for a walk' (Hayes, Strosahl, & Wilson, 1999). Julia's task was to walk out of the building to the next street and back whilst letting her voices 'do their own thing'. In the exercise, her therapist walked just behind her, playing the role of her voices by commenting on her actions and giving commands to return before the goal was reached. After a few practices, she felt buoyed by her success and confident about not responding to her voices. A simple plan of how to cope was agreed, using self-instructions written on a card she carried: (1) When you notice voices, stop and think. (2) Try to name the pattern; e.g., 'It's the voices commenting on what I'm doing', (3) Mindfully disengage asking yourself, 'What do I want to do in the situation? Keep 'walking' and leave the voices alone!' At completion of therapy, she rated this work as having been the most helpful.*

Minimizing and replacing maladaptive strategies

Three common maladaptive responses to voice, and a coping strategy for each, are briefly considered in this section. *Safety behaviours* are actions aimed at avoiding anxiety-related situations. Although such avoidance may bring short-term relief, it prevents the person from mastering the situation or discovering that their fears are exaggerated or unfounded (e.g., not going out for fear that voices will criticize), and the avoidance becomes self-perpetuating.

Strategy:

> *Name and gently confront fears.* Identifying the pattern, discussing the fears, and building confidence in strategies that are effective in the situation, through graded practice, can be a way to proceed.

Self-harming strategies frequently have as their objective of coping either voice cessation (e.g., ear-stuffing; head banging), tension reduction (e.g., cutting of skin), or self-soothing (e.g., smoking tobacco; using illegal drugs). As well as having health risks, these may in addition be maladaptive because of avoidance or by focusing attention internally rather than on the real world.

Strategy:

Discuss risks and alternatives. Working with the person to recognize the risks and develop effective alternatives can be an important part of a coping intervention.

Angry engagement (e.g., yelling back at the voice) is a common pattern of interaction, especially where voices are frequent or predominantly abusive. Typically such interactions increase the likelihood that voices will remain—an emotional response by a voice-hearer will frequently be followed by an expectation (and sometimes fear) of a response from the voice, increasing the likelihood of the encounter being prolonged.

Strategy:

Disengagement. Strategies include exposing the pattern and observing that the voice is more likely to stay; and, if relevant, characterizing the voice as a bully and discussing strategies for managing bullying including disengagement and decatastrophization.

Working with triggers and the environment

Where the assessment has identified situational, emotional, or stimulation-related antecedents, these may be a focus for collaborative or sometimes unilateral intervention.

Strategies:

1. Create *optimal stimulation* levels: Avoid both sensory monotony (e.g., lying awake in bed, nothing to do) and sensory overload (e.g., being overwhelmed by the noise and chaos of a busy shopping centre).

2. Reduce or *manage specific triggers.* The presence of voices has been associated with anxiety and fluctuations of daily stress (Myin-Germeys & van Os, 2007). Some triggers for voices (e.g., anxiety about being in crowds) may require support or therapy to manage.

3. Avoid and *interrupt preoccupation* and engulfment. Absorption in voices and other internal psychotic processes risks elaboration and reinforcement as well as reducing opportunities for rewards from engagement in the real world. Preoccupation can be minimized by activity scheduling, arranging visitors, and engaging environments (e.g., day programs). Activities that involve *competing auditory or verbal stimuli* (e.g., using a personal music player; conversation with others) can be used for prevention as well as interruption when voices are a problem.

Reduction of triggers that give rise to hallucinations (e.g., listening to TV) and changing environments (e.g., low external stimulation) can be done independently of insight. The case of Robert illustrates a simple attempt to change the environment, and to enhance verbal control of behaviour.

Robert *Robert, a 40-year-old man in a residential facility had heard voices many times a day for the past 20 years, and had little insight that they were part of a mental health problem. The referral noted two concerns about his voices—their contribution to his self-absorption and withdrawal, and their occasional prompting of inappropriate behaviour. Every few months, Robert would wait outside the house of a woman he erroneously believed to be one of the voices to politely ask her to stop harassing him. This had led to a court order that prohibited him from her street. Although co-operative with treatment and at times quite distressed by voices, he could not contemplate the possibility of directing any action towards them, saying that the voices 'wouldn't like that' or that he might 'miss something important'. Treatment centred on reducing preoccupation by structuring his day and encouraging him to listen to the radio and favourite music. Staff informally monitored his voice experiences, being alert for any comments connecting the voice with the woman. They took these and other natural opportunities to remind him of the court order, for example by prompting his recall that he had been apprehended by the police and found it stressful. Over time, he settled into a more active pattern of activity and did not visit the house.*

Implementing a coping strategy approach for voices

The implementation approach is outlined below in numbered steps starting from those more likely to be used earlier. However, the 'steps' are simply a guide—in practice, the selection and ordering of steps should be prompted by the formulation, and capitalize on opportunities that arise as the work progresses. The preventive and environmental strategies that families and clinicians may use where insight or co-operation are currently barriers to collaborative work are added at the end.

The starting phase

1. *Engage and assess.* For some voice-hearers, it is a relief to discuss in detail their experiences with someone who obviously understands; however, others can be wary of disclosing a symptom, or be instructed by their voice to keep what it says as a 'secret'. The assessment tasks presented in Table 12.1 can be commenced at first contact but do not need to be completed before goal setting and initial interventions begin—building an effective working relationship and a purpose for meeting should be the priority in initial sessions.

2. *Set goals together.* Agreeing on a goal for working with voices helps to clarify the relationship and to focus both hallucinator and therapist on relevant actions, including monitoring whether the therapy is helpful. Examples of agreed goals are 'reducing distress' or 'not letting the voices interfere with my life'. Remember that medication-resistant voices are relatively impervious to change, so avoid agreeing with proposed goals about stopping voices, instead reframe them in terms of reducing distress, or getting on with life regardless of what the voices may say.

3. *Identify precipitants.* Clinical assessment or self-monitoring may identify stressors or environments that are associated with voices onset. Stressors may be situational (e.g., going to church, sitting in my room), and they probably work through the associated

emotional states (e.g., anxiety, loneliness), thus, assessing the emotional response to the situation as well as identifying any trigger can be helpful. Try to change these where this is viable (e.g., problem-solve the anxiety about going to church, phone a friend or relative when home and feeling lonely).

Implementing core interventions

4. *Commence disengagement strategies.* As early as possible, maximize the opportunities for the voice hearer to step back from the experience and notice it as a phenomenon, especially where the automatic response is engulfment or engagement with voices. The assessment process provides natural opportunities for this through the person describing their experiences and through monitoring. Focusing can build on this, and for some people, building skill in mindful distancing may be a key coping strategy.

5. *Identify, normalize, and 'label' natural coping strategies.* Note that coping is a natural thing to do and give examples of different strategies reported by other hallucinators, particularly problem-focused strategies. Labelling of behaviour supports the process of distancing and can build a shared vocabulary about working with voices (e.g., 'When you heard the voice this morning, did you deliberately do anything to cope/to feel better/to make the voice go away?' 'I'd call going outside and having a cigarette a *coping strategy*')

6. *Reinforce promising natural coping strategies.* Support strategies that seem to be adaptive, in order to build self-efficacy (e.g., 'Did you do anything to cope when you were at the football with your dad and you heard those voices? ...So you were able to survive by taking a few slow breaths and talking with your father, even though you were worried about the people behind you! That's great—tell me how you managed to do it...'). Where a promising strategy is in the person's repertoire, try to enhance its effectiveness by more routine implementation, fine-tuning its execution, troubleshooting any difficulties, strengthening via in-session practice, and broadening the repertoire by addition of alternative versions.

7. *Introduce or improve emotion-focused coping.* Discuss coping strategies used by the client, noting whether each strategy is aimed at emotion-focused coping, problem-focused coping, or prevention. The success of the person's emotion-focused strategies can be reviewed at this point, and for promising strategies, any barriers to implementation identified and addressed (see below). Where the person has a limited repertoire of effective strategies, introduce them to the three groups of emotion-coping strategies and encourage them to try out at least one new strategy from each.

8. *Introduce or improve strategies likely to reduce voices.* Check whether any natural coping strategy used by the client is likely to have an inhibiting effect on hallucinations via subvocalization or by increasing the prominence of external auditory stimuli. If likely to be accepted by the person, explain the mechanism of action in order to foster generalization of the principle of subvocalization or competing auditory stimuli.

9. *Reduce maladaptive strategies.* This work may commence early if the person is aware of the risks or ineffectiveness, but may need to wait until engagement has strengthened and some initial successes have been achieved if the maladaptive patterns are central.

10. *Work with triggers and the environment.* This can be integrated at any point, and where insight is poor, the work can proceed without explicit links to voice reduction, as described earlier.

Maximizing learning

11. *Encourage a learning approach.* Consider framing the therapy as a process of learning about voices and how to get on with life. This can support useful therapy elements including (1) a trial-and-error approach to finding effective strategies, (2) the use of personalized workbooks, which take the person through exercises such as identifying goals, evaluating coping strategies, monitoring for triggers and recording homework tasks (e.g., Coleman & Smith, 1997), and (3) psychoeducative input about coping and the relative effectiveness of strategies, which, depending on the client, may be explained in scientific terms or as ways to cope that others have found helpful.

12. *In-session demonstration and rehearsal of coping* is recommended. However, this may be anxiety provoking for those who have performance anxiety, low self-esteem, thought blocking, or for those whose voices are too powerful for the person to dare to so publicly move against them. Very easy in-session steps that disconfirm expectations of trouble from voices can build confidence (e.g., 'Let's start by just planning what might be good to do, and see how you go… OK, so you noticed the voice have a go at you about that—did you survive it? …you have put up with much worse that—great! Let's have a practice of the reading-out-loud strategy..')

13. *Cue recall of strategies.* Hallucinators sometimes fail to use a strategy in their repertoire, because they do not recall it in the situations where it is relevant. This may be because of engulfment in the voice experience or because the strategy is situation-specific (e.g., singing or whistling are usually only applicable when one is alone—they may cause social embarrassment when on the bus!). Listing strategies the person finds effective alongside situations where each can be used may enhance memory. Carrying such strategy lists on cue cards means that only the presence of the list needs to be recalled on the spot, rather than all strategies.

Addressing complexities

14. *Troubleshoot barriers to strategy use.* Potentially effective coping strategies, both natural and new, may be impeded by implementation barriers. The SACMOV model suggests three barriers to be alert to. The *perceived difficulty* of a useful strategy may mean that it is rarely tried (e.g., ignoring unfair comments by voices). *Self-efficacy* can also be a barrier (e.g., having little confidence about one's performance may get in the way of starting a conversation), as can a pessimistic *expectancy of outcome* i.e., predicting that the strategy probably will not work (e.g., 'The voice will probably just say

worse things if I do that'). Problem-solving, support, and experimentation can all be helpful in addressing barriers.

15. *Extend the coping repertoire.* Where auditory hallucinations are problematic, trialling of coping strategies across several types is encouraged (e.g., 'Would you like to hear of some coping strategies that other people have found helpful for voices?') A printed list of strategies and their consumer-rated usefulness can be a good discussion starter (e.g., Fig. 12.2).

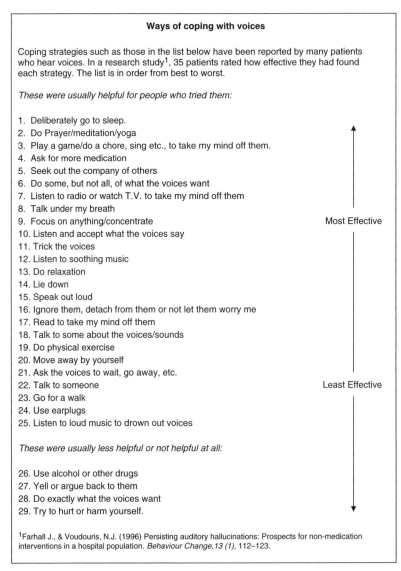

Ways of coping with voices

Coping strategies such as those in the list below have been reported by many patients who hear voices. In a research study[1], 35 patients rated how effective they had found each strategy. The list is in order from best to worst.

These were usually helpful for people who tried them:

1. Deliberately go to sleep.
2. Do Prayer/meditation/yoga
3. Play a game/do a chore, sing etc., to take my mind off them.
4. Ask for more medication
5. Seek out the company of others
6. Do some, but not all, of what the voices want
7. Listen to radio or watch T.V. to take my mind off them
8. Talk under my breath
9. Focus on anything/concentrate
10. Listen and accept what the voices say
11. Trick the voices
12. Listen to soothing music
13. Do relaxation
14. Lie down
15. Speak out loud
16. Ignore them, detach from them or not let them worry me
17. Read to take my mind off them
18. Talk to some about the voices/sounds
19. Do physical exercise
20. Move away by yourself
21. Ask the voices to wait, go away, etc.
22. Talk to someone
23. Go for a walk
24. Use earplugs
25. Listen to loud music to drown out voices

These were usually less helpful or not helpful at all:

26. Use alcohol or other drugs
27. Yell or argue back to them
28. Do exactly what the voices want
29. Try to hurt or harm yourself.

Most Effective

Least Effective

[1]Farhall J., & Voudouris, N.J. (1996) Persisting auditory hallucinations: Prospects for non-medication interventions in a hospital population. *Behaviour Change, 13 (1),* 112–123.

Fig. 12.2 Coping list for discussion with patients.

Issues and directions

Limitations of the coping strategies literature

In many ways, the coping literature on voices is limited as a guide to practitioners. First, although there are some helpful observations about the extent and nature of coping strategies and their effectiveness, most studies are descriptive and make no attempt to control for phases of disorder or situational factors. For example, voices in psychosis may be problematic because their unrelenting frequency is so distracting or because their content evokes distressing responses, but the coping literature gives no guide as to what strategies may be most relevant to different phenomenological presentations. Neither does the literature cast much light on why voices continue to be problematic even when hallucinators can report strategies for coping. Are the strategies ineffective? Are useful strategies not retrieved in the stress of the encounter with the voice? And exactly what are coping strategies directed at? Are hallucinators primarily directing their efforts at stopping the voice, as the strategy effectiveness measures seem to assume, or is the primary objective of coping, the management of difficult emotions in the presence of a persisting stressor? These are questions that are very pertinent for clinicians to ask to understand and enhance the process of coping. In this chapter, we have suggested a model to structure clinical formulations to address such issues.

What is the aim of treatment of voices?

A treatment goal of reduction or cessation of voices dominates the research literature and is often assumed by hallucinators and workers to be the ultimate goal of treatment, but this view can be limiting, for several reasons. First, voice reduction is but one possible pathway to the more important goal of living a more fulfilling life, and the hallucinators whose symptoms persist (and their supporters) need to be focused on getting on with life, and using coping strategies in the service of this goal, rather than being overly preoccupied with voice reduction. Second, a minority of voice hearers with psychoses appraise their voices as primarily benevolent—these voices may be experienced as a guide or companion, and may not be something the person wishes to (or needs to) relinquish, although they may be associated with poorer social functioning (Favrod, Grasset, Spreng, Grossenbacher, & Hode, 2001). Given the investment of some consumers in their 'positive' voices, the therapeutic aim may be to retain or even utilize positive voices whilst weakening negative voices. The decision about this will rely on a judgement about what is the best pragmatic route to improved adaptation. Finally, for hallucinators who are quite unwell, and those with limited resources for adaptation, reduction of distress, and where possible, acceptance and coping with ongoing symptoms may be valuable adaptive outcomes.

The effectiveness of strategies

Enhancement of coping strategies for voices is frequently adopted as a therapeutic approach, yet the efficacy of strategies is still surprisingly under-researched, and few therapeutic packages specifically report the outcomes of coping enhancement for voices.

Our model suggests that the approach to evaluation has been very limited—asking voice hearers about the effectiveness of lists of strategies suffers from limitations of self-report, but more importantly, it ignores the different objectives of coping and situational factors that may make the difference between an action being effective or not (e.g., yelling back at a voice may be rated by one person as highly effective, because it helped them feel better in the short-term, or interrupted the voice, whereas it may be rated by another as ineffective because the voice always returns and is more critical).

For clinicians, two directions are suggested by this literature. Given that a large variety of strategies is claimed as at least moderately effective by voice hearers, a trial-and-error approach makes sense, perhaps utilizing lists of strategies reported by other voice hearers (e.g., Fig. 12.2) to help engage the client in choosing new actions. Given the evidence that strategies apparently utilizing competing auditory stimuli, distraction, and subvocalization may inhibit processes underpinning voice activity or conscious awareness of it, strategies with these elements should have some priority.

Styles of adaptation

The research on coping with voices has focused on strategies, but adaptation may be more fundamentally determined by coping style. The factors identified in factor analytic studies (O'Sullivan, 1994; Farhall & Gehrke, 1997) and the notion of 'orientation' to voices referred to by Ramanathan (1984) seem to capture at a more general level some fundamentally different styles of response to voices. Interestingly, these styles appear to be variations of active and passive engagement and disengagement; the disengaged styles echoing the 'acceptance' of voices orientation of good copers described by Romme and Escher (1989). Research is needed to establish what styles of adaptation are most adaptive and the extent to which these may be modified or learned through therapy.

Simple model: Complex phenomenon

The model of coping and the steps for implementing coping enhancement may appear to be a straightforward approach to therapy. It is certainly true that the essential ideas of stress–appraisal–coping theory are logical and the notion of enhancing naturally occurring strategies easy to learn. However, this does not mean that implementation is always easy. Hallucinations are very powerful experiences—they are perceptually compelling (it is hard to ignore them), they may appear unpredictably, and consumers often are 'listening' for them. This means that simple coping and distraction techniques may be less effective than expected, unless they are crafted to compete effectively with the salience of the hallucinatory experiences. In addition, the content of hallucinations (and delusions) is not random—often it appears to be a distortion of emotionally salient material such as unfinished interpersonal business, doubts about sexuality, fearful and guilt-ridden themes relating to past events, and exposure of, or reactions against, inadequacy and threats to identity or integrity of the person. In this context, the formulation should seek to understand why particular material is present and consider whether other therapeutic assistance may be needed to address emotionally important material, possibly at the same time as the symptom-focused work described here.

There may be a complex relationship between the person and the voice, especially where the voice has been present for long periods (Benjamin, 1989; Soppitt & Birchwood, 1997). Such relationships may be reflective of other relationships in the person's life, especially those in which the person has been subordinated (Birchwood, Meaden, Trower, Gilbert, & Plaistow, 2000). A further complexity is the web of beliefs in which hallucinations are typically embedded. Such beliefs may directly interfere with even the notion of coping ('It's wrong to interrupt voices—they are a gift from God').

Command hallucinations (see Meaden, Birchwood & Trower, this volume) that instruct the hearer to take risky or dangerous actions can be stressful for the hearer and those around them. However, because the risk of compliance is greater where the voice is appraised as positive as opposed to being a threat (Shawyer *et al.*, 2008), engaging the hallucinator through an assumption that they wish to 'cope' with the commands may be misguided, and other strategies such as values clarification (Hayes, Strosahl, & Wilson, 1999), belief modification, or external controls may be required.

What if more than coping is needed?

The simplicity and flexibility of a coping strategy approach underpin a wide applicability, which is attested to by the range of contexts in which it has been reported (self-help, integrated into case management, group programs, CBT for psychosis, comprehensive hallucinations treatments, etc). However, the complexities raised in the preceding section illustrate that there are limits to what a coping-only paradigm can offer, and coping strategy enhancement may need to be supplemented by belief modification, psychoeducation, or therapy driven by formulations about the content or function of the voices. Other chapters in this book illustrate a range of alternative and additional treatments.

References

Allen, H. A., Halperin, J., & Friend, R. (1985). Removal and diversion tactics and the control of auditory hallucinations. *Behav Res Ther*, **23**(5), 601–605.

Bach, P., & Hayes, S. C. (2002). The use of acceptance and commitment therapy to prevent rehospitalization of psychotic patients: A randomized controlled trial. *J Consult Clin Psychol*, **70**(5), 1129–1139.

Benjamin, L. S. (1989). Is chronicity a function of the relationship between the person and the auditory hallucination? *Schizophr Bull*, **15**(2), 291–310.

Bick, P. A., & Kinsbourne, M. (1987). Auditory hallucinations and subvocal speech in schizophrenic patients. *Am J Psychiatry*, **144**(2), 222–225.

Birchwood, M. (1986). Control of auditory hallucinations through occlusion of monaural auditory input. *Br J Psychiatry*, **149**, 104–107.

Birchwood, M., Meaden, A., Trower, P., Gilbert, P., & Plaistow, J. (2000). The power and omnipotence of voices: Subordination and entrapment by voices and significant others. *Psychol Med*, **30**, 337–344.

Buccheri, R., Trygstad, L., Kanas, N., Waldron, B., & Dowling, G. (1996). Auditory hallucinations in schizophrenia. Group experience in examining symptom management and behavioral strategies. *J Psychosoc Nurs*, **34**(2), 12–26.

Buccheri, R., Trygstad, L., Dowling, G., *et al.* (2004). Long-term effects of teaching behavioral strategies for managing persistent auditory hallucinations. *J Psychosoc Nurs*, **42**(1), 18–27.

Carr, V. J., & Katsikitis, M. (1987). Illness behaviour and schizophrenia. *Psychiatr Med*, **5**(2), 163–170.

Carter, D. M., Mackinnon, A., & Copolov, D. L. (1996). Patients' strategies for coping with auditory hallucinations. *J Nerv Ment Dis*, **184**(3), 159–164.

Chadwick, P., Birchwood, M., & Trower, P. (1996). *Cognitive therapy for delusions, voices and paranoia.* Chichester: Wiley.

Chadwick, P. (2005). Mindfulness groups for people with psychosis. *Behav Cogn Psychother*, **33**, 351–359.

Coleman, R., & Smith, M. (1997). *Working with voices!* Merseyside: Handsell Publications.

David, A. S., Woodruff, P. W., Howard, R., *et al.* (1996). Auditory hallucinations inhibit exogenous activation of auditory association cortex. *NeuroReport*, **7**, 932–936.

Done, D. J., Frith, C. D., & Owens, D. C. (1986). Reducing persistent auditory hallucinations by wearing an ear-plug. *Br J Clin Psychol*, **25**, 151–152.

Drury, V., Birchwood, M., Cochrane, R., & Macmillan, F. (1996). Cognitive therapy and recovery from acute psychosis: A controlled trial. I. Impact on psychotic symptoms. *Br J Psychiatry*, **169**, 593–601.

Falloon, I. R. H., & Talbot, R. E. (1981). Persistent auditory hallucinations: Coping mechanisms and implications for management. *Psychol Med*, **11**, 329–339.

Farhall, J., & Voudouris, N. J. (1996). Persisting auditory hallucinations: Prospects for non-medication interventions in a hospital population. *Behav Change*, **13**(1), 112–123.

Farhall, J., & Gehrke, M. J. (1997). Coping with hallucinations: Exploring a stress and coping framework. *Br J Clin Psychol*, **36**, 259–261.

Farhall, J., & Cotton, S. (2002). Implementing psychological treatment for symptoms of psychosis in an area mental health service: The response of patients, therapists and managers. *J Ment Health*, **11**(5), 511–522.

Farhall, J., Greenwood, K. M., & Jackson, H. J. (2007). Coping with hallucinated voices in schizophrenia: A review of self-initiated strategies and therapeutic interventions. *Clin Psychol Rev*, **27**, 476–493.

Favrod, J., Grasset, F., Spreng, S., Grossenbacher, B., & Hode, Y. (2001). Benevolent voices are not so kind: The functional significance of auditory hallucinations *Psychopathology*, **37**, 304–308.

Fowler, D., Garety, P. A., & Kuipers, E. (1995). *Cognitive behaviour therapy for psychosis.* Chichester: Wiley.

Fowler, D., Garety, P. A., & Kuipers, E. (1998). Cognitive therapy for psychosis: Formulation, treatment effects and service implications. *J Ment Health*, **7**(2), 123–133.

Frederick, J. A., & Cotanch, P. (1995). Self-help techniques for auditory hallucinations in schizophrenia. *Issues Ment Health Nurs*, **16**, 213–224.

Gallagher, A. G., Dinan, T. G., & Baker, L. V. J. (1995). The effects of varying information content and speaking aloud on auditory hallucinations. *Br J Med Psychol*, **68**, 143–155.

Gaudiano, B. A., & Herbert, J. D. (2006). Acute treatment of inpatients with psychotic symptoms using acceptance and commitment therapy: Pilot results. *Behav Res Ther*, **44**(3), 415–437.

Green P. (1978). Defective interhemispheric transfer in schizophrenia. *J Abnorm Psychol*, **87**(5), 472–480.

Green, M. F., & Kinsbourne, M. (1990). Subvocal activity and auditory hallucinations: Clues for behavioural treatments? *Schizophr Bull*, **16**(4), 617–625.

Haddock, G., Bentall, R. P., & Slade, P. D. (1996). Psychological treatment of auditory hallucinations: Focusing or distraction? In G. Haddock & P. D. Slade (Eds.), *Cognitive-behavioural interventions with psychotic disorders* (pp. 45–70). London: Routledge.

Haddock, G., Slade, P. D., Bentall, R. P., Reid, D., & Faragher, E. B. (1998). A comparison of the long-term effectiveness of distraction and focussing in the treatment of auditory hallucinations. *Br J Med Psychol*, **17**, 339–349.

Hayashi, N., Igarashi, Y., Suda, K., & Nakagawa, S., (2007). Auditory hallucination coping techniques and their relationship to psychotic symptomatology. *Psychiatry Clin Neurosci*, **61**(6), 640–645.

Hayes, S. C., Strosahl, K. D., & Wilson, K. G. (1999). *Acceptance and commitment therapy: An experiential approach to behavior change.* New York: Guilford Press.

Herrmann-Doig, T., Maude, D., & Edwards, J. (2003). *Systematic treatment of persistent psychosis (STOPP): A psychological approach to facilitating recovery in young people with first episode psychosis.* London: Martin Dunitz.

Hogarty, G. E., Kornblith, S. J., Greenwald, D., *et al.* (1995). Personal therapy: A disorder-relevant psychotherapy for schizophrenia. *Schizophr Bull*, **21**, 379–393.

Jenner, J. A., Nienhuis, F. J., Wiersma, D., & van de Willige, G. (2004). Hallucination focussed integrative treatment: A randomised controlled trial. *Schizophr Bull*, **30**(1), 133–145.

Johns, L. C., Hemsley, D., & Kuipers, E. (2002). A comparison of auditory hallucinations in a psychiatric and non-psychiatric group. *Br J Clin Psychol*, **41**, 81–86.

Kingdon, D. G., & Turkington, D. (1994). *Cognitive-behavioral therapy of schizophrenia.* New York: The Guilford Press.

Lamontagne, Y., Audet, N., & Elie, R. (1983). Thought-stopping for delusions and hallucinations: A pilot study. *Behavioural Psychotherapy*, **11**, 177–184.

Lazarus, R. S., & Folkman, S. (1984). *Stress, appraisal, and coping.* New York: Springer.

Liberman, R. P. (1988). *Social and independent living skills. Symptom management module.* Los Angeles: Clinical Research Center for Schizophrenia and Psychiatric Rehabilitation.

Liberman, R. P., Kopelowicz, A., & Young, A. S. (1994). Biobehavioral treatment and rehabilitation of schizophrenia. *Behavior Therapy*, **25**, 89–107.

Margo, A., Hemsley, D. R., & Slade, P. D. (1981). The effects of varying auditory input on schizophrenic hallucinations. *Br J Psychiatry*, **139**, 122–127.

Maxwell, J. (2008). *Coping with hearing voices: Augmenting family carer responses with psychological management strategies.* Doctor of Psychology Thesis, School of Psychological Science, La Trobe University, Bundoora, Australia.

Morley S. (1987). Modification of auditory hallucinations: Experimental studies of headphones and earplugs. *Behavioural Psychotherapy*, **15**, 240–251.

Myin-Germeys, I. & van Os, J. (2007). Stress-reactivity in psychosis: Evidence for an affective pathway to psychosis. *Clin Psychol Rev*, **27**(4), 409–434.

Nayani, T. H., & David, A. S. (1996). The auditory hallucination: A phenomenological survey. *Psychol Med*, **26**, 177–189.

Nelson, H. E., Thrasher, S., & Barnes, T. R. E. (1991). Practical ways of alleviating auditory hallucinations. *Br Med J*, **302**, 327.

O'Sullivan, K. (1994). Dimensions of coping with auditory hallucinations. *J Ment Health*, **3**, 351–361.

Perlman, L. M., & Hubbard, B. A. (2000). A self-control skills group for persistent auditory hallucinations. *Cogn Behav Pract*, **7**(1), 17–21.

Pinto, A., La Pia, S., Mennella, R., Georgio, D., & DeSimone, L. (1999). Cognitive-behavioural therapy and clozapine for clients with treatment-refractory schizophrenia. *Psychiatr Serv*, **50**(7), 901–904.

Ramanathan, A. (1984). A study of coping with auditory hallucinations in schizophrenics. *Indian J Psychiatry*, **26**(3), 229–236.

Rector, N. A., & Beck, A. T. (2002). Cognitive therapy for schizophrenia: From conceptualisation to intervention. *Can J Psychiatry*, **47**(1), 39–48.

Romme, M., & Escher, A. (1989). Hearing voices. *Schizophr Bull*, **15**(2), 209–216.

Shawyer, F., Farhall, J., Sims, E., & Copolov, D. (2005). Command hallucinations in psychosis: Acceptance and disengagement as a focus of treatment. In M. Jackson & G. Murphy (Eds.), *Theory and practice in contemporary Australian cognitive and behaviour therapy: Proceedings of the 28th AACBT Conference* (pp. 5–14). Melbourne: Australian Association for Cognitive and Behaviour Therapy.

Shawyer, F., Mackinnon, A., Farhall, J., *et al.* (2008). Acting on harmful command hallucinations in psychotic disorders: An integrative approach. *J Nerv Ment Dis*, **196**(5), 300–308.

Sims, E. (1998). *Factors influencing the implementation of coping strategies for auditory hallucinations.* Australia: Honours Thesis, School of Psychological Science, La Trobe University.

Singh, G., Sharan, P., & Kulhara, P. (2003). Role of coping strategies and attitudes in mediating distress due to hallucinations in schizophrenia. *Psychiatry Clin Neurosci*, **57**, 517–522.

Slade, P. D. (1994). Models of hallucination: From theory to practice. In A. S. David & J. C. Cutting (Eds.), *The neuropsychology of schizophrenia*. London: Lawrence Erlbaum Associates.

Soppitt, R. W., & Birchwood, M. (1997). Depression, beliefs, voice content and topography: A cross-sectional study of schizophrenic patients with auditory verbal hallucinations. *J Ment Health*, **6**, 525–532.

Tarrier, N. (1987). An investigation of residual psychotic symptoms in discharged schizophrenic patients. *Br J Clin Psychol*, **26**, 141–143.

Tarrier, N., Harwood, S., Yusopoff, L., Beckett, R., & Baker, A. (1990). Coping strategy enhancement (CSE): A method of treating residual schizophrenic symptoms. *Behavioural Psychotherapy*, **18**, 283–293.

Tarrier, N. (1992). Management and modification of residual positive psychotic symptoms. In M. Birchwood & N. Tarrier (Eds.), *Innovations in the psychological management of schizophrenia: Assessment, treatment and services* (pp. 147–169). Chichester: John Wiley & Sons.

Tarrier, N., Beckett, R., Harwood, S., Baker, A., Yusupoff, L., & Ugarteburu, I. (1993). A trial of two cognitive-behavioural methods of treating drug-resistant residual psychotic symptoms in schizophrenic patients: I. Outcome. *Br J Psychiatry*, **162**, 524–532.

Tarrier, N., Yusupoff, L., Kinney, C., *et al.* (1998). Randomised controlled trial of intensive cognitive behaviour therapy for patients with chronic schizophrenia. *Br Med J*, **317**, 303–307.

Tarrier, N., Kinney, C., McCarthy, E., *et al.* (2001). Are some types of psychotic symptoms more responsive to cognitive-behaviour therapy? *Behav Cogn Psychother*, **29**, 45–55.

Tsai, Y.F., & Ku, Y.C. (2005). Self-care symptom management strategies for auditory hallucinations among inpatients with schizophrenia at a veterans' hospital in Taiwan. *Arch Psychiatr Nurs*, **19**(4), 194–199.

Wahass, S., & Kent, G. (1997). Coping with auditory hallucinations: A cross-cultural comparison between western (British) and non-western (Saudi Arabian) patients. *J Nerv Ment Dis*, **185**, 664–668.

Wiersma, D., Jenner, J. A., van de Willige, G., Spakman, M., & Nienhuis, F. J. (2001). Cognitive behaviour therapy with coping training for persistent auditory hallucinations in schizophrenia: A naturalistic follow-up study of the durability of effects. *Acta Psychiatr Scand*, **103**, 393–399.

Wykes, T., Parr, A.-M., & Landau, S. (1999). Group treatment of auditory hallucinations. *Br J Psychiatry*, **175**, 180–185.

Wykes, T., Hayward, P., Thomas, N., *et al.* (2005). What are the effects of group cognitive behaviour therapy for voices? A randomised control trial. *Schizophrenia Research*, **77**, 201–210.

Zubin, J., & Spring, B. (1977). Vulnerability: A new view of schizophrenia. *J Abnorm Psychol*, **86**, 260–266.

Chapter 13

Personal history and hearing voices

Marius Romme and Sandra Escher

To position our chapter, we would like you to understand that our studies have focused on the experience of 'Voices and Visions' as people perceive them. As a consequence, we use their language and, for example, never talk about 'hallucinations' but rather about 'hearing voices'. In psychiatry, the word 'hallucination' is easily equated to a symptom of an illness. Although recent reviews about hallucinations acknowledge that they occur in healthy people (Aleman & Larøi, 2008), in psychiatric practice, voice hearers still come up against an unjustified psycho-pathological way of thinking (Romme *et al.*, 2009). Several epidemiological population surveys show that about 4% of the population experience voices and only a relatively small group is hindered by these experiences. Tien (1991) found that only about one-third suffer from them and are in need of some form of help. Van Os *et al.* (2001) showed that a far smaller part could indeed have fitted within the psychosis categories of the DSM.

Based on epidemiological studies, we work with the assumption that hearing voices, as such, is not a psycho-pathological phenomenon or a symptom of an illness, but rather a human variation in coping with emotions. Voices *per se* are a normal human reaction to trauma or stressful circumstances. However, it is the inability to cope with traumatic experiences and voices that might lead to illness. It is therefore up to the voice hearer to undertake a journey in which his/her experience is the starting point.

In this chapter, we would like to discuss the theoretical background behind our approach, how we gather information about the experience itself, how this information is used in a psychological formulation of the person's problems, what voice hearers themselves tell us about their recovery, and how all this information can be used in a therapy plan.

Our theoretical background stems from social psychiatry, which is a science that studies mental health problems in the context of their socio-emotional background. We were familiar with the fact that many mental problems are reactive patterns to socio-emotional problems in daily life and/or problems in the person's past and his/her upbringing. In our first study in 1987 (Romme & Escher, 1987), we already found a high percentage (70%) of trauma at the onset of voice hearing. By studying the experience more intensively, it became clear that this phenomenon is mostly a reactive pattern to very troublesome life experiences such as trauma or emotional neglect. This idea has more recently been acknowledged in many studies. Read *et al.* (2005) reviewed 180 studies and concluded that 'psychosis can be a reaction to traumatic experiences given the prevalence of such experiences in people with psychosis and the links to the form and content of psychotic experiences'. In this overview, there are several studies in which it also becomes clear that traumatic experiences are more prevalent in people with a history of serious mental illness like schizophrenia and manic-depressive psychosis than in the normal population (Mueser *et al.*, 1998). There are also some studies in which traumatic experiences are shown to be of causal importance with hallucinations (Spauwen *et al.*, 2006).

When linking life stories and voices, we feel in tune with the work of Watkins (2008) who wrote about hearing voices as a human variation, and White (1996) who developed a method he called 'Re-authoring lives'. White describes quite clearly the relationship between people's voice hearing and their life story and shows that voice hearers can gradually retake ownership of their lives when they learn about this relationship. This opinion is confirmed by the voice hearer Coleman (1997) who also describes the relationship between his voices and his life story in his process of recovery. He reports how in learning to cope with the traumatic experiences that were at the roots of his voice hearing experience, he was able to recover from the distress caused by his voices. It enabled him to take control of his life again.

Over the years, we have interviewed over 350 voice hearers within five different studies (Romme & Escher 1989, 1993; Romme, 1996; Escher, 2005; Romme *et al.*, 2009). In three of these studies, we compared voice hearers who were patients with those who never received care. In all of these studies, in about 70 to 80% of the voice hearers who became patients, their voices were related to endured and mostly long-term serious problems in their lives, which they experienced as traumatic. In our studies, we focused on the links between the kind of trauma and emotions involved and the characteristics of the voices. In particular, we specifically observed the importance of focusing on the experience itself in order to enable people to learn to cope with their voices, to accept them, and to stimulate the voice hearer to learn to cope with the problems that lay at their roots. This means coping with the memories of traumatic experiences and distorted emotions that are the consequence of these. Voices in patients must be seen as a signal of problems but should certainly not be the only point of interest in the mental healthcare of voice hearers. Although it is often thought that our research population was highly selective, the study of comparing 'healthy voice hearers' with 'patient voice hearers' (Romme, 1996; Honig *et al.*, 1998) was done with voice hearers who were still in hospital or only in the care of an out-patient department for chronic psychiatric patients with a background of psychosis and hospitalization. They were willing to talk about their voices because we were really interested in their experience and they did not risk getting more medication or encounter any further negative approaches when talking about their voices. The same applies to many people taking part in the recovery study (Romme *et al.*, 2009), these people suffered many years of rather senseless hospitalization and treatment with medication. Also a number of the children in the children's study had 'suffered' psychiatric treatment (Escher *et al.*, 2004).

Experience-based approach

Hearing voices is a very confusing experience. As Antje Muller explains (Romme *et al.*, 2009): 'I started hearing voices when I was in the third week at this new school. I had some real difficulties with mathematics. I had never had that before. I had already been sitting at my desk for 3 hours and simply did not know where to start. I got very agitated, when I heard a very clear voice saying: 'are you stupid?' After that, the voice laughed in a very unpleasant way. I did not know what was happening so I looked around me, but there was no one there. After half an hour, I thought I had imagined it. A day later, 'he', the voice, came back. It was during a mathematics lesson, and I was staring at my desk. The same voice said to me, 'there is no need to have a close look. You will never be able to understand this'. After that, he started to berate me. He belittled me. He told me that I was not able to do anything. After some minutes, two further voices joined him and they said the same things. So they were like a choir. Thereafter, they were there, not always talking but sometimes making noises. When they spoke, they always said the same things. The voices stayed with me for the next 13 years'. This lady has since recovered and is the Chair of the German Hearing Voices Network in Berlin.

Voice hearers are often not inclined to talk about their voices as they have experienced that most people do not listen to them. On the other hand, professionals are not trained to talk about the experience itself or to relate the experience to a person's life story. Over time, we have learned the value of a systematic approach and to make a psychological formulation (Dallos & Johnstone, 2006) or construct (Romme & Escher, 2000) a relationship between voices and life story. We observed that we needed an instrument and therefore developed an interview based on our experiences with voice hearers, the 'Maastricht Interview with voices' (Romme & Escher, 2000).

The interview conditions

Safety and trust

There are several conditions in order to properly interview a voice hearer about his/her experience—the first condition is safety. The voice hearer must feel safe and trust the interviewer. The interviewer should be aware of his/her own attitude towards the voice hearing experience and communicate his attitude with the voice hearer. If an interviewer is convinced that hearing voices is a symptom of a disease or is afraid of what he might hear, this will influence the process. Voice hearers might be reluctant to share information about their experience. Acceptance of the experience by the interviewer is an important condition.

Normalization

The interviewer should be aware of the fact that hearing voices as such is not a sign of madness. Voice hearing is apparent in the normal population, and one can learn to cope with the voices. Since the experience is confusing and the world around easily interprets hearing voices as a sign of madness, this easily results in a lowering of self-esteem. Therefore, the voice hearer needs to be supported with regard to their self-esteem. In psychiatry, hearing voices is commonly interpreted as a symptom of an illness like, for example, schizophrenia, a chronic illness with little hope of a cure and being able to function well in society, so the voice hearer needs to be given hope, which is an important support component. Talking about voices in a normalizing way (also see Garrett, this volume) may break down these anxiety-provoking prejudices. However, the interviewer should also explain to the voice hearer that talking about these voices can stir up emotions. As such, this is normal and one should not be afraid of this. It might be of help to organize someone who can support the voice hearer during the 24 hours after the first voices interview, just in case the voice hearer wants support.

Relationship

Before the interviewer starts the interview, he/she should attempt to develop a relationship with the voice hearer by expressing interest in the voice hearer as a person, not as an interview subject, but as an interesting person. Like Eleanor who talked about her new psychiatrist, 'I went back to Bradford and my new psychiatrist was Pat Bracken and that was a massive help. The very first time I met him, he said to me, 'Hi Eleanor, nice to meet you. Can you tell me a bit about yourself?' So I just looked at him and said 'I'm Eleanor and I'm a schizophrenic'. And in his quiet, Irish voice, he said something very powerful, 'I don't want to know what other people have told you about yourself, I want to know about you'.

Interview skills (Romme & Escher, 2000)

The interviewer needs to develop the following skills:

1. The ability and willingness to focus on the voice hearer's experience, remembering that it is the voice hearer who is the expert. This holds true for patients and non-patients.

2. Willingness to accept that the experience is real.

3. The ability to refrain from interpreting the information while interviewing.

4. The ability to take a journalistic approach to asking questions. For instance, when the person says that he has been subjected to long-distance x-rays, resist the temptation of asking questions for diagnostic purposes (e.g., Do you really believe in being subjected to long distance x-rays? Being bombarded with x-rays?), but rather ask, 'who is spreading the x-rays? What are their motives? How do you know this? How are they influencing you? etc.', until the picture of the experience is complete (the difference is exploring the experience in relation to the person who experiences the voices or believes he does versus looking for confirmation of diagnostic convictions). Voice hearers feel the difference very well and can tell you the difference so ask them for a change.

The Interview (based on the Maastricht hearing voices interview; Romme, 1996; Romme & Escher, 2000)

The interview consists of 12 sections, of which we will only discuss those that are particularly relevant to the psychological formulation or to construct the relationship with the life story.

1. The nature of the experience. This question draws a picture of the voices and offers the voice hearer a chance to talk freely about the subject. The questions also give information about whether the voices are being attributed to someone or something else or not. The answers are often informative about the identity of the voices.

    Questions:

    1-1 I would like you to tell me about the experience of hearing voices. How many voices do you hear? Do you hear sounds as well? Do you see visions, or feel being touched?

    1-2 Can the sounds you hear also be heard by other people? Can you explain why?

    1-3 Where do the sounds/voices come from? Where are they located? In your head, by your ears left/right/both, or somewhere else within your body?

    1-4 Are your voices coming from your own person or are they from somebody or something else? Can you explain why?

    1-5 Are you able to carry on a dialogue with your voices or communicate with them in any way?

2. Characteristics of the voices. This establishes how many voices are being heard and whether this has changed over time. It goes into more detail, listing each voice: name, age and gender, frequency, and the way in which it usually speaks (critical or supportive). It notes whether the voice bears resemblance to anyone the voice hearer knows.

    2-1 Do you hear one or more voices? How many? Has it always been like this?

    2-2 Are you able to indicate who the voices belong to and/or the names you have given them? Their age? Gender? In what way do they speak to you, in what kind of tone, and how frequently? Example of a registration:

No.	Name	Age	Gender	Tone/content	Frequency
1	Green	20	Female	Friendly, helpful	3 times a day
2	Purple	40	Male	Friendly, positive	Have to call
3	Blue	18	Male	Abusive	Once a week
4	Red	40	Female	Abusive	Every day
5	Child	8	Female	Scared	Twice a week

    2-3 Does the manner or tone of the voices remind you of someone you know or used to know? If yes, who?

3. The history of hearing voices. The questions take the voice hearer back to the first onset of the different voices and identify the different periods when the voices were active. It tries to find out whether anything in particular was happening at these different moments. It runs through a list of events and circumstances that might have preceded the first time or that may have influenced changes in hearing the different voices. It also establishes whether the voice hearer can connect the voices to one or more of the events listed. One should go through the entire list, as often people do not talk about emotional or stressful circumstances spontaneously.

3-1 Let us return to the time when you first started hearing voices. How old were you when you first heard voices? Can you remember at what age you started hearing each voice? During which further periods in your life did you hear voices?

3-1 Can you describe, for every voice, the circumstances during which you first heard them?

3-3 We have put together a list of the kind of circumstances and situations that people might experience in their lives. Which of these life events have happened to you? At what age did you experience them? Was it or was it not related to the start of hearing the voices or did it change or did it not change the nature of the voices? The list includes 25 questions, for example, about stressful changes in the voice hearer's life, about illness and death, about love and sexuality, and about religion, spirituality, and mystic or cosmic experiences.

3-4 If one or more of these circumstances is related to the moment, did you begin hearing voices or did the nature of the voice start to change (from being friendly to becoming negative), could you tell me more about this please?

4. What triggers the voices? Triggers might be defined as 'whatever provokes the voices in daily life'. This set of questions also investigates what puts a stop to them. It reveals whether certain times, places, situations, or activities act as triggers. It also endeavours to establish whether people know why this happens. This also applies to the feelings that seem to give rise to the voices.

4-1 Have you noticed whether the voices tend to be present when you take part in particular activities or that they arise in a certain kind of circumstances? Can you describe what these are? (For example, shopping, watching TV, cooking, being alone, being in a crowd, etc.)

4-2 Are there particular times (day, night, weekend, particular hours) when the voices are present or not present? Do you have any idea why?

4-3 Have you noticed whether the voices come from certain objects, like the TV, radio, or computer? From which objects?

4-4 How do you feel when the voices are triggered?

4-5 Have you ever noticed whether the voices are present when you feel certain emotions? Let us check this list: insecurity, fear, doubt, in love, anger or aggression, your own sexual feelings, the sexual feelings of others, jealousy, grief, fatigue, sad or depressed, happy, and lonely. Can you describe how the voices react? (For instance, are they comforting and helpful, or frightening and unhelpful?) Do they have an effect on the emotion you are feeling, for instance making you more or less depressed, or more or less happy?

5. What do the voices say? It asks about the voices that are friendly and positive and will gather some verbatim examples of what they say. It also looks at the negative voices, those that threaten, make nasty comments, indulge in name-calling, evoke unpleasant thoughts, or become very noisy. Moreover, it looks at the subjects, themes, or people the voices talk about.

    5-1 Do you hear positive (friendly) voices? What do they say? Please give an example of the exact words they use.

    5-2 Do you hear negative (unfriendly) voices? What do they say? Please give an example of the exact words they use.

    5-3 Do the voices talk about specific subjects/persons? Can you describe them? What do the voices say? Do those subjects concern you as well?

6. How do you explain the origin of the voices? It explores the voice hearer's own explanation of their voices. Each possible option is checked on a list. It asks about the frame of reference, i.e., the theory the hearer has about the origin of the voices, like reincarnation, illness, telepathy, etc.

7. What impact do the voices have on the way you live? It establishes the way in which the voices want to influence the hearer and what effect they have on the hearer and other people. This is also an opportunity to discuss how and in what way the voices affect behaviour, which then becomes more understandable. It also establishes whether any voices scare the hearer or make him/her happy and whether they interfere with the daily life of the hearer, and it asks how they do this. In this way, it explores the power the voices have and the power they are given by the voice hearer.

8. The balance of the relationship. This section examines whether or not the voice hearer and voices have an equal relationship. The more equal and open the relationship, the less inconvenient the voices are. This section also estimates the power of the voice hearer in relation to the voices (see Trower *et al.*, this volume).

9. Coping strategies (see Farhall, this volume). This covers everything the hearer does to try and deal with the voices and to retain his/her own freedom. It is not about what they do in obedience to the voices. The interviewer has to go down a list, which is categorized into cognitive strategies, behavioural strategies, and physical strategies. Then the interviewer comes to a conclusion with the voice hearer, going over what he/she mostly does and discusses using more passive or active strategies and the effectiveness of the strategies used.

10. Childhood experiences. The purpose here is to find out whether there have been any traumatic experiences or experiences of emotional neglect in the past, especially in early childhood. The order of these problems runs from less to more intrusive.

10-1 Was your childhood pleasant or stressful? Can you tell me about it?

10-2 Did you feel safe at school, in the streets, and at home? If not, please explain why.

10-3 As a child, were you ever mistreated? If so, how?

10-4 As a child, did you ever receive strange punishments? For example, being locked in a toilet or being tied up?

10-5 Have you ever, as a child or a teenager, been yelled at or belittled?

Did you experience the feeling of not being wanted or did you feel that you were never able to do anything right? Were you free to express your emotions at home?

10-6 Have you ever witnessed the maltreatment of another family member?

10-6 Have you ever been sexually abused by a member of your family or someone else?

10-8 Have you ever had sex against your will? A situation in which you were unable to resist or to escape from?

11. Treatment history. This explores the chronological history of healthcare treatment received. It looks at the treatment provided and the satisfaction with it and establishes what alternative treatments have been tried.

12. Social network. It lists the people the voice hearer maintains contact with and with whom he may or may not talk about his/her voices.

13. Questions. This gives the voice hearer the opportunity to volunteer any further information or to ask questions. Maybe there is an issue that is not discussed, which is important for the voice hearer to talk about.

The report

When the interview has finished, the interviewer writes a report summarizing the information given under each heading in a way that can be easily remembered. The voice hearer is then asked to read the report and comment on it. Possible gaps or misunderstandings are discussed. Participating in this way can be a first step in eliminating emotional and cognitive avoidance that is so common with voice hearers. The written report of their experiences can also stimulate the voice hearer to discuss and find other strategies for dealing with voices and emotions. The interview can also reveal practical and social issues that may be hindering recovery.

Corstens *et al.* (2008 p. 325) stipulate, 'We have often found that the interview itself was a big step in the process of recovery because the voice hearer became aware of the meaning of their voices; the relationship with their emotions and important issues in their lives, and felt stimulated to try other coping strategies. The interview often has a therapeutic effect. We emphasize that the systematic use of the interview is necessary to structure the experience and become aware of important aspects of the voice hearing experience'.

The construct or psycho-social dynamic formulation

Making sense of voices acknowledges the connection of the voice hearing experience with the life story between which the voices express various links. As Corstens *et al.* (2008) state 'In order to retrieve the relationship between the voices and the life events, 'the code' of defence needs to be broken (i.e., what the voices say may not adequately represent their purpose). This 'code' in patients hearing voices often involves a destructive way of communication and an exaggerated and negative way of expressing individual emotional problems'.

This systematic and open search for meaning leads to a psycho-social dynamic formulation that we (Romme & Escher, 2000) have called 'the construct'.

Two questions are to be answered from the information in the report in order to formulate the construct:

1. Who do the voices represent?
2. What problems do the voices represent?

Who do the voices represent?

In traumatic events, other people as well as emotions are involved, which the person finds difficult to cope with. How the voices relate to the voice hearer often resembles the identity and the characteristics of significant individuals related to the trauma in a literal or in a metaphorical way.

One example is that of Lisette's name of her voice 'Stephan' that metaphorically expresses the identity of her 'stepfather', who abused her. Many voice hearers recognize the characteristics of their voice(s) as being the characteristics of their 'traumatizer(s)'. The content of the voice might directly or metaphorically tell us what is said to the person like the example of 'Mien' who was trying to tell her mother about her abuse by the village priest at the age of seven. Her mother did not believe her and became angry and said 'you are a no-good' an expression her second woman's voice also used.

The identity and characteristics combined with the content give the most information about who the voices represent (often people involved in the trauma), but also possibly an emotion or warning connected to the traumatic situation as is demonstrated in Jolanda's voices, we will elaborate on this example further later on in this chapter.

What problems do the voices represent?

This question refers to the circumstances or events that lie at the roots of the voice hearing experience. The problems, situations, and events were so overwhelming that they exceeded the individual's coping strategies. We have already given examples of sexual abuse. How to cope with trauma depends also on childhood experiences. In childhood, we learn how to cope with stress in life and with internal and external conflict. Many voice hearers have been emotionally strangled in their youth (emotional neglect) or during their education (like with bullying). We will give examples of the relationships between characteristics of the voices and the trauma suffered in the second half of this chapter. The more vulnerable a person is, the more problematic it will be for this person to cope with stressful events.

The history of the voices (that is, the circumstances in which they started or got worse as well as the triggers and the content) and childhood experiences provide most information about the kind of problems the voices represent.

An example of the information needed for a construct

Jolanda is a thirty year-old woman who hears three voices.

The identity of the voices. Each voice has its own name: Nina, Eva, and Hanna.

The characteristics of the voices. All three voices are women. Nina is seven years old, cries a lot or shouts if Jolanda does not want to listen to her. Eva is nineteen and thinks of Jolanda as worthless and is aggressive towards her most of the time. Hanna is of the same age as Jolanda and is a positive voice that helps her.

The history of the voices. Nina came when Jolanda was seven years old, which is also the age when she began to be sexually abused by an uncle. This abuse lasted till she was twelve years old. Eva showed up when Jolanda was nineteen years old. At that age, Jolanda wanted her parents to help her to officially accuse the uncle and start a trial. While they initially agreed, her parents changed their minds and withdrew just before the formal accusation. That is when the voice of Eva appeared. Hanna entered the stage when Jolanda was undergoing therapy. This voice helps Jolanda to cope with the other voices.

The content of the voices. Nina wants to tell Jolanda what happened with her when she was abused and will cry or shout when Jolanda does not listen to her. Eva accuses Jolanda of not being strong enough and not being persistent when she should defend herself against other people. Eva brutalizes Jolanda and tells her to kill herself because she is 'such a wimp'. Hanna gives advice, such as not to listen to the other voices and to look for something that distracts her.

Triggers. For Nina, triggers are visits to Jolanda's parents who live on the same street as Jolanda's uncle who abused her. Confrontations with sexuality in her life also trigger Nina. Triggers for Eva are when Jolanda has to take a stand and does not dare to do that or when Jolanda visits her family and tries to convince her father to change his mind or when she talks to men, because Eva does not want her to relate to men. Hanna appears when the other voices, especially Eva, are very aggressive and Jolanda is afraid of them or thinks that she will do what Eva is telling her to do.

Childhood history. Jolanda enjoyed a very protective upbringing where she did not learn how to stand up for herself and was not allowed to be angry. However, she was sexually abused when she was seven years old.

The construct

Who do the voices represent? The voices Nina and Eva do not represent other people, but represent Jolanda's emotions, which were, and still are, troublesome and related to the sexual abuse when Jolanda was seven (Nina) and to the aggression she felt but could not effectively express when Jolanda was 19 (Eva). Hanna represents the helping part of Jolanda herself.

What problems do the voices represent? Jolanda agrees that all the information points to her difficulties with coping with the sexual abuse in her past.

'*Breaking the code*' is not an isolated activity of the professional but results from collaboration between voice hearer and professional. The 'code' can also be broken (or 'construct' generated) in a group of voice hearers and professionals; it can be very useful for an individual to hear the range of associations that come out of such a group. Experienced voice hearers can be of great support in this process and can act as professional helpers (Corstens *et al.*, 2008).

From theory to practice

Through the interview, we developed a format that is useful for the recovery of the voice hearer as it helps to relate the voices to the individual life story. The positive contribution of accepting and making sense of voices in recovering from the distress of voices and taking control of one's life again was the focus of our last study (Romme *et al.*, 2009).

In this most recent study of 50 voice hearers, we selected voice hearers who recovered from the distress associated with their voices. They took control of their lives again by changing their relationship with their voices. They made choices that enabled them to socially function well again. In this study, we focused on the steps people take to recover and on the links between the traumatic experiences and the characteristics of the voices.

In this latest study, we observed that in order to recover from the distress with voices, it is important for the voice hearer to recognize the relationship with those traumatic experiences. It is even more important that they recognize their distorted emotions as a consequence of what happened to them and to learn to cope with these emotions.

We will first report on the traumas and links with the voices and then report on the steps taken to recover.

The kind of traumas related to hearing voices

In our study with 50 voice hearers who recovered, we were told about the following traumatic experiences. Some people experienced more than one kind of trauma.

1) Sexual abuse	18 (Three of them combined with physical abuse)
2) Emotional neglect	11 (Plus two being counted within sexual abuse)
3) Adolescent problems	6
4) Severe (actual) stress	4
5) Being bullied	2 (Plus two being counted within sexual abuse)
6) Physical abuse	2 (Plus three being counted within sexual abuse)
7) Not clear	7
Total	*50*

With the exception of severe (actual) stress, all traumatic experiences were suffered in childhood. They were either directly related to the beginning of the voice hearing experience or the voices came later during a stressful situation that activated the memory of a childhood emotion. The onset of the voice hearing and the two different kinds of triggers are understandable when we take into account the differentiation between

1. The influence of traumatic experiences creating vulnerability in emotional crises or psychosis.
2. The stress or personally significant events that cluster before onset or relapse.

It is easier to study each of them with people who have recovered, since they have more insight into the impact of their traumatic experiences and emotions on their hearing voices experience as well as on their emotional crises periods compared to many patients. An example:

The vulnerability part

Lisette tells in Romme and Escher (1989), 'I have been sexually abused by my stepfather from the ages of 12 to 15. I was 17 when I heard the voice for the first time. I lived with my mother and stepfather at the time and there were great tensions in the house, and I was worrying a lot about my incest past.

I never spoke about this with anyone. I just tried to suppress all these memories. I do not think that anyone perceived what was going on in me, but I was hindered by it a lot. The voice was very critical and commented on everything I did, nothing was ever good enough. Whenever a memory of the incest came up, I dissociated and could find myself back anywhere else without knowing how I came there'. Dissociation is also a kind of escape away from an emotion, and in such instances, people can literally go away and Lisette could end up at the beach for example, without knowing how she got there. In the case of Lisette, her voices and dissociation served to suppress all memories of the incest.

The actual stress part

Lisette also tells, 'I never wanted any help until two years ago (at the age of 32). I wanted help because at my daughter's second birthday party, my stepfather gave a niece a smack. It was as if the sound of the smack woke me up, and I became conscious of the incest by my stepfather. I started to experience strange things such as blackouts and flashbacks of the incest.

The stress or personally significant events before the onset or relapse:

> In response to threatening experiences and the overwhelming emotions related to trauma, people react with dissociation or repression of emotions. Such responses are often built on an upbringing of emotional neglect and denial of emotions. Typically, hearing voices is the end result of the sequence: trauma, overwhelming emotions, provoking dissociation or repression, extra provocation of emotions, coping fails, and hearing voices start (Corstens *et al.*, 2008).

Voices expressing traumatic experiences

How do voices express traumatic experiences or what are the links?

We will give examples of links based on the main topics discussed in the interview and used to make a psychological formulation or construct about the relationship.

1. Identity of the different voices

2. Character of the different voices, such as sex, age, and way of speaking

3. History, i.e., when and in what circumstances the voices started or changed

4. Content of the voices or what do they say or tell the voice hearer

5. Triggers or what triggers the voices in daily life

Sexual abuse and the links to the voices

Sexual abuse and identity of the different voices

With sexual abuse, the identity of one of the voices is quite often the abuser. *Flore*, for example, says, 'With me there has never been confusion about my voices. I recognized the voice—it was the abuser'.

The identity can also be a metaphor for the abuser such as in the case of Lisette whose voice called himself Stephan, and *Lisette* discovered for herself that it was a metaphor for her stepfather who abused her.

The identity can also be a name given by the voice hearer as 'this name' has certain characteristics and a function in relation to the traumatic event like with *Jolanda*. One of her voices she calls 'Nina', who is still a child of seven. This was the age when her sexual abuse by her uncle started, and Nina reminds her of what happened at the time. If *Jolanda* does not listen to her, Nina starts to cry, which is even worse than being reminded. This is triggered when *Jolanda* starts having bodily contact with someone, even in case of, e.g., a friendly kiss.

Sexual abuse and the character of the different voice

With *Jolanda*, we saw that the identity and the character of her voice Nina were related to the sexual abuse. When a voice is experienced as a child of seven, then we automatically ask what happened when the voice hearer was at that age her/himself. Voices like Nina do not get older, but they stay the age of the time the trauma started.

With *Lisette*, we saw that the way the voice talked to her was the same as the abuser talked to her, i.e., always being critical. Voices can also be helpful like with *Jeanette* who was abused when she was twelve by an outsider who pulled her from her bicycle, she says, 'At the moment of the abuse, I started to hear two voices, two adult men, who were nice to start with. They took me serious in my anxieties and loneliness'.

Sexual abuse and personal history

Many sexually abused voice hearers report that their voice(s) started at the time of the abuse and such was the case with Jeanette. This was also the case with *Mien* who tells us,

'I started hearing voices when I was seven, just before my first holy communion (a Roman Catholic Church event in childhood). It was at that time that the sexual abuse by the priest of the church started'.

With others, it started somewhat later but was related to the abuse like with *Flore* who states, 'I started hearing a voice when I was 14. This was at the time when I started my protest behaviour, which ended the abuse'.

Sexual abuse and triggers

We have just discussed this in *Jolanda's* example with her voice called Nina (see Sexual abuse and identity of the different voices).

Sexual abuse and content

With sexual abuse, the abuser often tells the voice hearer that he or she seduced him in order to abuse the voice hearer (Coleman, 1997). The abuser also often tells how bad or worthless the abused is (see the Danish film 'Festen', directed by Thomas Vinterberg). Therefore, the content reflects these issues. For example, in the case of *Mien*, she hears two voices, one of which she recognizes as the voice of the abuser. This voice tells her, 'You are a devil's child'. The second voice, which she recognizes as the voice of her mother, tells her, 'You are a no-good; you are a failure; be happy with the leftovers'.

However, it is also possible that the voices remind the person of what has happened like, for example, with Nina who tells *Jolanda*, when there is a chance of bodily contact, 'you know what has happened, walk away from him'. Nina also said, 'don't get into the car' when *Jolanda* had driving lessons for her driver's license with a male instructor.

Sexual abuse and influence

With *Jeanette*, her two voices were nice to her after the abuse but then she says, 'The voices did not become awful overnight but gradually they (the voices) ended up being the only ones who understood me and supported me. In this way, they gained more and more control of me. I became dependent on them, asking them for advice. Then they started giving me tasks to complete. First just simple tasks and when I obliged, they were nice to me. Then they told me that I was subordinate to them. That became very creepy. When I did not do something well, according to them, I had to run up and down the stairs three times'. This is what we often see, that the voice hearer gives too much power to the voices. Like *Debra* stated, 'All the power the voices had, I gave it to them'.

The impact of the voices is for the most part not directly related to the trauma but more to the way the person reacts to the trauma and to the voices, for example, not talking about the trauma with anyone and in this way taking a greater risk of giving power to the voices.

Being bullied and the links between this trauma and the characteristics of the voices

It would take up too much space in this chapter to give extended examples of all the kinds of traumas we observed in our research, so we will only give one further example—the links between the trauma of being bullied over a long period of time and the characteristics of the voices. The voices can imitate the bullying situation (1) because of the actual stress that can trigger an existing vulnerability, (2) because of their characteristics, (3) because of situations that can trigger them, (4) because of the words they use, and (5) because of the influence voices have on the bullied person. In this example, it is good to also listen to the metaphoric way in which voices express themselves.

Karin: 'I was 26 when I first started hearing voices. I was in Mexico in the bathroom of a house I was sharing with three other students and they were talking behind my back'. This was the actual acute stress to which Karin was quite sensitive, because she had been bullied all along during her school years, which had made her very insecure, especially when in contact with peers (the vulnerability part).

Karin talks about the characteristics of her voices, 'I heard many different voices. The strongest and most negative came from the people I used to go to school with. I recognize the people who bullied me'. She also talks about the triggers, 'The most important trigger is when I go out into crowded places, like pubs, in a busy street or on a bus'. This trigger sounds like a metaphor for situations in which bullying takes place. When you are bullied, it happens in a crowded place that you are overwhelmed by. Also, the words can be seen as referring to the bullying experience when *Karin* says, 'The voices say things like she is a nutter, she's disgusting, she failed her A-levels' The same holds for the impact of voices, which can be seen as metaphoric. *Karin* says, 'Voices made me afraid and tearful and had the ability to strip me of my dignity and self respect'. Her powerlessness towards the voices also seems metaphoric for bullying. *Karin*: 'I could not make them go away'.

All traumatic experiences that voice hearers related to their hearing voices show many links with their voices not only relating to the situation, but also to the emotions involved as a consequence.

How do voice hearers recover?

From our study with 50 voice hearers who recovered from the distress with their voices and who took control of their lives again, we selected those issues that were described as important in recovering from the distress with voices, and also those reported repeatedly. We will give an overview and an example of each of the issues:

1. *Meeting someone who takes an interest in the voice hearer as a person*

   It seems very important to meet someone who takes an interest in the voice hearer as a person. Voice hearers have often experienced a negative approach by others because of their hearing voices.

   Ron: 'Any recovery story has a beginning and for me the beginning was my meeting Lindsay Cooke, my support worker; it was her who encouraged me to go to the self-help group in Manchester at the start of 1991. It was her, not me, who believed that a self-help group would benefit me. It was her who saw beneath my madness and into my potential. It was her faith in me that kick-started my recovery'.

Eleanor: 'I went back to Bradford and my new psychiatrist was Pat Bracken and that was a massive help. The very first time I met him he said to me, 'Hi Eleanor nice to meet you. Can you tell me a bit about yourself?' So I just looked at him and said 'I'm Eleanor and I'm a schizophrenic'. And in his quiet, Irish voice he said something very powerful, 'I don't want to know what other people have told you about yourself; I want to know about you'.

2. *Giving hope, showing a way out, and normalizing the experience*

Meeting someone who takes an interest in the voice hearer as a person is often combined with this 'someone' providing an alternative and giving hope. Voice hearers talk about this as an important combination at the start of their recovery.

Like *Ron* saying, 'It was her (my support worker) who encouraged me to go to the hearing voices self-help group in Manchester at the start of 1991. It was her, not me, who believed that a self-help group would benefit me'.

Several stories tell about the importance of meeting people who managed to normalize their experience. Like with *Mien*, 'My psycho-therapist told me I was not mad but that they (the voices) were related to my past. That it is a rather normal experience you can talk about with others. It helped me to realize that hearing voices is a rather normal experience, that you can talk about them and voices express what is happening with you. It is something that belongs to me'.

3. *Meeting people who accept the voices as being real*

Being interested in the person and asking about what has happened in their lives is one way of showing acceptance of the voices and being open enough to talk about them. We see in the stories that it looks like a condition *sine qua non* for recovery to meet people who accept voices as a reality for the voice hearer.

Ron Coleman writes about this: 'Anne Walton, a fellow voice hearer, who at my first hearing voices group, asked me if I heard voices. When I replied that I did, she told me that they were real. It does not sound like much, but that one sentence has been a compass for me showing me the direction I needed to travel and underpinning my belief in the recovering process'.

4. *Becoming actively interested in your experience*

When one just sees hearing voices as a symptom of an illness, there is not much reason to go into detail about their background in daily life. In contrast, when one discovers the relationship a voice has with what has happened to you in your life, this gives the voice hearer an argument to become active and gives the professional a handle to become helpful.

Ami tells, 'I came across an advertisement on a billboard that somebody would give a lecture about hearing voices, a lecture given by Liz Bodil (a mental health professional who heard voices herself and at the time was leading the hearing voices network in Stockholm and was promoting the accepting voices approach in Sweden). This was the turning point. She also sold books. I read that book (about accepting voices) in one night. I just felt this was for me. This described my experience and also told me that there is a reason for voices.

5. *Recognizing your voice as personal*

   Voices are mostly talked about in general terms. The other issue is that if voices are negative, you reject them. It really is a big step to recognize them as personal, belonging to you.

   Daan tells 'I thought I was bad because the voices called me all sorts of names. Later, I realized that the voices were related to the physical abuse because they have the characteristics of those who abused me. Then I perceived that the voices became more or less intrusive depending on the situation I was in. They become bad when there are conflicts in the house. So they become a kind of mirror of the living situation'.

6. *Changing the power structure between you and your voices*

   This seems to be a necessary prerequisite for recovery. Reorganizing the way of coping might help for instance by giving the voices a certain time in the day and sending them away if they come at any other time. Setting limits.

   A. *Reorganizing the way of coping*

   Stewart: 'I was already able to talk back to my voices with my thoughts, but I learnt to make a specific time of day, the evening, when I would focus, and simply tell the voices 'later' if they came at another time'.

   B) *Freeing oneself from the victim role*

   Jeanette W: 'In therapy I learned to say to myself you are responsible to the extent you feel hurt. It is not only the one who hurts you, but also how heavily you take it to heart'.

   C) *Address the demons of your past*

   Peter B: 'When I looked at my life, the demon of my past was my abuser. I would still see her in Sheffield on a regular basis, walking in the street. When I saw that girl, I would run away in real fear. Then one day, I decided I would address this demon of my past. I would not run away. When I saw her down the street, my first idea was to run. My heart was beating, but I kept eye contact with her. I kept walking closer to her. She turned her eyes and looked the other way. I then felt I had altered the balance of power. I did not have to fear her anymore. It was actually meaningless'.

   D) *Challenging the power of the voices*

   Eleanor says, 'I realized that the fear I felt had created this vicious circle of avoidance and isolation. I tentatively began to test out what the voices claimed. One night he said. I want you to cut off your toe, and if you do not, I'll kill your family. It was the hardest thing I've ever had to do but I said just do it. It was a terrible night but nothing happened, so I realized he didn't have much power'.

E)   *Taking back power*

> *Debra*: 'I realized that the only power the voices had was the power I gave them. They needed me to perform tasks and speak to certain people; without me, they were impotent. I approached the voices as I would approach any relationship and began to put parameters around how and when they could contact me'.

7)   *Making choices*

Making choices is important for recovery on different levels during the whole process. It is very basic like staying alive, to find people as friends to belong to, to develop oneself, to find a purpose in life. *Debra*: 'I decided I needed to take the risk of inviting real people into my world and cautiously and clumsily this became my new quest. I eventually got to the stage where I began to venture out from my home. I continued my education, went to university, made friends, and gained employment'.

8)   *Changing the relationship with your voices*

It seems very important in the recovery process to change the relation with one's voices, and therefore it looks like it is a condition *sine qua non*. We will give some examples of how voice hearers managed to change the relationship with their voices in a more special way.

Ami says, 'My relationship with my voices changed when I learned to see them as a signal of my problems and when I learned to react positively to them. When the voices said to me 'look at her, what a disaster', I looked in the mirror and thought they are right 'I should dress properly'. From a negative influence it became a stimulus'.

Antje says, 'I then met a therapist—a woman with whom I discussed my voices and she gave me very concrete hints about how to talk to a voice. I had no idea myself. I started in an aggressive way and the voices reacted with aggression. The therapist taught me to talk to the voices in a friendly way. And when I tried, my voices reacted in a friendly way, which was strange to me. She also taught me to speak to the voices very slowly. After three or four weeks talking to the voices three or four times a day in this friendly, slow way, they slowed down and became quieter'.

Therapy differentiated according to the three phases in the recovery process

Based on the recovery study results, we earlier discussed the steps voice hearers took to recover, but from our earlier studies, we also learned that one has to distinguish between different phases in the recovery process (Romme & Escher, 2000). As a therapist or counsellor or another voice hearer, you have to adapt your interventions to these phases.

1.   In the first phase, the voice hearer is overwhelmed by the strange experience of hearing voices and becomes afraid of the voices. In this phase, normalizing and being shown a way out are important, as well as exercising techniques to get more control and become less anxious.

2. In the second phase, when more control has been gained, people are stimulated to get themselves interested in the phenomenon of hearing voices and learn about the personal aspects of one's voices and taking back power. In this phase, the links between the voices and the life story are explored and a construct can be made. Therapeutically speaking, it is important to work through the emotions involved with the traumatic experiences in their lives, which brings us to the next phase.

3. In the third phase, we speak of stabilization. There is more control, more insight, and making choices and taking back power are important issues. These will make it possible to change one's relation with the voices and to accept one's own emotions. Interventions are oriented to stimulating the voice hearer to make choices, to take back power with regard to making choices, which are necessary to function in society according to one's own choice. Support is the greatest need as well as creativity to find a place in society. A place in society is necessary to stimulate self-esteem, self-awareness, and self-worth.

The therapy plan

To simplify the issues as described above, we will formulate the therapy plan in a way that is rather easy to understand. From the information of the construct, a treatment plan can be developed, focusing on three goals: (1) to identify the most hindering aspects of the voices, to choose a strategy, and to practice this method, (2) to improve the voice hearer's relationship with difficult emotions and to adopt alternative coping mechanisms for dealing with those emotions, and (3) to deal with the historical events that have been difficult to accept and to work through the associated anxiety and guilt.

Dealing with difficult voices

Voices can command, demand, and be destructive. Often, they disturb the life of the voice hearer all day long and they imprison the voice hearer into isolation, passivity, and destructive activities. Voices tend to get stronger when the individual sets no limits. Most voices threaten when the voice hearer tries to disobey them. Voices have their own strategies to keep the voice hearer within their power. The relationship between voices and voice hearer reflects the power relation in the trauma situation. The voice hearer can develop new strategies to address the voices, and he/she has to learn to set his or her own limits. This allows the voice hearer to have more power or control. Create a first turning point by

1. Giving reassuring information can decrease the anxiety level considerably.

2. Creating hope in a situation that appears devastating will empower the voice hearer.

3. Acquiring more control through anxiety reduction and decreasing the frequency of the voices are the first goals.

Interventions for this purpose are described in most of the literature about cognitive-behavioural therapy and in most of the chapters in this book. We learned about a number of interventions from voice hearers, which are described in Romme and Escher (2000;

chapter 10). A hearing voices support group can be helpful as well for these purposes. In a hearing voices group, voices are accepted as real, one is not stigmatized because of hearing voices, but appreciated because of trying to cope with them. One learns coping strategies from other voice hearers and one is encouraged to use one's own qualities in coping with life, etc. This increases a person's self-esteem, while traditional psychiatric care breaks down this self-esteem, as a result of identification with an illness with little hope for cure due to becoming the passive victim of this disease, etc.

Anti-psychotic medication, however, hardly ever achieves a lasting effect on voices (Honig *et al.*, 1993; see Sanjuan *et al.*, this volume). It reduces the person's emotionality, which is useful in the short-term, but diminishes recovery effects because coping with emotion is not learned. Alternatively, benzodiazepines can be prescribed (short term) to diminish anxiety. If depression triggers the voices, antidepressants may also help.

Finding new ways of dealing with difficult emotions

Often, certain emotions are severely repressed in voice hearers. Examples are anger, guilt, and sexual feelings. The anger of the voices represents the anger of the voice hearer, which he/she does not recognize as his/her own. Practicing expressing these emotions in social situations—as is done in assertiveness training or support with socializing—helps the voice hearer to express difficult emotions. This can also be stimulated in hearing voices support groups. It is about building up resilience.

Many voice hearers express the need to build another identity—to find a new way of relating to others. In this process, stimulation is needed to take back power from the voices and work towards a turning point in which the voice hearer realizes that all the power the voices have is the power he/she gives to them. Voice hearers can be stimulated to test their voices by asking, 'can the voices do anything on their own without the help of the voice hearer?' They will discover that the answer is 'No'.

They can then practice disobeying their voices and discover that threats will not be carried out.

An example Eleanor gives, 'I tentatively began to test out what the voice claimed. I began to realize that nobody else could see or hear him—what does that tell me? Having realized this, I decided to try and push it a little bit further. Does he have the influence that he claims? He says that he can do all this stuff, that he can kill my family, can he though? One night he said, I want you to cut off your toe, and if you don't, I'll kill your family'. It was the hardest thing I've ever had to do but I said, 'go on then, just do it'. It was really eerie because during these instructions his voice had been painfully loud. It was really frightening. I sit there thinking oh my God, what is he going to do? But I stuck to my word, and what I did was sit outside my parent's room all night, from nine at night to seven in the morning and nothing happened'.

This can then become the basis of changing the relationship with their voices and look for their positive intentions as, for example, warning the voice hearer or simulating the voice hearer like with Ami: 'My relationship with my voices changed when I learned to see them as a signal of my problems when I learned to react positively to them. When they said to me, "look at her, what a disaster", I looked in the mirror and thought they are right, "I should dress properly". From a negative influence it became a stimulus'.

Or with Eleanor, 'I began to put boundaries in place, saying things to him like "do not talk to me before 8 o'clock in the evening because I will not talk to you". I then learned that the contempt and loathing that he expresses has actually to do with me in that it reflects how I feel about myself. He is like a very external form of my own insecurities, my own self-doubt'.

Accepting the past and working through associated anxiety and guilt

As already stated, voice hearers have often suffered from traumatic experiences. They often re-experience traumatic memories, partly in their voices and partly in their emotions, and react by avoiding overwhelming emotions in blocking of emotions or developing symptoms such as depersonalization, de-realization, numbing (often interpreted as so-called 'negative symptoms'), amnesia, re-enactments, and nightmares. Many people who are identified as 'psychotic' do not receive ordinary psycho-therapeutic intervention based on the false belief that talking to them about their voices (or other 'psychotic symptoms') will worsen their symptoms. It is important that the therapist or counsellor is used to dealing with strong transference reactions. It is also important to create a supportive social environment in a hearing voices network, self-help groups, and other social support that increases the ability to work through traumatic memories, as well as difficult and overwhelming feelings like anxiety, guilt, and despair. We still think that the best description of what is needed to work through the emotions involved in traumatic experiences is described in 'Trauma and recovery' by Judith Herman (1992). She differentiates some important phases like (1) accepting what has happened has really happened, (2) working through disturbing emotions, and (3) reconnecting. These are very important purposes within a healing, supportive relationship that will give more self-esteem, self-awareness, and self-worth to the traumatized person.

Reconnecting with the world around

During the whole process, it is important to stimulate the voice hearer to make choices. From the beginning, the therapist should stimulate the voice hearer to use his/her qualities. From the beginning, learning small techniques to connect with others and using acceptable excuses when the voice becomes too loud, like for example, going to the toilet and telling them to come back tonight and to get lost for now, or using a mobile telephone as a smoke screen.

Most important is joining a support group to slowly learn to talk about one's experience, feel accepted as a voice hearer, and learn that your experience is something special belonging to you.

During the next phases, choosing activities in the daily world is important to overcome the threat of being a failure instead of a person with certain qualities. In mental healthcare, there is a tendency to protect the voice hearer but that works like medication—it inhibits development. In a recovery process, development is more important than cure, and support is more important than protection (Escher *et al.*, 2004). The recovery process is also quite seriously handicapped, when the person is not able to accept that what has happened in his/her life has really happened, as working through the emotions is then blocked. The shame about what has happened is a factor and even more so when the person wants to keep a good relationship with the one(s) who also traumatized the voice hearer. This is also described by Topor (2001) as managing the contradictions. Some people are emotionally neglected by their parents, which was not the purpose, but part of the effect of their upbringing/education. This can happen when upbringing/education focuses on forbidding and not on stimulating, on being critical instead of stimulating, and in inhibiting the expression of emotions instead of learning to cope with emotions. Because the purpose was positive, it is not recognized by educators as emotional neglect and on the other hand the voice hearer as an adult also does not like to give up his/her relationship with the educators. These kinds of contradictions are quite inhibiting in a recovery process. An open attitude is not possible for the voice hearer who is afraid of losing the positive sides of the relationship or keeping old power structures in place instead of differentiating what was wrong and what was right and to become more adult in the relationship.

Sometimes what has happened was so awful that it is difficult to accept that it did happen and the voice hearer remains in doubt also because of the discrepancy between the purpose of education of the educator and the reality of expressing this role. Some traumatized people become very sad about this discrepancy of having had such educators.

It is also more difficult to recognize emotional neglect for the voice hearer. For example, being forbidden to express emotions as a child is not felt as a conscious problem. However, later the outcome might be that the person cannot cope with emotions that become difficult when a real emotion-provoking situation presents and the person is then not able to react emotionally and instead might get confused. Also when a person is continually criticized, this is not felt as emotional neglect but as an imprint of not being good at all. This also can make the person very insecure, which in turn is also a reason to doubt oneself and to remain in one's own shadow: unable to make choices, to change the power structure, to change the relationship, and to recognize one's own emotions expressed by the voices. All of which are metaphoric for the relationships with emotional neglect.

Discussion

The Maastricht approach to hearing voices offers an alternative to the traditional attitude in psychiatry where eradication of the voices is the aim. Making sense of voices, however, is a systematic way of exploring the relationship between the voices and a person's experiences in life, because voices are meaningful personal phenomena. People can only be supported to recover fully when the reality of hearing voices is also accepted by others and the meaningfulness is explored. The aim is not eradication, but changing the relationship between them and the problems that lay at their roots.

These few sentences already indicate that there are quite some differences versus the approach of the general mental health professional. They were taught not to talk about voices and also do not know how to talk about them. They are not used to working systematically with instruments that are absolutely necessary to explore the meaningfulness, since otherwise one stumbles on the anxiety-laden and often chaotic way voice hearers talk about their voices, because they never learned to talk about them.

Another difference with the cognitive psychological approach is the conviction that hearing voices is a symptom of an illness. In spite of overwhelming evidence from epidemiological research, mental health professionals stick to their illness concepts and this makes full recovery impossible as well. It is therefore that we spend most of our time supporting voice hearers' organizations instead of trying to change professionals. The evolution of ideas about hearing voices is similar to how mental health looked at homosexuality in the fifties. Voices are also a human variation in expressing or coping with emotions. Positive voices express positive emotions and are experienced as inspirational. Negative voices express negative and conflicting emotions and are seen as threats.

The approach can be used with all types of voice hearer populations, though the success depends on a number of conditions.

1. The voice hearer has to leave the illness conviction of this experience and that is very difficult when all around him/her the focus is on the illness concept.

2. It is more difficult to recover when the traumatic experiences were experienced before the age of seven or when the cumulative trauma experience is high (Ensink, 1992). Also severe emotional neglect over long periods and from a very young age makes recovery more difficult.

3. Limits to recovery are mainly the consequence of the seriousness of the problems that lay at the roots of the voice hearing experience. The degree of emotional neglect can be a great handicap to full recovery. We then see that the voices are, in fact, not the biggest problem, but instead the degree of emotional neglect in learning to cope with emotions (Romme et al., 2009).

4. Based on experience, we believe that voice hearers who have a very technical explanation for their voices like for example 'microwave transmission of human speech by military forces' are less inclined to explore their emotions involved with their voices and so will be less open for the personal interaction part with their experiences.

Over the last 10 years, the cognitive psychological approach and therapy with voice hearers has been very beneficial, but only to a certain degree. The experience is accepted as the person's reality and there is a tendency for normalization, but many therapists still want the person to get rid of their voices. We think that this is because cognitive psychology focuses more on the thought processes and explanations than on the voices as expressing emotions. It would be interesting to study how far learning to cope with emotions is of more or less value in coping with voices than to change the explanation for one's voices. Cognitive psychology might also look more at the associated negative emotions that voices elicit in individuals rather than analysing which conflicting emotions are expressed by the voices as the consequence of traumatic experiences or emotional neglect.

References

Aleman, A., & Larøi, F. (2008). *Hallucinations: The Science of Idiosyncratic Perception*. Washington, DC: American Psychological Association.

Coleman, R. (1997). *Recovery: An Alien Concept*. Fife: P & P Press.

Corstens, D., Escher, A., & Romme, M. (2008). *Accepting and working with voices: The Maastricht approach*. In Andrew Moskowitz, Ingo Schafer, & Martin J. Dorahy, Psychosis, Trauma and Dissociation. Chichester: John Wiley and Sons; Wiley-Blackwell pp. 319–333.

Dallos, R., & Johnstone, L. (2006). *Formulation in psychology and psychotherapy: Making sense of people's problems*. London: Routledge.

Escher, A., Morris, M., Buiks, A., Delespaul, Ph., Van Os, J., & Romme M. (2004). Determinants of outcome in the pathways through care for children hearing voices. *International Journal of Social Welfare*, **13**, 208–222.

Escher, A. (2005). *Making Sense of psychotic experiences, Ph.D. Thesis*, University of Maastricht.

Ensink, B.J. (1992). *Confusing realities: A study on child abuse and psychiatric symptoms*. Amsterdam: VU University Press.

Herman, J.L. (1992). *Trauma and recovery*. New York: Basic Books.

Honig, A., Romme, M., Ensink, B., Escher, S., Pennings, M., & de Vries, M. (1998). Auditory hallucinations, a comparison between patients and non-patients. *J Nerv Ment Dis*, **186** (10), 646–651.

Mueser, K.T., Goodman, L.B., Trumbetta, S.L., *et al.* (1998). Trauma and posttraumatic stress disorder in severe mental illness. *J Consult Clin Psychol*, **66**(3), 493–499.

Read, J., van Os, J., Morrison, A.P., & Ross, C.A. (2005). Childhood trauma, psychosis and schizophrenia: A literature review with theoretical and clinical implications. *Acta Psychiatr Scand*, **112**, 330.

Romme, M. (1996). *Understanding voices*. Fife: P & P Press.

Romme, M., & Escher, S. (1987). Leren omgaan met het horen van stemmen. *Maandblad Geestelijke Volksgezondheid*, **718**, 825–831.

Romme, M., & Escher, S. (1989). Hearing voices. *Schizophr Bull*, **15** (2), 209–216.

Romme, M., & Escher, S. (1993). *Accepting Voices*. London: Mind.

Romme, M., & Escher, S. (2000). *Making sense of voices*. London: Mind.

Romme, M., Escher, S., Dillon, J., Corstens, D., & Morris, M. (2009). *Living with voices*. Ross-on-Wye: PCCS Books in association with Birmingham City University.

Spauwen, J., Krabbedam, L., Lieb, R., Witchen, H., & van Os, J. (2006). Impact of psychological trauma on the development of psychotic symptoms: Relationship with psychosis proneness. *Acta Psychiatr Scand*, **188**, 527–533.

Tien, A.Y. (1991). Distribution of Hallucinations in the population. *Soc Psychiatry Psychiatr Epidemiol*, **26**, 287–292.

Topor, A. (2001). *Managing Contradictions. Recovery from Severe Mental Disorders*. Sweden: Akademitryck AB.

van Os, J., Hanssen, M., Bijl, R.V., & Vollebergh, W. (2001). Prevalence of psychotic disorder and community level of psychotic symptoms. *Arch Gen Psychiatry*, **58**, 603–668.

Watkins, J. (2008). *Hearing voices: A common Human Experience*. Australia: Michelle Anderson Publishing.

White, M. (1996). *Power to our Journeys*, in American Family Therapy Academy Newsletter, 11–16.

Chapter 14

Self-help approaches to hearing voices

Rufus May and Eleanor Longden

We must become confident in our own abilities to change our lives; we must give up being reliant on others to do everything for us. We need to start doing these things for ourselves. We must have the confidence to give up being ill so that we can start being recovered.

Coleman (2004, p.15)

Self-help refers to approaches to healing and recovery from emotional distress, which focus on the endeavours of the individual to help themselves. In the context of hearing voices,[1] self-help both refers to groups where voice hearers mutually assist each other and to the autonomous actions of the voice hearer to take back control over their lives. To write a chapter about self-help strategies in a clinical textbook has its challenges. The self-help movement offers a challenge to traditional approaches of professional help giving, emphasizing the expertise that lies within the individual. Self-help strategies are creative, continuously evolving, and less amenable to the traditional types of evidence base as conventional approaches to the experience of living with voices. However, self-help techniques are very compatible alongside professional help-giving methods, as are self-help groups. Why are self-help movements required? The traditional psychiatric paradigm has emphasized medical remedies, which require a fairly passive response from the recipient. Hospital treatment, which many voice hearers have been given to reduce their distress, has traditionally encouraged the patient to passively adapt to the routines of the hospital ward and pharmacological treatment. A self-help ethos offers a shift of emphasis from the passive to the active. It says we can change our attitudes and experiences by making choices and taking action.

This chapter will outline the emancipatory philosophy of the hearing voices movement before outlining the group and individual approaches to self-help that have emerged over the last 20 years. We will look at the three stages of voice hearing and likely self-help strategies that will complement these stages.

---

[1] While 'auditory hallucinations' is a preferred phrase in the professional literature, we feel the term 'hearing voices' is more neutral and 'user-friendly' and as such is preferred here.

'The freedom to hear voices': The hearing voices movement

Since its launch in the late 1980s, inspired by the innovative work of Romme and Escher (1989a, 1990, 1993, 2000), the hearing voices movement has proposed that self-help initiatives and the 'expertise of experience' be given equal status to academic and professional wisdoms. While not denying that voice hearing is often distressing and demoralizing, the hearing voices movement disputes such psychological turmoil is indicative of organic pathology. Rather than a meaningless mental illness requiring eradication and 'cure' at the hands of a pharmaceutical arsenal, voice hearing is deemed significant, decipherable, and intimately entwined to a hearer's life story (see Romme & Escher, this volume). As an alternative to the traditional attempt to silence or cure the person of voices, understanding, accepting, and integrating their emotional meaning is suggested as the recovery response. Voices are characterized as messengers, which communicate important information about genuine problems and emotional traumas in the person's life. Therefore, it simply does not make sense to shoot the messenger; conversely, helping the person to listen to the voices without anguish is a more authentic long-term solution than extinguishing them and 'ignoring' the message. To recover from distress, the person must learn to cope with both their voices and the original problems at the heart of the experience. Moreover, the ethos of the hearing voices movement is to accept a diverse range of explanations for voice hearing and support the person to find empowering ways to use these understandings—if an individual claims to be communing with God, and finds the experience valuable, no efforts are made to divest them of it, but discover what it means to them.

The philosophy of 'accepting voices' (e.g., Romme & Escher, 1989a, 1990, 1993, 2000) was developed in close collaboration with voice hearers. It proposed that (a) voice hearing is a normal human experience, which is widely prevalent in the general population, (b) has a personal meaning in relation with life history whose meaning or purpose can be deciphered, and (c) is best considered a dissociative experience and not a psychotic symptom. The fact that many voice hearers have suffered from trauma is a neglected aspect of the voice hearing experience and psychosis in general (e.g., Read & Ross, 2003; Read, van Os, Morrison, & Ross, 2005; Moskowitz & Corstens, 2007). Thus, in addition to emphasizing understanding the purpose/meaning of the voices, a specific treatment model for working directly with a person's voices—emphasizing their dissociative nature—has been developed by adapting the Voice Dialogue Method (Stone & Stone, 1989) for working with voice hearing (e.g., Corstens, Longden & May, in press; Moskowitz & Corstens, 2007). In contrast, Western clinical psychiatry sees voices as symptoms of an illness, a meaningless pathological phenomenon (Leudar & Thomas, 2000; Smith, 2007). As such, its only goal is eliminating the voices; it has little to offer voice hearers who seek help beyond medication. However, from Romme and Escher's perspective, rejecting the meaning of the voices is the same as rejecting the person.

Paul Baker, a British community development worker who was present when Romme and Escher publicly delivered their findings for the first time, later recorded: 'Fundamental to this approach…has been its emphasis on partnership between voice hearers themselves and professionals…this was a refreshing change from most of the approaches I had come across before which rarely—if ever, gave such importance to the views of those who had actually experienced the mental health difficulties under consideration' (Baker, 1989, p.11). Mark Greenwood, a colleague of Baker's, was affected by his enthusiasm and organized a trip to visit Romme at his home in Maastricht. He was equally impressed, 'We could see why Paul was getting so excited…we immediately grasped the significance of it' (quoted in James, 2001, p.47–48). Romme (2000) has since likened the 'emancipation' of voice hearer's to the civil right movements of the 1960s, in which medicine wields a yoke of cultural, social, and psychological oppression. From Romme's perspective, psychiatry must change its attitudes toward voice hearing in the same way it changed its attitudes towards homosexuality—learning to respect and support the experience rather than 'cure' it. The hearing voices movement affirms this protesting stance, and the approach has become progressively more powerful and influential, dispersing across Europe, Australia, Japan, and elsewhere in the form of research, forums, conferences, publications, and self-help groups. These activities evoked, induced, and ultimately became embedded in what is now referred to as 'the hearing voices movement', a philosophical and social trend in which networks of voice hearers organized outside the psychiatric system seek and elaborate ways to support one another, empower themselves and work towards recovery in their own ways. The foundation of such networks have created possibilities for acknowledging and supporting voice hearers and, crucially, spread the forgotten revelation that people can learn to live with their voices. Accepting and making sense of voices has thus become a new paradigm, constructively creating new ways of recovery. From a political perspective, the hearing voices movement has also become an alternative to traditional psychiatry, where those who were traumatized by oppressive approaches could find acknowledgement and personal attention. Thus, the hearing voices movement has challenged the political power of psychiatry. However, in contrast to the anti-psychiatry movement (e.g., Szasz, 1961; Laing & Esterton, 1964), voice hearers themselves have gained the right to be heard, and a social movement has developed in which 'experts-by-experience' have been able to challenge the psychiatric system.

Hearing voices groups

Hearing voices groups are forums in which individuals who share the experience of voice hearing can gather together to gain support, exchange coping strategies and reduce feelings of stigma, isolation, and distress (see Romme & Escher, 1989b; Coupland, 2000; Downs, 2005; Dillon, 2006). This is a strategy with important theoretical and pragmatic justifications. According to Coleman (2008, p.9),

> We all know and probably fear the stereotyped voice hearer…There is a well-worn joke about talking to yourself being the first sign of a nervous breakdown and it is certainly a behaviour that is likely to have the label of 'mad' stamped on it—and no one likes to think of themselves as mad. Unsurprisingly then, hearing voices is not generally talked about because it is thought of as a socially stigmatizing and unwanted experience.

This sense of fear and shame can be so ingrained that it can impair the development of effective therapeutic relationships with mental health professionals (Strauss, 1989; Martin, 2000; Coffey & Hewitt, 2008) on the grounds that many clinicians 'don't know how to relate respectfully to someone who hears voices' (Corstens, Escher, & Romme, 2008, p.321) and therefore cannot engage in meaningful discourse about the experience. Furthermore, research suggests that the levels of social support available has an important impact on how distressing voice hearing is experienced (Hewitt, 2007). Crucially, research suggests not only does social isolation appear to exacerbate voices (Garety, Kuipers, Fowler, Freeman, & Bebbington, 2001), supportive social environments are a protective factor that moderate stressors, which could otherwise induce relapse (Romme and Escher, 1993; Ventura & Liberman, 2000). This is important, given the strong associations between emotive, high-stress environments, and voice severity (Kopelowicz, Liberman, & Zarate, 2002).

This discrepancy between professional (illness-orientated) indices of well-being and service-user concerns (standard of living and lifestyle) means less formal, more eclectic approaches to self-help and self-management are both appropriate and promising strategies (Repper, 2000; Hewitt, 2007; Coffey & Hewitt, 2008). Through the group, a social network can be restored, which provides meaningful dialogues, diminishes the negative emotions provoked by the voices, and provides a forum whereby individuals can articulate their unique and purposeful perspectives on both their experience and its effective management—which may differ from the views of psychiatric professionals. As well as voice hearers themselves, the group may also include their relatives, friends, and allies, and empathic professionals may request permission to attend meetings in order to increase their own aptitude for assisting and supporting their clients. Often members will utilize the group for different purposes and in different ways. For this reason, it is generally not helpful to evaluate groups in terms of measurable outcomes, such as how many attend, as this will inevitably fluctuate as people's needs, requirements, and personal circumstances change (Downs, 2005). Generally, most members will find considerable comfort and reassurance simply in the group's existence, even if they use it intermittently. Groups vary in their emphasis on mutual support, exploring emotional issues, and education and campaigning work and can often complement individual psychotherapeutic support by providing people with the confidence to work more deeply on the emotions and narratives underlying their voice hearing experiences.

Self-help groups aim to provide appropriate support and resources for voice hearers to understand and cope with their experiences, 'a safe-haven where people feel accepted and comfortable' (Downs, 2005, p.5). Voice hearing, by definition, is a lonely experience—for not only can no one else hear the voices, the sense of shame and stigma engendered by societal attitudes means individuals are often left limited options for articulating their experiences and seeking support (Corstens, Escher, & Romme, 2008). Thus, providing a space where feelings can be discussed freely and without censure often proves hugely empowering. The knowledge that other group members have had similar experiences and have learned ways to cope with them is both normalizing and gives the individual huge levels of confidence and solidarity. Silence can be a handicap, and Escher (1993) has interviewed many voice hearers in order to elucidate the advantages of speaking about one's voices to a compassionate audience. Her findings can be summarized as the following:

1. Engaging with the experience can help identify patterns, such as linking negative or difficult feelings to a critical voice.

2. Discussion can stimulate acceptance of the voice hearing experience and help cultivate a healthy identity as someone who hears voices.

3. By recognizing and exploring possible meanings, individuals may begin negotiating and improving their relationship with their voices.

4. It can be affirming and validating for individuals to recognize their own situation in the experiences of others.

5. Whereas avoidance can evoke feelings of powerless and anxiety, talking can reduce isolation and fear.

While mental health professionals can assist in organizing this kind of self-help, it needs to be a genuinely shared and collaborative process with voice hearers themselves. In contrast to clinical perspectives, in which self-help is often organized in terms of diagnostic categories (e.g., schizophrenia, bipolar disorder), the English Hearing Voices Network (HVN) advocates groups that are simply organized on the basis of shared experience (voice hearing) regardless of psychiatric status. While professionals may be involved in an advisory capacity, or to provide resources and infrastructure in partnership with voice hearers, the group is led by shared decisions of all its members. Group members seek solutions within their own frame of reference or understanding without pressure to conform to medical or even psychological explanations. This means that there is an ethos within groups that different understandings of voice hearing are acceptable and that there is no one right way to understand the experience. There is also an emphasis on voice hearers taking responsibility for running self-help initiatives wherever possible. For example, HVN (which comprises of over 180 groups) now has a board of trustees entirely comprised of voice hearing individuals, whereas previously there were a greater proportion of academic and clinical professionals involved in its leadership. Within groups, members are encouraged to be active participants and are seen as having unique understanding and expertise about their own experiences. This can often be developed within a dialogical context, where different understandings of voice hearing are valued and exchanged. This atmosphere of mutual support and collective involvement enables former recipients of care to get involved in providing empowering and safe spaces for other voice hearers. Safety is ensured by agreeing ground rules around confidentiality, mutual respect, equal opportunities, respect for different understandings, and limiting access to non-voice hearers who just want to attend to 'observe'. Groups become places where people's courage to face their fears is generated. As Reeves (1997) describes, this courage enables people to commence on a journey of self-discovery.

In the weekly running of such groups, the democratic principle is for members to share decision-making in terms of how the group is run and what initiatives it adopts.

In the UK, over the last 20 years, hearing voices groups have primarily been a place for support and a forum for sharing self-help strategies. Yet as crucial as this function is, there has also been an equal emphasis on information dissemination, in which conferences, training courses, newsletters, and self-help literature are widely distributed to create productive partnerships with professionals, relatives, and other societal groups. Furthermore, this kind of outreach work has helped promote tolerance, awareness, and positive explanations for voice hearing as well as spread the ethos of the hearing voices movement to a wider audience (Downs, 2005).

Within groups many helpful processes occur. Launch events and publicity actions, done in conjunction with local and national media, informs a broader population about the resources available. A diverse range of coping strategies are regularly discussed and exchanged, and groups can often generate their own literature about this and distribute it to interested parties in the wider community. In relation to aggressive and bullying voices, voice hearers are encouraged to learn how to resist destructive commands and realize they have a choice over their actions. Grounding, expressive and calming exercises are often explored within groups to enhance people's coping abilities—not only to deal with the voice hearing experience itself in a meaningful way, but also the challenging thoughts and feelings, which often accompany it. Guest speakers from different spiritual, social, and professional perspectives can broaden the awareness of group members. People have the opportunity to learn to see their voice hearing as symbolic and meaningful. Within groups, there is an educational opportunity to learn about different ways of understanding voice hearing, including emotional, political, philosophical, cultural, and spiritual understandings. Groups are also a space to find out about current research findings relating to voice hearing. In addition, they are a place where people support each other to deal with the prejudice and misunderstanding voice hearers often experience in community and psychiatric settings. Within groups, people tell their stories about who they are and what they have been through, thus developing a stronger sense of autonomy, identity, and self-determination. A space is also created where people can hear reassuring and empowering stories about how others have transformed their relationships with their voice hearing experiences and their emotions.

In our experience of facilitating and attending self-help groups, this pooling of collective resources and abilities is an immensely positive, affirmative, and empowering phenomenon. For this reason, we have included the following three stories to both illustrate the power of collective discussion and debate and to serve as inspiration and motivation for people to expect more from themselves and their lives:

Example one: 'David'

David, a 45-year-old man who had been diagnosed with schizophrenia and received treatment for 20 years, came to the hearing voices group for the first time. That week there was a discussion about bullying, and how domineering voices often relate to bullying relationships people have experienced in the past. The next week, David spoke of the profound effect this had on him—no one had ever suggested possible links between his voices and his life experience before. He explained he had experienced sexual abuse as a child and how it made a lot of sense that his voices were linked to these experiences. He then described some of his voice's communications. As well as criticizing him, it urged him to seek revenge on authority. It spoke about the class system and said that when the time was right, he would be able to wreak revenge on people in power. Within the group, we discussed the importance of interpreting menacing voices in a symbolic rather than literal way as well as the concept of 'soft revenge' (i.e., restoring justice in society without re-enacting violence on others). Realizing that his voices related to disempowering experiences in his childhood (and his own need to address this injustice) gave David more confidence to resist direct commands from his voices and plan ways to get more involved in raising awareness about the damaging effects of childhood sexual abuse. David also brought other examples of the content of his voices to the group. For example, if they said 'you are useless' we discussed whether this was an indication David himself desired to be more active. This lead to him thinking about ways to get more involved in voluntary work.

In such a situation, it seems that the group can become an empowering place for people to think about the content of their voices and how this might relate to their own feelings, needs, desires, and aspirations. The fact that this process is witnessed by others in a group setting can add to the power of the realizations people have and resolutions they make to act in new ways.

Example two: 'Catherine'

Catherine was a young mother and a survivor of torture who was seeking asylum and a regular member of her local hearing voices group. When she first came to the group, she was extremely socially isolated. For six months, she heard the voice and saw the image of a fellow prisoner (who had died when they were both incarcerated) standing by her bedroom window. In the group, she described the guilt she felt about his death. Despite being reassured in the past that the perpetrators, not her, were responsible for her friend's death, these feelings of remorse had never left her. Because she found the image extremely frightening, Catherine slept in her lounge and could not go into the bedroom. The group suggested she write a letter to her friend and explain her feelings and sadness about his death. She did this, however, the image remained. In connection with the group, Catherine took part in a series of drama sessions that used improvization and drama-games to explore power relationships and voice hearing. Catherine also began attending a college after being told by another group member about a free crèche service at the college to access this. One day, shortly after a self-help group where we had concentrated on the value of facing your fears, Catherine decided to confront the image. Holding the hand of her young son, she walked up to it and touched it. Afterwards, the image vanished and has never reappeared.

The power of social connectedness of both attending the self-help group and later the college and drama group allowed Catherine to build up her confidence in being able to face her fears and find new ways to understand her trauma experiences, which her voice hearing and visions represented.

Example three: 'Nigel'

Nigel, a 29-year-old man, came to the group for the first time whilst an in-patients. Because the group had a guest speaker that week, I [Rufus] was aware we had not focused on coping strategies as much as we normally do when a new member arrives, so I offered to spend some time with Nigel afterwards exploring his experiences. Nigel heard two voices. One, which he had heard for five years, sounded like a 50-year old man, was critical, and often ordered him to self-harm. When asked if there was anyone in his life who had intimidated him in the way the voice did, Nigel identified a geography teacher who used to hit the desks with a ruler in a threatening way. Nigel reflected that maybe this was a significant experience of a formidable authoritarian figure in his life and the voice therefore reflected many of the characteristics of this character. This voice had started shortly after Nigel had a major operation in which he thought he was going to die. I explained that sometimes we may subconsciously invite figures in our minds to come and help us at difficult times. Nigel related to this to a memory of when he was very ill in hospital, thinking the doctors were trying to kill him. In his dream-like state, he had requested 'the devil' to help him survive. Nigel had read Faust (who sells his soul to the devil in return for youth and power) when he was younger and considered that he might have used this story as a blueprint to recruit a powerful fighting spirit for help. I explained that he could change the 'contract' with this figure in order to reclaim his fighting energy and learn to stand up for himself.

We explored this possibility with me encouraging him to have a conversation with his voice. Nigel had never conversed with it before, but with my support, asked the voice why he had appeared. The voice said, 'To help you survive'. Nigel then asked it why it told him to cut himself, to which it replied 'To show people how strong you are'. I then asked Nigel to ask the voice if it wanted him to stand up for himself and express his needs more: 'Yes', the voice said, 'That is what I have been trying to tell him for years'. Nigel then asked the voice 'So you ask me to self harm when you are frustrated that I have not stood up for myself?' The voice agreed this was the case. We then did some assertiveness exercises and shadowboxing to enact Nigel defending himself. The voice commented to Nigel that it particularly liked the boxing. I suggested he write a letter to the voice, acknowledging how it had helped him have a fighting spirit when physically ill but now the arrangement/contract needed to change as he wished to reclaim his fighting spirit and learn to stick up for his needs and to invite the voice to support him in this endeavour. We discussed how he could learn to interpret his voice not as a bully but as someone who is trying to teach him to assert himself more and defend his boundaries more.

The second voice was female and aged about 25. She was less negative than the first voice and only spoke about Nigel rather than to him. Nigel said that he also felt aged 25, despite chronologically being 29. We reflected that the shock of the operation had prevented him from developing emotionally. I asked Nigel if anybody fitted the description of the voice. Nigel explained that he had a female friend who had died in a car-crash about the time of his operation, which made him feel guilty that she had died while he had survived. I explained how survivor guilt is very common in such situations and suggested he write a letter to his 25-year-old self, explaining that he was entitled to live and that the best way to honour his friend's life was to live his own to the full. I also suggested he take up a self-defence practice and read Non-Violent Communication literature to help him learn to express his feelings assertively. The final suggestion was for Nigel to regularly come to the hearing voices group in order to meet other people who had changed their relationship with their voices.

This example shows how individual (psychotherapeutic) work complements self-help group work. We have found that the sense of acceptance (or normalization) one gets from attending a group gives people the courage to face and set boundaries with their voice hearing experiences and find new ways to integrate the emotions the voices represent into their lives. Nigel was soon discharged from hospital and became a regular member of the group as he rebuilt his confidence and began to plan ways to return to employment.

White (1996) has chronicled his experiences of self-help group facilitation under the title 'Power to Our Journeys', in which members describe how the sense of acknowledgement, justice, solidarity, and 'lightness of being' the group provided helped rekindle their love of life. Similarly, Ron Coleman, whose own triumph from the anguish of voice hearing is well documented (e.g., James, 2001; Laurance, 2003; Coleman, 2004), uses a travel analogy to describe the journey back to reclaiming one's life. Although painful and arduous, the voyage is considerably eased by a good map of the terrain, and this is something self-help groups can provide. The support and guidance offered by others who have travelled similar journeys is not about providing an instant solution, but motivating and inspiring members into learning to understand themselves. According to Romme and Escher (2000, p.116), this approach is enabling in that 'energy is freed up to allow people to be themselves [beyond the group]…an important prerequisite to gaining a new balance and social integration'. In the quest to change from 'victim to victor' (Coleman & Smith, 2006) practical healing from distress goes hand-in-hand with learning to understand one's self and experiences—personal input being the most powerful tool for change.

Practical self-help initiatives

Voices can threaten, disturb, command, and capture voice hearers in a demoralizing cycle of dependence, isolation, and destructive activities. Furthermore, their influence tends to increase when the person pacifies them and sets no boundaries (Chadwick & Birchwood, 1994). Fortunately, there are many strategies voice hearers can use to challenge the voices, impose their own limits and thus regain some control. As noted by Watkins (1998), a crucial source of distress and discontent for many voice hearers relates to the fear of losing control. Given the peculiarly invasive quality that voices possess, this is an understandable imperative; being constantly invaded and imposed upon brings its own breed of helplessness. Thus, a repertoire of methods for decreasing distress and regaining control is a key principle in any voice hearer's self-help strategy (e.g., Carter, MacKinnon, & Copolov, 1996; Coleman, Smith, & Good, 2003; Perron & Munson, 2006; Farhall, this volume). However, many mental health practitioners are unaware of effective coping strategies for managing distressing voices or how to teach them to their clients (Coffey & Hewitt, 2008). Furthermore, while the traditional service response is to refute the existence of voices and re-orientate clients towards a more impartial, objective reality, voice hearers themselves will often express a desire to utilize coping strategies in a bid to reclaim their sense of personal autonomy and control (Coffey & Hewitt, 2008). These imperatives are a crucial self-help strategy, as the attainment of such mastery over adverse experience is deemed an essential part of recovery not only from distressing voices (Honig, Romme, Ensink, Escher, Pennings, & Devries, 1998) but from mental health problems more generally (Young & Ensing, 1999).

The following table illustrates a range of self-help techniques that have been generated and discussed by members of the hearing voices in Bradford support group (to which the authors are affiliated) over the past few years. A certain amount of trial-and-error learning is germane to successful coping, as each individual must learn what suits them best and is most appropriate for their particular needs and circumstances. Furthermore, as voice hearing is an experience that occurs within the context of a person's whole life, a holistic, flexible approach to coping is the most apposite and useful. Thus, the following categories are a good example of the considerable creativity and resourcefulness individuals can draw from in order to mitigate and ease their distress (Table 14.1).

Mindfulness

Mindfulness is an extremely compatible tool for self-help groups and individual self-help endeavours, as it is a skill that is enhanced in group settings, yet for optimal efficacy needs to be regularly practiced by the individual in an independent manner. Mindfulness is increasingly being used for psychological approaches to voice hearing and other experiences that can be seen as 'psychotic' (e.g. Chadwick, Taylor, & Abba, 2005; Abba, Chadwick, & Stevenson, 2008). Acceptance and Commitment Therapy (e.g., Fletcher & Hayes, 2005) and dialectical behavioural therapy (e.g., Robins, 2002) are two techniques for working with voice hearers that place mindfulness at the heart of the method.

Table 14.1 Helpful and unhelpful strategies for coping with distressing voices

Distraction techniques	◆ Watch films—comedy or inspirational.
	◆ Read comedy novels or joke books.
	◆ Listen to music.
	◆ Tidy the house.
	◆ Shopping.
	◆ Phone a friend.
	◆ Gardening.
	◆ Exercise, e.g., playing sport, walking the dog, running, dancing, swimming.
	◆ Wear ear-plugs.
	◆ Reading aloud.
	◆ Puzzles/crosswords/sudouko.
	◆ Arts and crafts.
	◆ Watch TV.
	◆ Cooking.
	◆ Humming or singing.
	◆ Playing board games/cards/computer.
Relaxation strategies	◆ Give yourself permission to relax.
	◆ Recognise and acknowledge fears, then consciously let go of them.
	◆ Prayer.
	◆ Meditation.
	◆ Massage/acupuncture/yoga.
	◆ Focus on your breathing/breathe deeply.
	◆ Listen to guided relaxation CDs.
	◆ Listen to soothing music.
	◆ Relax each muscle individually.
Self-care and comfort	◆ Keep a list of achievements and strengths or a list of positive things other people have said about you.
	◆ Positive self-talk and self-forgiveness.
	◆ Look at comforting items, e.g., e-mails, love letters, birthday cards, and photos.
	◆ Take a warm, scented bath.
	◆ Wear comfortable clothes.
	◆ Get help with practical problems, e.g., housing, finances.
	◆ Remember that situations/feelings frequently change—'This too shall pass'.
	◆ Record positive statements onto a CD.
	◆ Eat a healthy diet.
	◆ Do something nice for 'me' each day.

(Continued)

Table 14.1 (continued) Helpful and unhelpful strategies for coping with distressing voices

	♦ Keep in frequent contact with support network, even if feeling okay.
	♦ Buy/pick fresh flowers.
	♦ Change the sheets on your bed.
	♦ Get a pet, or help care for someone else's.
	♦ Hold a safe, comforting object.
	♦ Holidays.
	♦ Humour.
	♦ Plan the day to ensure there aren't long periods of time with nothing to do.
	♦ Sleeping.
	♦ Create a personalised crisis plan when you are feeling well.
	♦ Having good support around you.
Making sense of the experience	♦ Keep a record of what the voices are saying.
	♦ Talk about the voices to someone you trust.
	♦ Join a self-help group or set one up.
	♦ Identify the voices—number, gender, age, etc.
	♦ Identifying triggers, e.g., situations, emotions, other people…
	♦ 'Voice dialoguing'—let someone you trust speak directly to the voices.
	♦ Talk to the voices, find out how they feel.
	♦ Write poetry/prose regarding feelings.
	♦ Paint/draw emotions.
	♦ Accepting that the voices themselves are not the problem, they are the result of a deeper, underlying problem. Your task is to find out more.
	♦ Acknowledging the association between trauma or significantly stressful life events and the voice hearing experience.
Challenging the voices	♦ Refuse to obey commands, or delay obeying them.
	♦ Ask the voices to justify their comments.
	♦ 'Time sharing'—schedule a time for them, and refuse to listen until that ♦ time.
	♦ Mentally visualize a barrier between yourself and the voices.
	♦ Set boundaries—refuse to speak with negative voices unless they are respectful.
	♦ Making deals, e.g., 'be quiet now and I'll listen later'.
	♦ Selective listening—only listening to the positive/least negative voices.
	♦ Using positive voices as allies.
	♦ Talk back to them (use a mobile phone if in public).
	♦ Examine the validity of what they say, e.g., Have they said the same things before? Do their predictions always come true? Is it possible to ignore them with no obvious consequences?

(Continued)

Table 14.1 (continued) Helpful and unhelpful strategies for coping with distressing voices

Unhelpful strategies	◆ Being over-medicated and medication side-effects.
	◆ Prejudice and stigma.
	◆ Being labelled with a psychiatric diagnosis.
	◆ Being told not to talk about voices because they are 'not real'.
	◆ Professionals rejecting your explanation for your voices.
	◆ Insomnia.
	◆ Other people having low expectations for you.
	◆ Being lonely and isolated.
	◆ Not having information.
	◆ Feeling negative and hopeless.

The roots of mindfulness are in Buddhist psychology, which has been developed over the last 3,000 years. We often use mindfulness at the beginning or end of self-help groups. It helps relax group members and re-orient them to their surroundings after discussing what can be challenging and emotional subjects that are related to the content of group member's voices. The aim of mindfulness is to develop an accepting approach to thoughts and feelings, and through understanding, these experiences develop more detachment and choice about how they influence us. Mindfulness aims to anchor the mind in 'the here and now' and promote a warm and compassionate approach to difficult events and experiences. The writings of Kabat-Zinn (2001, 2005) and Nhat Hanh (2002, 2005) have been instructive self-help texts for many people using hearing voices groups. The following are mindfulness exercises that individuals within the hearing voices self-help movement report finding of benefit:

Mindful breathing

There are many mindful breathing exercises. Counting the breath involves counting each in-breath and out-breath: 'Breathing in one, breathing out one, breathing in two, breathing out two', and so on up to five (or ten). If the person becomes distracted and loses count, they return to one again. This is continued for a set time, say ten minutes. Sitting calmly, focussing on the breath is another possible technique. Every time the person notices they have become distracted, they acknowledge the thought or feeling and come back to their breathing. If someone finds, they are too easily distracted, visualizing breathing in 'healing white light' and breathing out 'black smoke of negativity' is another exercise that can be used.

Alternate nostril breathing

Alternate nostril breathing involves the following exercise: hold one nostril closed and breathe in, then close the other nostril and breathe out, breathe back in the same nostril, close that nostril, and breathe out the other. Repeat for ten minutes.

Mindful walking

As we walk along the street, we can focus on each step whether we are breathing in or out, so we might be saying 'in, in, in, out, out, out', and so on. This technique can again reduce the number of thoughts flowing through our mind as we focus our concentration on our breathing. If indoors, we can do a slower meditation where we walk, very slowly, moving one foot forward in time with each in-breath or out-breath. If the person is practicing mindful walking on their own, they can invite someone they trust and respect to accompany them in their mind. For example, as someone is walking and he/she breathes in they can say, for example 'Ben, Ben, Ben', inviting their friend's presence to be with them; and as they breathe out say in their mind 'I am here, I am here, I am here', which also says that the person is there for their friend too (adapted from Nhat Hanh, 2002). A fourth type of mindful walking involves just walking slowly and focusing on each step and the environment as it is perceived through the senses. This can be very calming and grounding if we do it in a park or other more natural setting.

Adopting a non-judgemental approach to challenging thoughts seems also very applicable to voice hearing. Nhat Hanh (2002) recommends smiling towards challenging thought structures, which he describes as habit energies, saying, '*Hello habit energy, I know you are there but you cannot make me do anything I don't want to do. I acknowledge you are there but I am free from your influence*'. We can use this same non-judgemental but assertive attitude towards voices. From this position of tolerance, we can go on to understand what emotions and relationship issues the voices might be representing. This is similar to the attitudinal change recommended by Romme and Escher (2000): 'Changing the relation to the voices is to become respectful to them, not fighting against them but talking to them slowly and with warmth, which has as a consequence that they also change their approach. It can also be testing out their power and finding that they are not almighty at all'.

Phases of healing and recovery

Both trauma and recovery research and hearing voices literature suggests there are three phases of healing: safety, making sense of one's experiences, and social reconnection (e.g., Romme & Escher, 1993; Herman, 1992; May, 2004). Both group and individual approaches to self-help have embraced this therapeutic knowledge about what assists recovery. Within such groups, an individual can meet others who (in many ways) are further on in the recovery process, and this can be extremely motivating. The recovery stages of safety, 'making sense', and social reconnection are not a linear process. For example, a deep sense of understanding one's experiences may only come once someone feels grounded in a set of social relationships where they are valued and supported. The phases of recovery are more likely to be a circular, dynamic, and iterative procedure that people need to revisit as they move forwards and become more confident in relations to their voice hearing experiences and wider social relationships. A challenge for mental health professionals is to sensitively endorse and support such recoveries in a way that is guided both by the experiences of voice hearers and the developing literature in the area (Repper, 2000, 2002).

Phase one: Safety

Central to this preliminary stage is learning to cope with the intense anxiety that often accompanies the onset of voice hearing. In recognition of this, Romme and Escher (1993) have deemed the beginning of voice hearing as the 'startling stage', in lieu of its shocking and disorientating character. Even if voices are positive, the awareness that seemingly separate consciousnesses are imposing on our thoughts and feelings can be a deeply frightening, unsettling experience (e.g., Steele, 2002; Coleman, 2004). Furthermore, voice hearing's taboo status in Western society means it is often treated with mistrust and fear; the dread that others will not understand or accept us may fuel the voice hearer's sense of shame, stigma, and isolation (Leudar & Thomas, 2000; Romme, 2000; Longden, 2005; Coleman, 2008).

Thus, the key task in this stage is to normalize the experience, accept that one is hearing voices and then develop ways to regain a sense of control and calmness in order to deal with their intrusions. It is very important for the voice hearer to find trusting relationships to talk with about the voices (Romme & Escher, 1993) and self-help groups can be good safe space to meet others who will listen non-judgmentally and share similar experiences reducing a person's sense of isolation and alienation (Downs, 2005). Meaningful social activities can also be very grounding, and if established or resumed, can create significant levels of safety. Indeed, making social changes that reduce isolation or agitation, but increase one's sense of social participation can be significantly helpful at this stage. Self-help materials, normalization literature, and recovery stories can promote hope, optimism, and acceptance. Very useful, accessible resources of this type are readily available on Internet websites such as Intervoice (see Table 14.2). Medication is one means of reducing the fear and anxiety associated with voice hearing, although within the self-help movement many individuals make informed choices to seek other ways of reducing anxiety and coping with their distress (e.g., Longden, 2003; Hall, 2007; Harrow & Jobe, 2007). Where medication is used, it is also recommended people learn other, more active strategies to induce relaxation or productively process and channel anxiety into action. Thus, voice hearers learn to own their voices and take responsibility for their actions (Coleman & Smith, 2006). Distraction strategies can provide some initial relief, although their long-term benefit is not substantial and more active strategies are likely to be required to deal with voices more comprehensively. There are a broad range of relaxation exercises people can learn to use, including breathing exercises, self-massage techniques, yoga, and more general physical exercises. For example, Smith (2008) describes how spinning (an indoor form of high-intensity cycling) provided her with ways to cope with a difficult, critical voice. Walking in natural surroundings may be very effective as a way to reduce anxiety and mindfulness techniques, as described previously, have been found to be of great benefit. Positive affirmations may also be helpful (e.g., Hay, 2004) as well as literature from the emotional freedom technique (e.g., Lynch & Lynch, 2007).

Because preparation in advance of the voices beginning can be beneficial, anticipatory work such as identifying likely triggers (e.g., demanding social situations) and preparing ways to respond to the voices or implement coping strategies can be extremely helpful.

Table 14.2 Helpful organizations

Intervoice

An international network for training, education, and research into hearing voices. The organization also works across the world to spread positive and hopeful messages about voice hearing experiences.

www.intervoiceonline.org

The English Hearing Voices Network (HVN)

Offers information, support, and understanding to people who hear voices and those who support them. It also aims to promote awareness, tolerance, and understanding of voice hearing, visions, tactile sensations, and other unusual experiences. The site is full of resources around voice hearing, including newsletters, discussion forums, and links to support groups.

www.hearingvoices.org

Grampian Hearing Voices Network

Aims to relieve the distress and meet the needs of voice hearers, their friends, family, careers, and professionals by promoting the development of Hearing Voices Self-Help Groups throughout Scotland. Also aims to educate through the provision and distribution of training and research.

http://www.ghvn.blogspot.com/

Hearing Voices Network Australia

Aims to promote the acceptance of hearing voices and enable recovery for those in distress through providing self-help groups, education, and awareness.

http://www.rfwa.org.au/hvna.php

New Zealand Hearing Voices Peer Support Network

www.keepwell.co.nz

Stichting Weelank (Foundation Resonance)

The Dutch Hearing Voices Network.

www.stemmenhoren.nl

Netzwerk Stimmenhören

The German Hearing Voices Network

www.stimmenhoeren.de

Le Parole Ritrovate (The Words Recovered)

The Italian Hearing Voices Network.

www.leparoleritrovate.com

The Freedom Center

An American-based support and activism community for anyone experiencing mental health difficulties. Includes event lists, links, and advice around medication.

www.freedom-center.org

Such preparatory work allows a greater sense of confidence in dealing with voices when they commence, or become particularly challenging.

For many people, a crucial component of coping with voices is learning ways to express anger and other emotions. Where voices encourage or command aggressive behaviour, finding a non-violent way to express agitation can be very helpful (e.g., hitting a punch bag, drumming, writing angry letters that you don't have to send, and doing intense physical exercises or recruiting support from others to assertively address some experience of injustice.) A voice hearer who corresponds with one of the authors has learned that the symbolic action of screwing anger up into a ball and then blowing it away, or smiling at people she does not like helps her deal with her anger. Romme and Escher (2000) advocate listening carefully to what the voice says, wait a few moments, and then write down what it said. This is followed by thinking of and writing down ten different ways of expressing anger, which can then be implemented by the person. Another soothing technique that can be prepared for times of distress is for the person to mentally generate a compassionate figure, which they imagine is sending them warm feelings and attitudes such as understanding, sympathy, love, and reassurance. The figure can be real and known to the person or spiritual/imaginary (for example, individuals can devise their compassionate figure as an animal such as a lion, or an angel, or wise guide, etc). If desired, an object can be carried to symbolize this figure. Approaches of this nature have been used by Buddhists for hundreds of years and can provide the person with an alternative set of values to customary, destructive thoughts about the self. Recently psychologists such as Gilbert and Procter (2006) have clearly outlined the technique to combat feelings of shame and self-loathing, which difficult voices are often related to. Such visualization techniques can also be used to create positive voices, or individuals can visualize the self-help group in times of distress or carry a picture of the group.

Another important step is for the person to begin to set aside time to listen to the voices, rather than trying to avoid every confrontation with them (Corstens, Escher, & Romme, 2008). To this end, 'time-sharing' is an invaluable strategy whereby voice hearers arrange to have a specific time to listen to the voice and insist the voices wait until this scheduled time before listening to them (possibly writing down what they say). Such time-limited listening should be coupled with neglecting the voices at other times of the day. This can be combined with asking the voices for information or writing down what they say in order to understand them better and challenge the avoidance most people adopt when they are afraid of experiences. As well as helping acquire more distance and sense of choice, this strategy may be a progressive move towards dialoguing with the voice, a technique generally used in the 'making sense' stage. In contrast, for 'commentary-style' voices, which resist conversation, Romme and Escher (2000) suggest making 'simple replies' where individuals merely state whether or not they agree with the voices in a calm and assertive manner.

Phase two: Making sense of one's experiences

Once initial anxiety has been reduced, individuals may use the skills learned in the first stage to begin exploring the meaning of their voices more fully. Central to the 'making sense' process is paying detailed attention to the possible significance of the voices to the voice hearer with regard to both past and present, understanding the underlying emotions the voices represent and finding ways to manage these experiences. Essentially, this is about the person learning to use their voices as clues to inner conflict that need to be understood and channelled in new ways.

There are particular self-help techniques that are likely to aid this exploration. For example, keeping a record about circumstances under which the voices are heard, what they have to say and the nature of any triggers can assist in identifying patterns and making meaning. Such 'Voice Diaries' are excellent self-help tools not only for chronicling what the voices are saying, but as a space to reflect on one's own thoughts and feelings about it. Engaging in psychological therapy can help a person learn to interpret their voices more symbolically. Developing an ongoing personal narrative about the relationship between one's voices and one's life history, and communicating this to others, can be constructive and affirming. Similarly, a recent literature has begun to advocate the importance of exploring and privileging the relationships voice hearer's have with their voices (e.g., Hayward & May, 2007 ; Moskowitz & Corstens, 2007; Chin, Hayward, & Drinnan, 2008; Hayward, Denney, Vaughan, & Fowler, 2008; Corstens, May, & Longden, in press). Exploring the power and intimacy of these dynamics can help an individual gain a different perspective on what the voices are trying to communicate, as well as stimulate feelings of autonomy and control. At this point, it is very important for individuals to have opportunities to develop a full, healthy identity as someone who hears voices. Thus, the support and encouragement of groups can be very useful at this stage.

Certain emotions may be severely repressed in voice hearers so setting time aside to tune into one's emotion as desires and needs is likely to be of benefit. Likewise, learning emotional communication skills and trying them out in social relationships (e.g., Rosenberg, 2003) can help people learn to express and tolerate difficult, overwhelming feelings. In parallel to coping with the voices themselves, attention should be paid to the traumatic, underlying—and often unresolved—issues that originally evoked their presence. This should be carried out using psychotherapeutic interventions, which are very compatible with self-help initiatives. Therefore, it is good if self-help groups establish links with psychological therapists who can facilitate such emotional work on both group and individual levels.

Spiritual frameworks are consistently found to be helpful explanatory models for many voice hearers (Romme & Escher, 1993). As a consequence, self-help groups and initiatives are flexible in incorporating and valuing these perspectives (e.g., May, 2007a) and linking people to spiritual communities and also giving spiritual communities educational support around self-help approaches to hearing voices.

Phase three: Socially reconnecting

Recovery is about dealing with life and its difficulties. Voices challenge this process, but can also be adapted towards solving and understanding one's emotional obstacles and social dilemmas. Thus, through accepting the voices, talking about them, and finding positive ways to communicate with them, voice hearers can learn to have pride in their experiences, give their voices a personal and positive meaning, cope with them effectively, and create a life that the voices become part of—not the life that the voices dictate to them.

However, the shock of hearing voices—and the often catastrophic social reaction to the experience—means many people need to work hard and have good support before they are able to reconnect with valued activities and roles in society. This 'social inclusion' stage is as important and challenging as any other, given the prejudice and discrimination that exists currently towards voice hearing experience (e.g., Corrigan & Penn, 1997; James, 2001; Knight, Wykes, & Hayward, 2003). Therefore, initiatives that support this social recovery stage need more support and attention from social institutions. For instance, vocational activity may follow on from a process of emotional healing, or it may be a necessary progression that allows the person to feel safe enough to commence such healing and 'making sense' processes. As described, many individuals link their voice hearing to abuse and other experiences of injustice (see, e.g., Hammersley, Read, Woodall, & Dillon, 2007; Pearson, Smalley, Ainsworth, Cook, Boyle, & Flury, 2008; Andrew, Gray, & Snowden, 2008). In this social recovery stage, survivors often choose a 'survivor mission' that seeks to address these experiences in some restorative way and help prevent future psychological violence (Herman, 1992). Finding ways to contribute to the lives of others is also psychologically strengthening; finding roles that are valued by the self and others allows the nurture of self-confidence, which may have been severely damaged by periods of isolation and/or institutionalization. Some voice hearers may decide to contribute to the hearing voices movement by getting involved in community education initiatives; others can become role models by pursuing careers elsewhere whilst being open about their voice hearing. Social reconnection is also about educating the wider communities about the meaningfulness and acceptability of voice hearing. Therefore, in order to heal the denial and prejudice in wider society, many voice hearers have lead and participated in media projects that offer respectful and informative accounts of the voice hearing experience (e.g., Gunasena, 2004; May, 2007; Regan, 2008).

Conclusion

Because of their autonomous nature and resistance to traditional measures of evaluation and outcome, hearing voices self-help groups have not been systematically evaluated. However, hearing voices groups and the 'hearing voices approach' have now become more commonplace and accepted within mainstream mental health services (e.g., Wykes, Parr, & Landau, 1999; Coupland, 2000; Martin, 2000; Perron & Munson, 2006). Furthermore, their success can be measured by their popularity with voice hearers; in the UK, where there is a strong community development ethos, there are over 180 groups that have emerged over the last 20 years. Culturally, this phenomena is being increasingly recognized in newspaper stories and documentaries and dramas where the voice hearing experience is increasingly more accurately portrayed. There is also growing recognition of their efficacy in health care settings—for example, in the UK, a recent Healthcare Commission Report (2008) commended mental health trusts, which provided hearing voices groups in acute settings as offering 'appropriate and safe interventions' and advocated the wider availability of these resources in all psychiatric hospitals.

Self-help movements should not be seen as competing with therapeutic traditions, but complementary to them. Doubtless, some of the more personal dynamic work often required to integrate powerful emotions that voices represent is often something that cannot be supported by self-help initiatives alone and requires additional individual psychotherapeutic support. Nevertheless, the self-help ethos inspired by the hearing voices movement offers an emancipatory set of ideals where an individual can learn to see their voice hearing as an acceptable and meaningful experience. By embracing the experience through support from others and self-help approaches, voice hearing is reframed as both as an experience that one can live with and one that can inform us about our social lives and ways we can live together more peacefully. The 'Maastricht Approach', initiated by Romme and Escher, sees voices as a meaningful, interpretable experience originating within an individual's personal history and against a backdrop of overwhelming emotions in traumatic, threatening conditions. By working within this frame of reference, the purpose and meaning of the voices can be deciphered and communication with them promoted. Such a framework sits comfortably alongside spiritual frameworks that many voice hearers find helpful. Within the emancipatory approach, self-help techniques and personal narratives are seen as equal to academic and professional knowledge bases. Increasingly training events and resources are starting to reflect this power shift by increasing the involvement of people who hear voices more in their production. Thus, a new, more collaborative approach to therapy and ways of working to recovery is emerging. Within this equation, recovery and empowerment are the main objectives and self-help the guiding force. Integral to this is the promotion of social support through affirmative stories, positive information, and encouraging attitudinal change. Self-help movements can offer safe spaces for voice hearers to discover the power of mutual encouragement and creative ideas in order to reclaim control over both their voices and their lives. For professionals, we believe it is our duty to enable such cultures and opportunities through individual, societal, and political initiatives and support.

References

Abba, N., Chadwick, P., & Stevenson, C. (2008). Responding mindfully to distressing psychosis: A grounded theory analysis. *Psychother Res*, **18**(1), 77–87.

Andrew, E. M., Gray, N. S., & Snowden, R. J. (2008). The relationship between trauma and beliefs about hearing voices: A study of psychiatric and non-psychiatric voice hearers. *Psychol Med*, **38**, 1409–1417.

Baker, P. (1989). *Hearing Voices*. Manchester: the Hearing Voices Network.

Carter, D., MacKinnon, A., & Copolov, D. (1996). Patients' strategies for coping with auditory hallucinations. *J Nerv Ment Dis*, **184**(3), 159–164.

Chadwick, P., & Birchwood, M. (1994). The omnipotence of voices: A cognitive approach to auditory hallucinations. *Br J Psychiatry*, **164**, 190–201.

Chadwick, P., Taylor, K. N., & Abba, N. (2005). Mindfulness groups for people with psychosis. *Behav Cogn Psychother*, **33**, 351–359.

Chin, J. T., Hayward, M., & Drinnan, A. (2008). 'Relating' to voices: Exploring the relevance of this concept to people who hear voices. *Psychology and Psychotherapy: Theory, Research and Practice*.

Coffey, M., & Hewitt, J. (2008). 'You don't talk about the voices': Voice hearers and community mental health nurses talk about responding to voice hearing experiences. *J Clin Nurs*, **17**(2), 1591–1600.

Coleman, R., Smith, M., & Good, J. (2003). *Psychiatric First Aid in Psychosis: A Handbook for Nurses, Carers and People Distressed by Psychotic Experience* (2nd Edition). Fife: P&P Press Ltd.

Coleman, R. (2004). *Recovery: An Alien Concept* (2nd Edition). Fife: P&P Press Ltd.

Coleman, R., & Smith, M. (2006). *Working with Voices: Victim to Victor* (2nd Edition). Fife: P&P Press Ltd.

Coleman, R., (2008). *Working with Voices: A Working to Recovery Training and Education Manual.* Fife: P&P Press Ltd.

Corrigan, P. W., & Penn, D. (1997). Disease and discrimination: Two paradigms that describe severe mental illness. *J Ment Health.* **6**(4), 355–366.

Corstens, D., Escher, S., & Romme, M. (2008). Accepting and working with voices: The Maastricht Approach. In A. Moskowitz, I. Schafer and M. J. Dorahy (Eds.), *Psychosis, Trauma and Dissociation: Emerging Perspectives on Severe Psychopathology* (pp. 319–331). Oxford: Wiley-Blackwell.

Corstens, D., Longden, E., & May, R. (in press). *Talking With Voices.* Fife: P&P Press Ltd.

Coupland, K. (2000). The experience of focussed group-work for voice hearers experiencing malevolent voices. *Netlink, The Quarterly Journal of the Network for Psychiatric Nursing Research*, **16**, 3–4.

Dillon, J. (2006). Collective voices. *Open Mind*, **142**, 16–18.

Downs, J. (2005). *Starting and Supporting Hearing Voices Groups.* Manchester: The Hearing Voices Network.

Escher, S. (1993). Talking about voices. In M. Romme and S. Escher (Eds.), *Accepting Voices* (pp. 50–59). London: Mind Publications.

Fletcher, L. & Hayes, S. C. (2005). Relational frame theory, acceptance and commitment therapy, and a functional analytic definition of mindfulness. *J Ration Emot Cogn Behav Ther*, **23**(4), 315–336.

Garety, P. A., Kuipers, E., Fowler, D., Freeman, D., & Bebbington, P. E. (2001). A cognitive model of the positive symptoms of psychosis. *Psychol Med*, **31**(2), 189–195.

Gilbert, P. & Procter, S. (2006). Compassionate mind training for people with high shame and self-criticism: Overview and pilot study of a group therapy approach. *Clinical Psychology and Psychotherapy*, **13**, 353–379.

Gunasena, M. (Director). (2004). *Evolving Minds.* Undercurrents Films.

Hall, W. (2007). *Harm-Reduction Guide to Coming off Psychiatric Drugs.* A publication by the Icarus Project and The Freedom Center. Available online at: http://theicarusproject.net/alternative-treatments/harm-reduction-guide-to-coming-off-psychiatric-drugs.

Hammersley, P., Read, J., Woodall, S., & Dillon, J. (2007). Childhood trauma and psychosis: The genie is out of the bottle. *The Journal of Psychological Trauma*, **6** (2/3), 7–20.

Harrow, M., & Jobe, T. H. (2007). Factors involved in outcome and recovery in schizophrenia patients not on antipsychotic medications: A 15-year multifollow-up study. *Journal of Nervous and Mental Disorders*, **195**(5), 406–14.

Hay, L. (2004). *I Can Do It: How to Use Affirmations to Change Your Life.* London: Hay House Inc.

Hayward, M., & May, R. (2007). Daring to talk back. *Mental Health Practice*, **10**(9), 12–15.

Hayward, M., Denney, J., Vaughan, S., & Fowler, D. (2008). The voice and you: Development and psychometric evaluation of a measure of relationships with voices. *Clinical Psychology and Psychotherapy*, **15**, 45–52.

Healthcare Commission Report. (2008). *The Pathway to Recovery: A Review of NHS Acute in-Patient Mental Health Services.* London: The Healthcare Commission.

Herman, J. L. (1992). *Trauma and Recovery: The Aftermath of Violence from Domestic Abuse to Political Terror.* New York: Basic Books.

Hewitt, J. (2007). Critical evaluation of the use of research tools in evaluating quality of life for people with schizophrenia. *Int J Ment Health Nurs*, **16**, 2–14.

Honig, A., Romme, M. A. J., Ensink, B. J. M., Escher, S. D., Pennings, M. H. A., & Devries, M. W. (1998). Auditory hallucinations: A comparison between patients and non-patients. *The J Nerv Ment Dis*, **186**(10), 646–651.

James, A. (2001). *Raising our Voices: An Account of the Hearing Voices Movement.* Gloucester: Handsell Publishing.

Kabat Zinn, J. (2001). *Full Catastrophe Living: How to Cope with Pain and Illness Using Mindfulness Meditation.* London: Piatkus Books.

Kabat-Zinn, J. (2005). *Coming to Our Senses: Healing Ourselves and the World Through Mindfulness.* London: Piatkus Books.

Knight, M. T. D., Wykes, T., & Hayward, P. (2003). 'People don't understand': An investigation of stigma in schizophrenia using Interpretative Phenomenological Analysis (IPA). *J Ment Health*, **12**(3), 209–222.

Kopelowicz, A., Liberman, R. P., & Zarate, R. (2002). Psychosocial treatments for schizophrenia. In P. Nathan and J. Gorman (Eds.), *Treatments that Work: Evidence-based Treatments for Psychiatric Disorders* (2nd ed.), (pp. 201–228). New York: Oxford University Press.

Laing, R.D., & Esterson, A. (1964). *Sanity, Madness and the Family*, London: Penguin.

Laurance, J. (2003). Life Stories: Ron Coleman. In *Pure Madness: How Fear Drives the Mental Health System* (pp. 134–138). London: Routledge.

Leudar, I., & Thomas, P. (2000). *Voices of Reason, Voices of Insanity: Studies of Verbal Hallucinations.* London: Routledge.

Longden, E. (2003). Psychosis: Recovery and discovery. *Asylum: The Magazine for Democratic Psychiatry*, **14**(1), 27–28.

Longden, E. (2005). The dance of the lepers. *Asylum: The Magazine for Democratic Psychiatry*, **15** (1), 34–36.

Lynch, V., & Lynch, P. (2007). *Emotional Healing in Minutes: Simple Acupressure Techniques for Your Emotions* (2nd Edition). London: Thorsons.

Martin, P. J. (2000). Hearing voices and listening to those that hear them. *Journal of Psychiatric & Mental Health Nursing*, **7**, 135–141.

May R. (2004). Making sense of psychotic experiences and working towards recovery. In Gleeson, J. and McGorry, P. (Eds.), *Psychological Interventions in Early Psychosis* (pp. 245–260), London: Wiley.

May, R. (2007a). Reclaiming mad experience: Establishing unusual belief groups and evolving minds public meetings. In Stastny, P. & Lehmann, P. (Eds), *Alternatives Beyond Psychiatry* (pp. 117–128). Shrewsbury: Lehmann Publications.

May, R. (2007b). Mental Health Special Issue of The Independent on Sunday's, *The Sunday Review*, 18 March 2007. Independent News and Media LTD.

Moskowitz, A. & Corstens, D. (2007). Auditory hallucinations: Psychotic symptom or dissociative experience? *Journal of Psychological Trauma*, **6**, 35–63.

Nhat Hanh, T. (2002). *Be Free Wherever You Are.* London: Parallax Press.

Nhat Hanh, T. (2006). *Present Moment Wonderful Moment: Mindfulness Verses for Daily Living.* London: Parallax Press.

Pearson, D., Smalley, M., Ainsworth, C., Cook, M., Boyle, J., & Flury, S. (2008). Auditory hallucinations in adolescent and adult students: Implications for continuums and adult pathology following child abuse. *J Nerv Ment Dis*, **196**(8), 634–638.

Perron, B., & Munson, M. (2006). Coping with voices: A group approach for managing auditory hallucinations. *Am J Psychiatr Rehabil*, **9**(3), 241–258.

Read, J., & Ross, C. A. (2003). Psychological trauma and psychosis: Another reason why people diagnosed schizophrenic must be offered psychological therapies. *Journal of the American Academy of Psychoanalysis and Dynamic Psychiatry*, **31**, 247–268.

Read, J., van Os, J., Morrison, A. P., & Ross, C. A. (2005). Childhood trauma, psychosis and schizophrenia: A literature review with theoretical and clinical implications. *Acta Psychiatr Scand*, **112** (5), 330.

Reeves, A. (1997). *Recovery: A Holistic Approach*. Gloucester: Handsell Publishing.

Regan, L. (director). (2008). *The Doctor Who Hears Voices*. Kudos Films.

Repper, J. (2000). Adjusting the focus of mental health nursing: Incorporating service users' experiences of recovery. *J Ment Health*, **9**, 575–587.

Repper, J. (2002). The helping relationship. In N. Harris, S. Williams and T. Bradshaw (Eds), *Psychosocial Interventions for People with Schizophrenia* (pp. 39–52). Hampshire: Palgrave.

Robins, C. J. (2002). Zen principles and mindfulness practice in dialectical behavior therapy. *Cognitive and Behavioural Practice*, **9**(1), 50–57.

Romme, M. (2000). *Redefining Hearing Voices*. Based on a speech given at the launch of The Hearing Voices Network, Manchester, England, Summer 2000. Available online at: http://www.psychminded.co.uk/critical/marius.htm.

Romme, M., & Escher, S. (1989a). Hearing voices. *Schizophr Bull*, **15** (2), 209–216.

Romme, M., & Escher, S. (1989b). Effects of mutual contacts from people with auditory hallucinations. *Perspectief*, **3**, 37–43.

Romme, M., & Escher, S. (1990). Heard but not seen. *Open Mind*, (49), 16–18.

Romme, M., & Escher, S. (1993). *Accepting Voices*. London: Mind Publications.

Romme, M., & Escher, S. (2000). *Making Sense of Voices*. London: Mind Publications.

Rosenberg, M. (2003). *Non-Violent Communication: A Language of life*. London: Puddle Dancer Press.

Smith, D. B. (2007). *Muses, Madmen and Prophets: Rethinking the History, Science and Meaning of Auditory Hallucination*. New York: The Penguin Press.

Smith, J. (2008). Spinning. *Openmind*, **150**, 10–11.

Steele, K. (2002). *The Day the Voices Stopped: A Schizophrenic's Journey from Madness to Hope*. New York: Basic Books.

Stone, H., & Stone, S. (1989). *Embracing Our Selves: The Voice Dialogue Training Manual*. New York: Nataraj Publishing.

Strauss J. (1989). Subjective experiences of schizophrenia: Toward a new dynamic psychiatry II. *Schizophr Bull*, **15**, 179–187.

Szasz, T. (1961). *The Myth of Mental Illness: Foundations of a Theory of Personal Conduct*. London: Harper & Row.

Ventura, J., & Liberman, R. P. (2000). Psychotic disorders. In G. Fink (Ed.), *Encyclopedia of Stress* (pp. 316–326). San Diego: Academic Press.

Watkins, J. (1998). *Hearing Voices: A Common Human Experience*. Melbourne, Australia: Hill of Content Publishing Ltd.

White, M. (1996). Power to our journeys. *American Family Therapy Academy Newsletter*, Summer, 11–16.

Wykes, T., Parr, A., & Landau, S. (1999). Group treatment of auditory hallucinations: Exploratory study of effectiveness. *Br J Psychiatry*, **175**, 180–185.

Young, S. L., & Ensing, D. S. (1999). Exploring recovery from the perspective of people with psychiatric disabilities. *Psychosocial Rehabilitation Journal*, **22**, 219–231.

Chapter 15

Hallucinations in children and adolescents

Diagnosis and treatment strategies

Jean-Louis Goëb and Renaud Jardri

Introduction

Hallucinations are a common symptom in paediatric populations, which can be a transitory phenomenon but which can also constitute a serious cause of concern since it may be a sign of physical or mental illness. Available studies in the literature effectively established that hallucinations and delusions may occur in both clinical (neurological, psychiatric, or other pathologies) and non-clinical (i.e., normal) individuals, leading some authors to question the diagnostic specificity of these experiences during childhood (Larøi et al., 2006). It is important to mention that 'non-diagnostic hallucinations' can constitute normal features of child development related to psychological immaturity (Schreier, 1998; Sosland & Edelsohn, 2005; Edelsohn, 2006), and it seems most appropriate to first consider hallucinations as non-specific symptoms. In this way, much attention has to be drawn to the child's global clinical presentation and his/her social and familial context. Later on in the text, we will discuss that hallucinations may also be a symptom of psychosis or future emergence of the pathology. However, since early-onset psychosis is often difficult to diagnose, the question of whether to treat and how to treat remain debatable topics. Some authors proposed that since the diagnosis-specificity longitudinally improves, time and clinical evolution constitute the best diagnostic tools (Jeammet, 2000). Various clinical presentations may be characterized by disturbances in thinking and perception that are not clearly psychotic, accompanied by non-specific conduct disorders, such as recent, abrupt, or more insidious changes in sleeping, eating, global behaviour, or mood. A first prodromal period may last several years with non-specific signs such as deteriorating academic and social performance, emerging conduct problems, including delinquency and substance misuse or abuse, and pseudo-neurotic disorders (Biderman et al., 2004). In such prodromal cases, early treatment has been shown to be associated with better prognosis (McGorry et al., 2002; Yung et al., 2005). The non-identification of this syndrome can have devastating consequences, but on the other hand, systematic medication of children with hallucinations using anti-psychotic drugs in the emergency setting should be avoided until a complete exploration has been performed. Clinicians need to be aware of the wide range of differential etiological diagnoses, including medical (mainly metabolic and neurological), or psychiatric ones (schizotypy, schizophreniform disorders, early onset schizophrenia, mood disorders, traumatic life events such as sexual abuse, bereavement, bullying, post-traumatic stress disorder (PTSD), and other anxiety disorders, ADHD). Adequate explorations, monitoring, and therapeutic guidelines for hallucinatory experiences in children and adolescents will be considered in more detail.

Epidemiological data concerning hallucinatory experiences during childhood

The prevalence of hallucinations and/or delusions in the non-clinical population varies from 6% to 33% (Altman *et al.*, 1997; McGee *et al.*, 2000; Poulton *et al.*, 2000; Dhossche *et al.*, 2002; Yoshizumi *et al.*, 2004). Moreover, it has been proposed that the presence of hallucinations and delusions during childhood may increase the likelihood of various psychopathological conditions (but not exclusively psychotic disorders) later in life. In this way, some authors have found that higher scores on a composite measure of self-reported psychotic symptoms at age 11 in a general population setting may predict a diagnosis of schizophreniform disorder at age 26 (Poulton *et al.*, 2000). Dhossche and co-workers (2002) also found that hallucinations had a predictive value in a non-clinical sample, albeit they were found to be predictive for DSM-IV axis I disorders. In contrast, Garralda concluded that hallucinations had no prognostic value for psychosis or any other psychiatric disorder in a sample of child psychiatric outpatients with non-psychotic disorders (i.e., conduct and emotional disorders) (Garralda, 1984). Of course, variations in predictive measures in these studies might be related to differences in the assessed populations: inclusion of non-clinical (Poulton, Dhossche) versus clinical (Garralda) participants. We can suppose that the range of outcomes may be more restricted in clinical populations compared with non-clinical participants. This might be related to the fact that in clinical populations, the disorder is more or less already 'developed' or has already manifested itself to such an extent that there is a much less risk for the appearance of other disorders. On the contrary, in non-clinical individuals, there are many outcome possibilities, which depend on highly complex interactions between genetic, psychological, and social variables. Other methodological variations can explain differences between these predictive studies and deserve further comment. First, in the Dhossche and co-workers study, only hallucinations were assessed and adolescents were primarily included (mean age = 14 years), whereas hallucinations and delusions were grouped together to test children (mean age = 11 years) in Poulton and collaborators. Second, the time between the first (14 years of age) and last assessment (23 years of age) was 8 years in Dhossche *et al.* whereas the time between the first (11 years of age) and last assessment (26 years of age) was 15 years in Poulton *et al.* Third, the psychometric tools were different between the two studies. In Dhossche *et al.* the Youth Self-Report was used (i.e., self-report), whereas the diagnostic interview schedule for children (i.e., clinician-report) was used in Poulton *et al.* There might, therefore, have been a greater likelihood of detecting a (psychotic) disorder in the Poulton study since a broad range of (psychotic) symptoms were assessed, and furthermore since the age range between the first and second evaluation was greater (15 years), and finally since the first evaluation was quite early on (at 11 years of age). In contrast, the Dhossche *et al.* study was narrower in scope in that only hallucinations were assessed, the age range between the first and second evaluation was shorter (8 years) and participants were much older (mean age was 14 years of age). Finally and in spite of the importance of the above-mentioned studies in our understanding of the long-term evolution of hallucinatory experience during childhood, it is important to point out that the use of identical diagnosis criteria all across development is questionable since clinical presentation varies as a function of the child's mental and psychic capacities, acquired during childhood and early adolescence. Moreover, it is important to mention that many of these symptoms may be of a transient nature and therefore may disappear shortly after their apparition. Although auditory hallucinations are a sign of serious problems in daily life, a substantial number of children and adolescents experiencing hallucinations or delusions will not necessarily develop any major psychopathological conditions later in life (Escher *et al.*, 2004).

Clinical assessment of hallucinations in children and adolescents

Clinical manifestations

Hallucinations are classically defined as 'a false sensory perception not associated with real external stimuli' (Kaplan & Sadock, 1998). Patients may present with auditory, visual, tactile, gustatory, or olfactory hallucinations. Auditory hallucinations are usually experienced as voices, whether familiar or unfamiliar, perceived as distinct from the person's own thoughts (APA, 2000). Yale University's PRIME Research Clinic's (Prevention through Risk Identification, Management, and Education) scale of prodromal symptoms defines psychotic hallucinations as 'visions, voices, and other sensory events that are experienced as real and influence thinking, feeling, and behaviour at least minimally' (Miller *et al.*, 1999).

Some children speak easily and spontaneously about the voices they hear, but the question should be systematically, however tactfully, asked. Auditory Hallucinations have to be questioned even with deaf persons, despite the fact that there are many concerns regarding how clinicians and interpreters translate the concept of hearing voices that other people do not hear, and how deaf psychiatric persons with language dysfluency, who may not understand the concept of hallucination, understand the question (Glickman, 2007). In deaf or reticent/mutic persons, hallucinations can be suspected when people seem distracted, their eye gaze darting around, and sometimes communicating back to the voice they hear. Information should be gathered from a wide range of sources including family, teachers, and health and social services. In our clinical experience, whatever the diagnosis is, the frequency and the intensity of hallucinations fluctuate within the day, worsened by stress or separation, and may be absent for days or months

(Goëb & Delion, 2009a). Finally, the attention of the clinician should be drawn to the quality of the communication and affective patterns within the family. Familial difficulties may sometimes be considered as a result of the disturbed child. Conversely, characteristics of the parent or family may be relatively independent of the child's behaviour (Asarnow *et al.*, 1994) and worsen the child's mental state.

The assessment may be complicated by difficulties differentiating between immature responses that are typical in younger children and pathologic symptoms such as thought disorder and delusion. The presence of formal thought disorder may discriminate between children with schizophrenia and non-schizophrenic controls after the age of seven (Caplan *et al.*, 1990; Asarnow *et al.*, 2004). It is important to clearly distinguish these manifestations in children from other perceptual experiences such as hallucinosis (i.e., false perception but without adherence from the subject) or illusions (altered perception of a real object). Thus, the estimation of the degree of adhesion to the false perception is crucial to diagnose hallucinations. Moreover, and as already evoked, hallucinations occurring while falling asleep (hypnagogic) or waking up (hypnopompic) are considered within the range of normal experiences, as well as isolated experiences of hearing one's name called, or hearing non-verbal noises, such as footsteps or knocking, without any other verbal hallucinations. In addition, hallucinations may be a normal part of religious experiences in a certain natural context (APA, 2000; Sosland & Edelsohn, 2005). Finally, imaginary companions usually differ from psychotic hallucinations when they appear, interact, and disappear at the will of the child and pose no threat to the child and are often a comfort to him/her (Martin *et al.*, 2007).

Psychometric assessment in young people

A number of existing psychometric tools may complement the clinical assessment, assisting with diagnosis and symptom rating. The main one is the Schedule for Affective Disorders and Schizophrenia for school-age children [Kiddie-SADS], a semi-structured diagnostic interview designed to assess current episodes of psychopathology in children and adolescents aged 6–18 years, according to DSM-IV criteria (Kaufman *et al.*, 1997). It requires a complete conscious access from the child, who cannot be tested in cases of fever, delirium, or under the influence of a psychoactive substance. These points emphasize the necessity of a complete physical examination of the child to exclude incidental or causative medical conditions (for more on this see the section 'Complementary explorations of hallucinations during childhood' in this chapter). For this schedule, 'diagnostic auditory hallucinations' include experiences of hearing one or more voices saying at least one word other than one's own name. The schizophrenia section of the Diagnostic Interview Schedule for Children (DISC-C) (Costello *et al.*, 1982) includes items concerning both delusions and hallucinations: (1) 'Some people believe in mind reading or being psychic. Have other people read your mind?', (2) 'Have you ever had messages sent just to you through television or radio?', (3) 'Have you ever thought that people are following you or spying on you?', (4) 'Have you heard voices other people can't hear?', and (5) 'Has something ever gotten inside your body or has your body changed in some strange way?'. Other structured interviews specifically developed to assess child and adolescent psychiatric disorders could also help the clinician in the diagnosis procedure: the Child and Adolescent Psychiatric Assessment (CAPA) (Wamboldt *et al.*, 2001), the Diagnostic Interview for Children and Adolescents (DICA) (McQuaid, 2001), or the Child Assessment Schedule (CAS) (Hodges *et al.*, 1990) are some of them. The Maastricht voices interview for children (MIK) (Escher *et al.*, 2002) is a rating scale that contains several items in relation to the experience of hearing voices. This includes the number of voices, the frequency, the emotional tone, and possible triggers of the voices and in addition, the degree of coping the voices mobilize, attributions of voices (i.e., the presence of secondary explanations), and the presence of life events. Projective techniques can also complete diagnostic interviews for accessing the 'inner-life' of the child or adolescent when pre-psychotic states are evoked. These tasks are particularly useful with these patients since providing narratives to pictures may be more engaging than direct questioning. Projective tasks allow the means to capture how the child processes ambiguous information and how it interacts with the external world with its specific object-relationship (e.g., erroneous generalizations from details). Also assessed are child's privileged psychic defence mechanisms and various emotional aspects of the child's personality. The more widely employed tools are the Rorschach Inkblot test (Weiner, 2003) or the Thematic Apperception Test (Murray, 1943). Finally, a neuropsychological assessment including sensory perception, motor skills, attention, memory, language, and executive functioning may complete the evaluation. Reality and source monitoring tasks (Larøi *et al.*, 2004) and agency tests (Jardri *et al.*, 2009) are also useful. These neuropsychological tests are helpful to assess early elements of cognitive disorganization (Bishop & Holt, 1980).

Psychiatric causes for hallucinations in children and adolescents

Hallucinations can be associated with a variety of childhood psychiatric syndromes such as pervasive developmental disorders, early-onset schizophrenia, reactive psychoses, dissociative disorders, depressive disorders, severe social and psychological deprivation, conduct and emotional disorders, traumatic life events, PTSD, anxiety disorders, socially inept children with adjustment reactions, and Tourette's syndrome (Garralda, 1984; Schreier, 1999; Ulloa *et al.*, 2000; Lataster *et al.*, 2006). Similarly, in studies including non-clinical individuals, the presence of hallucinations or delusions are often accompanied with high levels of depression, anxiety, dissociation, phobias, etc. High levels of anxiety and depression are also important hallucination continuation factors (Escher *et al.*, 2004). During mood disorders with psychotic features, hallucinations are classically congruent with the mood state. As an example, in melancholia, children could hear guilty or persecutory voices, while a maniac phase would be more characterized by divine comments with grand projects. Bereaved children may also present with hallucinations of the deceased, especially when there is unresolved mourning (e.g., related to the deceased parent), at a time when children are in need of cognitive and emotional support from their caregivers (Yates & Bannard, 1988). Finally, hysteria, although rarely observed in children or adolescents, can contain visions, voices, or voluptuous tactile sensations with mystic or sexual themes. The absence of schizophrenic dissociation, a brutal emergence after an affective trauma, suggestibility, and reinforcement in presence of other persons can evoke such a diagnosis (Iyer *et al.*, 2008). Therefore, proposing intervention strategies for these co-existing conditions is crucial. Interestingly, some studies revealed that the effective treatment of co-morbid or co-existing psychopathological disorders in (adult) psychotic patients has positive effects on hallucinations and delusions (Good, 2002).

Hallucinations and delusions are major signs of schizophrenia, but are neither necessary nor sufficient to establish a schizophrenia diagnosis, since the symptoms tend to be non-specific, especially in the early stage of the disease (White *et al.*, 2006; Remschmidt & Theisen, 2005). Major depressive disorder is a common diagnosis that merits further discussion. Differential diagnosis is not easy since significant affective symptoms are commonly present in episodes of schizophrenia (Judd, 1998). Conversely, non-psychotic major depressive disorder may be accompanied by auditory hallucinations, sometimes with voices telling the subject to commit suicide. In a study of non-psychotic hallucinations in a psychiatric emergency service, 34% of the studied children had depression (Chambers *et al.*, 1982; Edelsohn *et al.*, 2003). Finally one major issue with early onset schizophrenia is to promptly provide adapted care, before the acute or insidious development of florid psychotic features, ideally during the prodromal period, when changes in behaviour and subjective experiences are noticed by the individuals themselves, and their family and friends. Early signs often include social withdrawal, depression, decreased energy, substance abuse, impaired concentration, avolition, anhedonia, irritability, aggressiveness, sleep, mood and anxiety disturbances, odd/unusual/eccentric behaviour or ideas, suspiciousness, odd ideas of reference, unusual perceptual experiences, and blunted or flat affect. Mood variations and social withdrawal may indicate the presence of psychological distress that often precedes or accompanies the insidious onset of psychosis, which are frequently associated with a longer duration of untreated illness (Bishop & Holt, 1980; Iyer *et al.*, 2008).

Complementary explorations of hallucinations during childhood

Before orienting patient to a psychiatric ward, clinicians need to be aware of the wide range of medical differential diagnoses. To address organic conditions, both a careful medical examination (including a neurological and psychiatric examination) and the administration of complementary tests are warranted to identify and rule out treatable medical disorders (see Table 15.1). Finally, when necessary, a pre-therapeutic clinical and para-clinical examination has to be carried out. Metabolic side effects (for example, increased risk for metabolic syndrome, including diabetes and weight gain) are common during anti-psychotic treatments. Patients with early onset schizophrenia may be at very high risk of obesity and related cardiovascular disorders such as metabolic syndrome (Goëb *et al.*, 2008b). To assess tolerance of anti-psychotics in this population, sex- and

Table 15.1 Complementary explorations in children and adolescents suffering from hallucinations

	Rationale
Routine baseline assessment	
Full blood count (FBC)	To detect pre-existing hematological disturbance before medication
Fasting blood glucose	To detect pre-existing glucose regulation problems
Urea and electrolytes	To assess glomerular excretion function and detect pre-existing electrolyte disturbances, especially hyperkaliemia or hyponatremia
Liver function	To assess catabolic function and potential liver incapacity
EKG	To exclude pre-existing cardiac conduction anomalies, especially prolongation of the QT interval
Drug screening	Urine +/− blood screening
Sensory Examination	Exclude a pre-existing ENT (audiogram) or ophthalmological disease (visual field)... which may provoke hallucinoses and hallucinations
Second-line assessment (depending on clinical signs and history)	
Prolactin level	To exclude pre-existing hyperprolactinemia before the use of anti-psychotic medication
Thyroid function	To screen for dysthyroidy
Fasting cholesterol level	To detect a pre-existing lipid metabolism dysfunctions before anti-psychotic medication
Electroencephalography with sleep deprivation	When seizure is suspected
Brain imaging (CT scan or MRI)	When focal neurological signs are present, when the level of consciousness is disturbed, or when patients present with headaches, or vomiting
Functional MRI (fMRI)	To assess the neural structures and networks involved in the hallucinatory process that can be used to guide rTMS therapy (RCT in course to validate such an approach)

age-adjusted body mass index (Z-scores of BMI), fasting blood glucose and cholesterol levels, and an EKG need to be performed. Clinical and blood monitoring should therefore be repeated twice a year and be accompanied with physical activity and dietetic counselling.

The main differential diagnoses in children and adolescents presenting with hallucinations are listed below. *Metabolic disorders* include thyroid and parathyroid disease, adrenal disease, Wilson's disease, porphyria, beri-beri, and electrolyte imbalance (Martin *et al.*, 2007). Some *genetic anomalies* such as Velo-cardio-facial Syndrome but also *serious infections*, such as encephalitis or meningitis or febrile illness can be associated with hallucinations in children. Tiffin (2007) gives a synthetic overview of the main blood examinations that should be performed routinely at baseline assessment in young people presenting with a psychosis. *Drug intoxications* have also to be screened in urine and blood samples. Substances that may be hallucinogenic include solvents, LSD, phencyclidine (PCP), mescaline and its by-products, psilocybine, cannabis, cocaine, and amphetamines including Ecstasy, opiates, and barbiturates. As an example, LSD commonly provokes synaesthesia, characterized by additional percept awareness between modalities, such as seeing a color when hearing a tone. Interestingly, the causal effect of cannabis on the development of psychosis has been frequently reported (Arsenauld et al., 2004) at least in at-risk persons. Prescribed drugs that may cause hallucinations include steroids and anticholinergic medications (belladone or anti-parkinson drugs). Dilated pupils, extreme agitation or drowsiness, and other signs of intoxication may be explored. Visual and tactile hallucinations during methylphenidate therapy that resolve with treatment discontinuation have also been reported (Gross-Tsur et al., 2004). Finally, a few antiepileptic medications such as lamotrigine have psychiatric side effects, notably hallucinatory experiences (Brandt et al., 2007). *Migraines* have been linked to hallucinations that usually appear during the migraine attack and when headaches are not present. Visual hallucinations are the most common in patients with migraines, but gustatory, olfactory, and auditory hallucinations have also been described (Schreier, 1998), sometimes to such an extent as to mimic Alice-in-wonderland experiences (Ewans, 2006). *Seizure disorder* (principally partial complex seizure) may be suspected when repeated episodes of hallucinations of a single modality are observed (Sosland & Edelsohn, 2005). Hallucinations may affect somatosensory, visual (occipital), auditory (temporal), olfactory (temporal or orbito-frontal), or gustatory (temporal) senses. They may be unformed, such as flashing lights or rushing noises, or may be formed or geometrical images or spoken words or music (Wyllie, 1993). Complex visual seizures can be characterized by 'dreamy-states' during which the subject experiences a feeling of 'déjà-vu'. Hearing auditory hallucinations are frequently seen in temporal and frontal epilepsy with other psychopathologic symptoms like psychomotor excitement, hostility, and suspiciousness (Adachi et al., 2000; Huppertz et al., 2002; Zwijnenburg et al., 2002; Kechid et al., 2008). It is also important to mention that organic lesions such as neoplasms can cause complex hallucinations. More generally, neurological lesions result in hallucinosis more than real hallucinations and can be notably observed in sensorial deficits or deafferentation syndromes (phantom limb phenomenon for example). Focal pedoncular lesions have also been shown to be associated with complex hallucinosis such as coloured visions as in a silent movie or musical percept. Finally, in sleep disorders such as narcolepsy, hypnagogic hallucinations can be observed, which emerge during pathological drowsiness.

Other complex medico-psychiatric syndromes should also routinely be envisaged. *Catatonia* is a rare but severe condition, which most frequently is related to psychiatric causes, but severe organic causes should be considered as well (Lahutte et al., 2008). The diagnosis is made based on at least two catatonic motor signs or one catatonic motor sign (catalepsy, stupor, posturing, waxy flexibility, staring, stereotypies, psychomotor excitement, automatic compulsive movements, muscular rigidity, echopraxia) combined with a nonmotor catatonic symptom indicative of severely impaired behavioural and emotional functioning (withdrawal, mutism, mannerism, echolalia, incontinence, verbigeration, refusal to eat) (Cohen, 2006). Agitated or prepubescent forms of catatonia also constitute differential diagnoses for psychotic or pseudo-hallucinatory episodes in children and adolescents. Organic conditions responsible for catatonia include infectious diseases, neurological conditions, toxic-induced states, and genetic conditions including Inborn Errors of Metabolism (IEM) such as urea cycle defects, homocysteine remethylation defects, and porphyrias. Catatonia, visual hallucinations, and aggravation of the psychotic symptoms under anti-psychotic treatments are atypical features that should point to an IEM, especially in patients with mild mental retardation or behavioural disorders without the presence of a clear psychiatric syndrome (Lahutte *et al.*, 2008; Sedel *et al.*, 2007). Systemic Lupus Erythematosus (SLE) is also a rare organic cause of catatonia in which hallucinations can be observed (Mara *et al.*, 2007). A rapid diagnostic test using Zolpidem can be used to assess participation of catatonia in the symptomatology (Thomas *et al.*, 1997). In such a case, catatonic symptoms may dramatically diminish within half an hour with Zolpidem.

Clinical observation

Part 1. (for follow-up information, see Part 2 at the end of the chapter)

Audrey, a 12-year-old girl, was hospitalized for a month in our department to evaluate *social inhibition with behavioural disorders*, along with repeated conflicts at school (sixth grade) and at home. She does not present any school backwardness, but her integration with other children and with her teachers is difficult. She lives with her father, her stepmother, her sister, and a stepbrother. Since her parents' divorce, when she was two, she has had no contact with her mother according to a judiciary decision after a social survey. Audrey's personality reveals numerous symptoms of *dependent personality disorder*: she thinks that her mother 'threw her away' and she expresses the fear that her father would do the same with her. Audrey has a *neurological history*. Two years ago, she presented a viral encephalitis with an undetermined aetiology, responsible for a right temporal necrosis visible on the MRI. As a relapse, Audrey also shows epilepsy, complicated by two epileptic attacks last year. She is treated with sodium valproate (2 × 500 mg/day) and topiramate (2 × 125 mg/day). After this encephalitis, child psychiatric follow-up treatment was initiated for non-specific disorders, with a post-traumatic aspect. Audrey also shows *psychotic symptoms*, detected during the admission interview and confirmed at the beginning of the hospitalization. Audrey presents auditory-verbal hallucinations, 'I hear my godfather talking to me at night to reassure me', and she presents with a mental automatism syndrome, 'I hear three voices, a woman, a man, and a child arguing'. Functional MRI (see below in this chapter) was negative (hallucinations appeared only a few times a day). Sometimes, these hallucinations are coupled with multi-everyday right temporal *headaches*.

> **Part 1. (for follow-up information, see Part 2 at the end of the chapter) (continued)**
>
> Treatment with amitryptiline (30 drops at night) was prescribed according to the neuropediatrist's proposal to relieve potential headaches with aura. *Rapid mood fluctuations* led us to evoke a mixed mood state. We noticed depressive elements with sadness, anhedonia, and motor slowdown. Audrey was very preoccupied with the fear of disappointing her father and resembling her mother who she thinks is 'crazy'. Audrey notes that her 'composition' changed since her encephalitis. Her school integration is difficult, and she complains about having less friends. Contrasting with these depressive elements, Audrey also shows manic symptoms like disinhibition, logorrhoea, disordered hyperactivity, sexualized comments, and an over-exaggerated physical proximity with the other hospitalized children.

Treatment strategies

Orientation and first intervention in the emergency setting

First, it is difficult to claim that one treatment strategy is more efficient than others, since studies have not directly compared their efficacy in children and adolescents with hallucinations. As already mentioned, the treatment of youth presenting with hallucinations in an emergency psychiatric service should be guided by a complete evaluation and differential diagnosis. One of the first interventions to be provided is to assess the risk of self-violence or harming others, especially in cases where adolescents experience command hallucinations. In such a context, the subject needs to be systematically reinsured in a quiet place and when necessary a non-specific anxiolytic medication may be prescribed, although avoiding benzodiazepine, which could paradoxically increase aggressive behavior in children. Risk factors for suicidality must be systematically looked for. A careful physical examination and a psychological interview with the child alone and with his/her parents should be then quickly proposed. When parents are not present, a telephone contact with key adult informants is necessary. First- and second-line complementary examinations have already been listed in Table 15.1. Since causal diagnosis are rarely made in the emergency setting, it is important that anti-psychotic drugs for children are not routinely prescribed, but rather to propose to reassess the symptomatology on the basis of regular monitoring. For some children, this follow-up can be ambulatory while for others a hospitalization (complete or day-care) is more appropriate, to avoid suicide attempts or to manage possible co-morbid substance abuse. Such hospitalizations provide the occasion to mobilize a complete network around the suffering child and parents including medical, social, and school professionals and to propose psychotherapeutic interventions. Co-morbidity but also the co-existence of psychosocial conditions is clearly a major issue. Therefore, proposing intervention strategies for these co-existing conditions is crucial. Finally, when necessary, low-dose pharmacological treatment should be introduced (see next sections). A management chart for hallucinations in young people is provided in Figure 15.1.

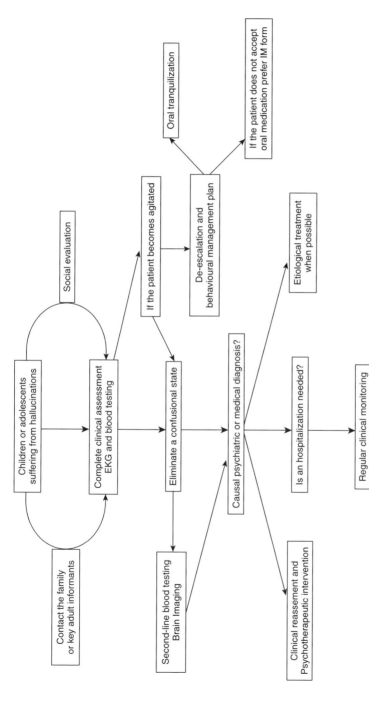

Fig. 15.1 Management Chart for Early-onset Hallucinations in the Emergency Setting. EKG: electrocardiogram; IM: intra-muscular administration.

Psychotherapeutic interventions

Interestingly, some psychotherapeutic programs have been developed with the objective to reduce distress associated with hallucinations or its frequency (but not always of its disappearance), but also to reduce the transition to psychosis in ultra high-risk adolescents. Numerous studies already explored the impact of individual or group Cognitive Behavioural Therapy (CBT) in the treatment of psychotic symptoms (i.e., see the meta-analysis by Zimmerman *et al.*, 2005; Smith *et al.*, this volume; Johns & Wykes, this volume). Moreover, CBT was found to be more effective in reducing psychotic experiences than case management and supportive psychotherapy after 6 months of treatment (Morrison *et al.*, 2004) and significantly reduced the rate of conversion to psychosis after adjustment for age, gender, family history, and baseline Positive and Negative Syndrome Scale scores, compared to monitoring without intervention (Sosland & Pinninti, 2005). Edelsohn (2006) also recently proposed that individual CBT could be used as a brief intervention in the emergency setting through an assessment of the patient's beliefs about hallucinations and helping them to identify alternative explanations for their symptoms. Asking the child what he or she thinks the hallucinations mean, what factors make the voice start or stop, etc. constitute the first step of the intervention, and where introducing coping strategies may be proposed subsequently. Coping strategies (see Farhall, this volume), defined as constantly changing cognitive and behavioural efforts to manage demands that exceed the subject's resources, constitute the second main approach in psychotherapy of hallucinations for children and adolescents. Chadwick and Birchwood (2001; also see Trower, Birchwood & Meaden, this volume) argue that the beliefs people have about voices (and not the voice activity *per se*) hold the key to understanding the affect and behaviour they generate. In particular, they have shown that voices believed to be malevolent provoked fear and anger and were resisted, whereas benevolent voices were associated with positive effect and were engaged. Moreover, voices construed as benign were associated with a greater diversity of coping strategies. Techniques attempting to weaken maladaptive (core) beliefs and strengthen more adaptive ones have been shown to have positive effects (e.g., reduced distress, improved coping) in (adult) patients (i.e., Bak *et al.*, 2001). Such an approach may also prove effective in younger patient groups and some studies (Escher *et al.*, 2003 and 2004) evidenced that teaching self-help methods, such as ignoring the voices by selective attention or distraction, is important. The baseline level of self-initiated coping should be assessed, since it has been shown that this is correlated to the degree to which these patients can defend themselves against the experience of being overwhelmed by the hallucinatory experience (Escher *et al.*, 2003). Escher and collaborators evidenced that an active problem-solving coping style was the most effective in providing more experience of control over the psychotic experience. Similarly, they showed that improving children's and adolescent's ability to cope with emotions may be helpful to make the voices discontinued (Escher *et al.*, 2004). In many cases of the last mentioned study, the voices were often related to problems in the individual's life history (divorce, physical illness, sexual abuse, etc.), and disappeared when these problems were solved and that the children's development took a positive turn, emphasing the importance of socio-environmental interventions. Finally, specific psychotherapeutic programs (e.g., Hallucinations-Focused Integrative Therapy (HIT); Jenner and van de Willige 2001; see Jenner, this volume) have also been developed for adolescents suffering from hallucinations, which integrate a number of different types of strategies (CBT, coping strategies, supportive counselling, psychoeducation). In Jenner and van de Willige (2001), 14 first-episode adolescents with both acute and chronic auditory hallucinations were assessed. At two consecutive months after treatment, nine patients were judged free of voices. Interestingly, this program had a good acceptability among the young patients, and the authors suggested it could help motivate those non-compliant adolescents to accept pharmacological treatment in later instances. In a randomized-controlled trial comparing HIT versus routine care, Jenner and collaborators (2004) also evidenced that hallucinations experienced by patients in the HIT group had significantly decreased levels of distress and the amount of interference hallucinations had on daily functioning decreased at 9 months, but that hallucination frequency and duration did not significantly decrease.

Finally, although the efficacy of Long-Term Psychodynamic Psychotherapy (LTPP) has not been examined in the literature (Jeammet, 1984, 2000, 2003), a recent meta-analysis reported that LTPP was an effective treatment for complex psychiatric disorders (Leichsenring & Rabung, 2008). Moreover, adapted psychotherapy remains of great interest for patients to alleviate their high levels of 'primitive' anxiety (such as fear of falling, exploding, and liquefying) going along with unimodal sensorial functioning and primitive level of sensory experiences (Meltzer, 1975; Haag, 2005). These primitive fears are usually described in autism (Delion, 2003), but they are also frequently seen in severe states of schizophrenia. Obviously, conventional psychoanalytical design is not appropriate in numerous cases of hallucinating children. Institutional care (Delion, 2005) and mediated relationship through various therapeutic activities (e.g., equitherapy, hydrotherapy, drawing or cooking activities) in a group context with other patients allow a novel investment of thought process (Bion, 1967). 'Packing' therapy is a therapeutic approach consisting of wrapping the patient with his underclothes several times a week with spin-dried towels (previously wet in water). The patient is then wrapped with blankets to help the skin warm up. There is no hypothermia, the skin's temperature returns to 37°C within a few minutes. The envelopment usually lasts 45 min. Three or four members of staff are always looking after the patient and are carefully attentive to the quality of the relation they experience with the patient. The wrapping and the warming up, which follows the initial chill, seem to help the patient achieve a greater perception and integration of his own body, allowing him to experience a growing sense of containment (Delion, 2003; Haag et al., 2005). Within a specific pluridisciplinary therapeutic program, this technique is usually proposed to treat autistic children with serious self-injurious behaviour, and who do not respond to usual psychotropic drugs (Goëb et al., 2007; Goeb et al., 2009b, in press). In clinical practice, this approach appears to be very useful to enter in contact with adolescents with schizophrenia suffering from hallucinations and self-injurious disorders.

Psychoeducative programs

Numerous studies suggest that very few children and adolescents reveal their hallucinations to their entourage. For instance, Dhossche and collaborators (2002) checked the number of parents who reported hallucinations in their children (all of whom heard voices) and the results revealed that there were five (<1%) positive reports of auditory and visual hallucinations. Furer and co-workers (1957) found that children were only mildly reluctant to talk about the voices they heard. In addition, they reported that the children's long-term therapists rarely knew about the hallucinations. Schreier mentions the fact that children in his study were 'at most, mildly reluctant to talk about the voices', and that they had simply not been previously asked (Schreier, 1999). Finally, in Chambers and collaborators (1982), only a third of the parents were aware of the symptoms their children reported. Based on these results, it is important to attempt to understand why children and adolescents are so reluctant to talk about these experiences. *Educational programs* have in this sense crucial clinical implications by providing information to patients, but also to their immediate entourage (e.g., family) and to others (e.g., health professionals). Indeed, family members appear to appreciate and benefit from the reassurance that hearing voices does not necessarily mean that they are crazy or that the child is suffering from schizophrenia or another psychotic condition. Evidence from meta-analyses of psycho-social treatment in adults with schizophrenia also provides strong support for family-based interventions (Pilling *et al.*, 2002). In light of evidence that hallucinatory experiences are experienced by a large majority of normally functioning individuals in the general population (i.e., van Os *et al.*, 2000), normalizing these experiences in children and adolescents may be highly fruitful. *Normalization* (see Garrett, this volume) refers to the process by which thoughts, behaviours, moods, and experiences are compared and understood in terms of similar thoughts, behaviours, moods, and experiences attributed to other individuals who are not diagnosed as ill (Kingdon & Turkington, 2005). Presenting normal circumstances in which subjects can have hallucinations may provide persons with alternative explanations of the hallucinatory experience and facilitate its reattribution. Normalization interventions in adult populations are successful in alleviating the distress associated with the presence of hallucinations and delusions and thus may also be effective in child and adolescent populations (i.e., Larøi *et al.*, 2006).

What is the role of anti-psychotic drugs in the treatment of hallucinations in the non-adult population?

The question of whether to recommend *pharmacological treatment* in children and adolescents with hallucinations also deserves further consideration. It is important to keep in mind that the diagnosis of prodromal schizophrenia can only be proposed from a retrospective point of view and is thus difficult to treat at an early stage even if some psychometric instruments, as the CAARMS (Comprehensive Assessment of At-Risk Mental States), had been proposed to identify individuals at high mental-state risk (Yung *et al.*, 2005). On the other hand, studies have focused on the prognostic benefits of early pharmacotherapy of pre-psychotic states (i.e., Yung *et al.*, 2006.). Moreover, practice parameters have been developed by the American Academy of Child and Adolescent Psychiatry to treat children when early-onset schizophrenia is diagnosed, which emphasize anti-psychotic medications in combination with psychotherapeutic, psychoeducational, and social support programs (McClellan *et al.*, 2001). Prescription in paediatric populations also implies good knowledge of the human physiological development (Bailly & Mouren, 2007). From a pharmacokinetic point of view, the drug's half-life within the child's body is reduced due to higher glomerular filtration and catabolic activity (liver enzymes have maximal activity around 10 years of age). Moreover, since the volume of distribution of the molecule is reduced, the drug's posology needs to be fractioned over the entire day and adjusted according to the child's weight. From a pharmacodynamic point of view, monoaminergic systems reach maturity only at the end of adolescence while the density of D1 and D2 dopaminergic receptors is enhanced in children, which can cause a higher sensitivity to the effects of anti-psychotics in these patients compared to adults. When such a treatment is proposed, anti-psychotics are generally first prescribed at low dosages and only one anti-psychotic is proposed (monotherapy). A posology increase can be proposed every 72 hours with an adequate monitoring. The therapeutic effect of the medication is usually assessed between 4 and 8 weeks of adequate treatment. In some cases, plasmatic dosages can help to adjust the posology for a better efficacy and tolerability.

Few studies have examined the efficiency of anti-psychotic drugs in the treatment of hallucinations in young persons compared to other paediatric pharmacological domains. A recent meta-analysis identified 15 Randomized Controlled Trials (RCT) (including a total of 209 children with schizophrenia) using typical or atypical anti-psychotics (Armenteros & Davies, 2006). This review evidenced that the average response rate among eight studies employing atypicals was 55.7% compared to 72.3% among 13 studies employing typicals. The fact that second-generation anti-psychotics did not show superiority compared to typical anti-psychotics in the non-adult population is in accordance with data from a meta-regression realized over 52 trials grouping 12,649 adults with schizophrenia (Geddes *et al.*, 2000). Nevertheless, it cannot be excluded that such an effect could be due to a selection bias since previous studies have proposed atypical anti-psychotics in second line only for patients showing a more severe symptomatology. Moreover, the main side effects reported were identical to what is usually described in adult populations: weight-gain, hyperprolactinemia, neurological symptoms (essentially dyskinesia and extrapyramidal syndrome), sedation, and biological disturbances. Acute dystonia seems more frequent during childhood, especially in boys during the first five days of treatment. Dopamine agonists, classically prescribed in adults when extrapyramidal side effects are present, should be used carefully in children and adolescents due to the risk of confusional state and increase in hallucinations. When induced-akathisia is observed, adjunctive clonazepam (Rosenberg *et al.*, 1994) or propanolol (Gogtay *et al.*, 2002) treatment has been shown to be effective in children. Adequate pre-therapeutic and monitoring explorations need to be instituted to ensure the best tolerability in children (i.e., Goëb *et al.*, 2008a). Since there are few short-term differences in response to the various anti-psychotic medications, side-effect profiles should guide the clinician's choice about which anti-psychotic to prescribe first (Ross, 2008). In another review of the use of anti-psychotic drugs in children (Kennedy *et al.*, 2007), only six studies (over a total of 2062 papers listed) met the quality criteria for inclusion, and only one of these RCT comparing haloperidol to clozapine found a superiority for the second-generation drug (Kumra *et al.*, 1996). The present consensus is to recommend second-generation anti-psychotics in children or adolescents rather than typical ones (Deniau *et al.*, 2008). Among these medications, risperidone, quetiapine, and olanzapine have been shown to be the most frequently prescribed in cases of first episode psychoses in children and adolescents (Castro-Fornieles *et al.*, 2008), but other more recent agents such as aripiprazole have also demonstrated good efficiency in such indications (Findling *et al.*, 2008). Some authors also suggested that long-acting injectable anti-psychotics should be preferred in cases of poor compliance to treatment (i.e., Parellada, 2006). Finally, when two distinct anti-psychotic drugs remain unsuccessful in reducing hallucinations in children or adolescents, clozapine can be an alternative medication (Remschmidt *et al.*, 2000). Clozapine can help children with severe refractory hallucinations but imposes a careful hematological monitoring due to increase risks for seizures, myocarditis, and agranulocytosis (Kranzler *et al.*, 2006). Indeed, a recent review confirmed superior effectiveness of clozapine in reducing symptoms of schizophrenia compared to typical anti-psychotic drugs but these benefits have to be weighed against the risk of the potentially dangerous white blood cell decline, which seems to be more frequent in children and adolescents than in young or middle-aged adults (Essali *et al.*, 2009).

What is the rationale for the therapeutic use of repetitive Transcranial Magnetic Stimulation in hallucinations before 18 years of age?

Transcranial Magnetic Stimulation (TMS) is a method of focal neural depolarization provoked by a time-varying magnetic field applied over a certain scalp position (see Aleman and Hoffman, this volume, for more details about this technique). When repetitively applied, rTMS can be used for therapeutic purposes. In a recent meta-analysis, Aleman and collaborators (2007) reported 10 studies of 1-Hz rTMS as a treatment of refractory auditory verbal hallucinations in adults suffering from schizophrenia (a total of 216 patients). They evidenced a mean standardized effect size of 0.76 providing some support for the efficacy of rTMS in such an indication. Interestingly, this method constitutes a dimensional treatment of hallucinations and can be used in combination with other therapeutic strategies, even if rTMS is actually proposed for patients suffering from schizophrenia with drug-resistant hallucinations. Only a few studies have explored the potential interest of the use of rTMS for hallucinations during childhood and no RCT studies have been carried out for this population. Tolerability of TMS treatment was assessed in persons less than 18 years in a meta-analysis that included 1,034 children and revealed no adverse effect or seizure (Quintana, 2005). This tolerability in children is reinforced in protocols using low-frequency magnetic fields to inhibit rather than to activate the cortex (Gilbert, 2008). Two case-reports used a low-frequency fMRI-guided rTMS paradigm to treat refractory auditory hallucinations in children. For this treatment, cortical activation maps obtained during the fMRI-scan were used to direct rTMS to the location where activity during hallucinations was maximal. One study evidenced a 47% improvement of the intensity and the frequency of hallucinations in an 11-year-old child, which was maintained during 6 weeks after rTMS treatment (Jardri *et al.*, 2007). The second study reported that rTMS treatment can also improve self-awareness capacities in a child, independently or in combination with a reduction of the frequency and the intensity of hallucinations, according to the chosen brain-target for neuromodulation (Jardri *et al.*, 2009). Even if these two reports seem encouraging, replication in larger groups and with a RCT design is needed to fully assess the impact of this therapeutic method in children and adolescents.

Clinical observation

Part 2

Audrey's health and relationship greatly improved during the 5 week hospitalization (including individual and group psychotherapy and medication adjustment), to such an extent that her father remarked that she was 'like before'. The hallucinations quickly disappeared, only giving way to the major depressive disorder, which also rapidly disappeared after the hospitalization and during follow-up. Antiepileptic treatments and amitryptiline were maintained.

Psychometric tests, realized a few weeks after the acute difficulties, showed an IQ close to the light deficiency zone (with heterogeneous aspects), as well as logical thought disorders, and non-specific attentional and spatial organization disorders. A project concerning her school orientation in a specialized institution was organized with her father and the school. Several months after her hospitalization, Audrey was still fine. As a conclusion, the initial complex symptomatology (which included hallucinations, depressive and manic elements in a child with headaches, and encephalitis neurological relapses) rapidly improved with adequate care and the retained diagnosis was atypical major depressive disorder.

Conclusion and future directions

Studies investigating the efficacy of various intervention strategies for hallucinations in children and adolescents are clearly needed. In practice, a hallucinating child first requires careful medical and psychiatric assessments. It is furthermore crucial to provide adequate care during this diagnostic period. Psychotherapy, institutional care (full time or sequential/day-care hospitalization), and non-specific (i.e., non-neuroleptic) anxiolytic medications may be prescribed in early stages. Psychotic symptoms may be treated with specific medications. Anti-psychotic medications should be given when there is a clear necessity to diminish hallucinations. Their utility (benefit and tolerance) should be questioned regularly. Mood stabilizers may be useful when psychotic symptoms occur in the context of a bipolar mood disorder. Particular attention should be paid to the parents' and siblings' reactions. Further studies are needed in order to better define the exact place that rTMS has as a treatment strategy for childhood refractory hallucinations. In our child and adolescent psychiatry department, we propose fMRI-guided rTMS treatment for drug-resistant hallucinations before third-line anti-psychotics, such as clozapine, are proposed. In the years to come, clinical trials should compare the efficacy of rTMS and anti-psychotic medications as first-choice intervention strategies for hallucinations in children and adolescents.

Acknowledgments

Emilie Dujardin (psychologist), Virginie Petit (psychologist), and Natacha Parsy (for help in translation).

References

Adachi, N., Onuma, T., Nishiwaki, S., *et al.* (2000).Takei N. Inter-ictal and post-ictal psychoses in frontal lobe epilepsy: a retrospective comparison with psychoses in temporal lobe epilepsy. *Seizure*, **9**, 328–35.

Aleman, A., Sommer, I.E., & Kahn, R.S. (2007). Efficacy of slow Transcranial Magnetic Stimulation in the treatment of resistant auditory hallucinations in schizophrenia: a meta-analysis. *J Clin Psychiatry*, **68**, 416–421.

Altman, H., Collins, M., & Mundy, P. (1997). Subclinical hallucinations and delusions in nonpsychotic adolescents. *J Child Psychol Psychiatry*, **38**,413–20.

A.P.A American Psychiatric Association. (2000). *Diagnostic and Statistical Manual of Mental Disorders.* 4th Edn. Text Revised. Washington, DC: APA Press.

Armenteros, J.L. & Davies, M. (2006). Antipsychotics in early onset schizophrenia: systematic review and meta-analysis. *Eur Child Adolesc Psychiatry*, **15**, 141–8.

Arsenauld, K., Cannon, M., Witton, J., & Murray, R.M. (2004). Causal association between cannabis and psychosis: examination of the evidence. *Br J Psychiatry*, **184**, 110–7.

Asarnow, J.R., Tompson, M.C., & Goldstein, M.J. (1994). Childhood-onset schizophrenia: a followup study. *Schizophr Bull*, **20**,599–617.

Asarnow, J.R., Tompson, M.C., & McGrath. E.P. (2004). Annotation: childhood-onset schizophrenia: clinical and treatment issues. *J Child Psychol Psychiatry*, **45**, 180–94.

Bailly, D. & Mouren, MC. (2007). *Les prescriptions médicamenteuses en psychiatrie de l'enfant et de l'adolescent.* Paris: Elsevier Masson.

Bak, M., van der Spil, F., Gunther, N., Radstake, S., Delespaul, P., & van Os, J. (2001). Maastricht assessment of coping strategies (MACS-I): a brief instrument to assess coping with psychotic symptoms. *Acta Psychiatr Scand*, **103**, 453–9.

Biderman, J., Petty, C., Faraone, S.V., & Seidman, L. (2004). Phenomenology of childhood psychosis: findings from a large sample of psychiatrically referred youth. *J Nerv Ment Dis*, **192**, 607–14.

Bion, W. (1967). *Second thoughts.* London: W. Heineman Medical Books.

Bishop, E.R .Jr, & Holt, A.R. (1980). Pseudopsychosis: a reexamination of the concept of hysterical psychosis. *Compr Psychiatry*, **21**, 150–61.

Brandt, C., Fueratsch, N., Boehme, V., *et al.* (2007). Development of psychosis in patients with epilepsy treated with lamotrigine: report of six cases and review of the literature. *Epilepsy Behav*, **11**(1), 133–9.

Caplan, R., Perdue, S., Tanguay, P.E., & Fish, B. (1990). Formal thought disorder in childhood onset schizophrenia and schizotypal personality disorder. *J Child Psychol Psychiatry*, **31**, 1103–14.

Castro-Fornieles, J., Parellada, M., Soutullo, C.A., *et al.* (2008). Antipsychotic treatment in child and adolescent first-episode psychosis: a longitudinal naturalistic approach. *J Child Adolesc Psychopharmacol*, **18**(4), 327–36.

Chadwick, P. & Birchwood, M. (1994). The omnipotence of voices: a cognitive approach to auditory hallucinations. *Br J Psychiatry*, **164**,190–201

Chambers, W.J., Puig-Antich, J., Tabrizi, M.A., & Davies, M. (1982). Psychotic symptoms in prepubertal major depressive disorder. *Arch Gen Psychiatry*, **39**, 921–7.

Cohen, D. (2006). Toward a valid nosography and psychopathology of catatonia in children and adolescents. *Int Rev Neurobiol*, **72**, 131–47.

Costello, A., Edelbrock, C., Kalas, R., Kessler, M., & Klaric, S. (1982). *NIMH Diagnostic Interview for Children: Child Version.* Rockville: National Institute of Mental Health.

Delion, P. (2003). *Le packing avec les enfants autistes et psychotiques.* Eres: Ramonville Saint-Agne.

Delion, P. (2005). *Soigner la personne psychotique: concepts, pratiques et perspectives de la psychothérapie institutionnelle.* Paris: Dunod.

Deniau, E., Bonnot, O., & Cohen, D. (2008). Drug treatment of early-onset schizophrenia. *Presse Med*, **37**, 853–8.

Dhossche, D., Ferdinand, R., Van der Ende J, Hofstra, M.B., & Verhulst, F. (2002).Diagnostic outcome of self-reported hallucinations in a community sample of adolescents. *Psychol Med*, **32**, 619–27.

Edelsohn, G.A., Rabinovich, H., & Portnoy, R. (2003). Hallucinations in non-psychotic children: findings from a psychiatric emergency service. *Ann N Y Acad Sci*, **1008**, 261–64.

Edelsohn, G.A. (2006). Hallucinations in children and adolescents: considerations in the emergency setting. *Am J Psychiat*, **163**, 781–5.

Escher, S., Romme, M., Buiks, A., Delespaul, P., & van Os, J. (2002). Independent course of childhood auditory hallucinations: a sequential 3-year follow-up study. *Br J Psychiatry*, **181** (Supplement 43), 10–8.

Escher, S., Delespaul, P., Romme, M., Buiks, A., & van Os J. (2003). Coping defence and depression in adolescents hearing voices. *J Ment Health*, **12**, 91–9.

Escher, S., Morris, M., Buiks, A., Delespaul, P., van Os J., & Romme, M. (2004). Determinants of outcome in the pathways through care for children hearing voices. *Int J Soc Welfare*, **13**, 208–22.

Essali, A., Al-Haj Haasan, N., Li, C., & Rathbone, J. (2009). Clozapine versus typical neuroleptic medication for schizophrenia. *Cochrane Database Syst Rev*, (1), CD000059.

Ewans, R.W. (2006). Cases studies of uncommon headaches. *Neurol Clin*, **24**, 347–362.

Findling, R.L., Robb, A., Nyilas, M., *et al.* (2008). A multiple-center, randomized, double-blind, placebo-controlled study of oral aripiprazole for treatment of adolescents with schizophrenia. *Am J Psychiatry*, **165**(11), 1432–41.

Furer, M., Horowitz, M., Tec, L., & Toolan, J. (1957). Internalized objects in children. *Am J Orthopsychiatry*, **27**, 88–95.

Garralda, M.E. (1984). Hallucinations in children with conduct and emotional disorders, II: the follow-up study. *Psychol Med*, **14**, 597–604.

Geddes, J., Freemantle, N., Harrison, P., & Bebbington, P. (2000). Atypical antipsychotics in the treatment of schizophrenia: systematic overview and meta-regression analysis. *BMJ*, **321**, 1371–6.

Gilbert, D.L. (2008). Design and analysis of motor-evoked potential data in pediatric neurobehavioral disorder investigations. In EM Wassermann, CM Epstein, U Ziemann, V Walsh, T Paus, SH Lisanby (Eds.), *The Oxford handbook of transcranial stimulation* (pp. 389–400). New York: Oxford University Press.

Glickman, N. (2007). Do you hear voices? Problems in assessment of mental status in deaf persons with severe language deprivation. *J Deaf Studies Deaf Education,* 12, 127–47.

Goëb, J.L., Bonelli, F., Jardri, R., Kechid, G., Lenfant, A.Y., & Delion, P. (2008a). Packing therapy in children and adolescents with autism and serious behavioural problems. *Eur Psychiatry,* 23, S405–6.

Goëb, J.L., Marco, S., Duhamel, A., *et al.* (2008b). Metabolic side effects of risperidone in early onset schizophrenia: a follow-up pilot study. *Prim Care Companion J Clin Psychiatry,* 10(6), 486–487.

Goëb, J.L., & Delion, P. (2009a). Clinical considerations introducing this special issue on childhood schizophrenia. *Neuropsychiatr Enf Adolesc,* 57(1), 2–5.

Goëb, J.L., Kechid, G., Jardri, R., *et al.* (2009b). Packing therapy is efficient in behavioural disorders in children and adolescents with autism. (Les enveloppements humides initialement froids (packings) sont efficaces dans les troubles graves du comportement chez les enfants et adolescents autistes.) *Neuropsychiatr Enf Adolesc,* 57(6), 529-534.

Good, J. (2002). The effect of treatment of a comorbid anxiety disorder on psychotic symptoms in a patient with a diagnosis of schizophrenia: a case study. *Behav Cognitive Psychother,* 30, 347–50.

Gross-Tsur, V., Joseph, A., & Shalv, R.S. (2004). Hallucinations during methylphenidate therapy. *Neurology,* 63, 753–4.

Haag, G., Tordjman, S., Duprat, A., *et al.* (2005). Psychodynamic assessment of changes in children with autism under psychoanalytic treatment. *Int J Psychoanal,* 86, 335–52.

Hodges, K., Gordon, Y., & Lennon, M.P. (1990). Parent-child agreement on symptoms assessed via a clinical research interview for children: the child assessment schedule (CAS). *J Child Psychol Psychiatry,* 31(3), 427–36.

Huppertz, H.J., Franck, P., Korinthenberg, R., & Schulze-Bonhage, A. (2002). Recurrent attacks of fear and visual hallucinations in a child. *J Child Neurol,* 17, 230–3.

Iyer, S.N., Boekestyn, L., Cassidy, C.M., King, S., Joober, R., & Malla, A.K. (2008). Signs and symptoms in the pre-psychotic phase: description and implications for diagnosis trajectories. *Psychol Med,* 38, 1147–56.

Jardri, R., Lucas, B., Delevoye-Turrell, Y., *et al.* (2007). An 11-year-old boy with drug-resistant schizophrenia treated with temporo-parietal rTMS. *Mol Psychiatry,* 12, 320.

Jardri, R., Delevoye-Turrell, Y., Lucas, B., *et al.* (2009). Clinical practice of rTMS reveals a functional dissociation between agency and hallucinations in schizophrenia. *Neuropsychologia,* 47(1), 132–8.

Jeammet, P. (1984). Expériences psychotiques et adolescence. *Adolescence ,*2, 31–5.

Jeammet, P. (2000). Les prémices de la schizophrénie. In: De Clercq M, Peuskens J (Eds.) *Les troubles schizophréniques.* Paris: De Boeck Université.

Jeammet, P. (2003). Existe-t-il une continuité entre les changements vécus au moment de l'adolescence et la schizophrénie débutante ? In: Fédération Française de Psychiatrie. *Schizophrénie débutante, Conférence de consensus.* Paris: John Libbey Eurotext.

Jenner, J.A., & van de Willige, G. (2001). HIT: hallucination focused integrative treatment as early intervention in psychotic adolescents with auditory hallucinations: a pilot study. *Acta Psychiatrica Scand,* 103, 148–52.

Jenner, J.A., Nienhuis, F.J., Wiersma, D., & van de Willige, G. (2004). Hallucination focused integrative treatment: a randomized controlled trial. *Schizophr Bull,* 30,133–45.

Judd, L.L. (1998). Mood disorders in schizophrenia: Epidemiology and comorbidity. *J Clin Psychiatry,* 16, 2–4.

Kaplan, H.I., & Sadock, B.J. (1998). *Synopsis of psychiatry*. 8th Edn. Baltimore: Lippincott Williams & Wilkins.

Kaufman, J., Birmaher, B., Brent, D., *et al*. (1997). Schedule for affective disorder and schizophrenia for school-age children—present and lifetime version (K-SADS-PL): Initial reliability and validity data. *J Am Acad Child Adol Psychiatry*, **36**, 980–8.

Kechid, G., Auvin, S., Jardri, R., Vallée, L., Delion, P., & Goëb, J.L. (2008). Hearing hallucinations in a 12-year-old child: psychotic disorders or temporal epilepsy? *Prim Care Companion J Clin Psychiatry*, **10**(4), 328–9.

Kennedy, E., Kumar, A., & Datta, S.S. (2007). Antipsychotic medication for childhood-onset schizophrenia. *Cochrane Database Syst Rev*, **18**, CD004027.

Kingdon, D.G., & Turkington, D. (2005). *Cognitive therapy for schizophrenia*. New York: Guilford Press.

Kranzler, H.N., Kester, H.M., Gerbino-Rosen, G., *et al*. (2006). Treatment-refractory schizophrenia in children and adolescents: an update on clozapine and other pharmacologic interventions. *Child Adolesc Psychiatr Clin N Am* ,**15**, 135–59.

Kumra, S., Frazier, J.A., Jacobsen, L.K., McKenna, K., Gordon, C.T., & Lenane, M.C. (1996). Childhood onset schizophrenia: a double-blind clozapine-haldol comparison. *Arch Gen Psychiatry*, **53**, 1090–7.

Lahutte, B., Cornic, F., Bonnot, O., *et al*. (2008). Multidisciplinary approach of organic catatonia in children and adolescents may improve treatment decision making. *Progr Neuro-Psychopharmacol Biol Psychiatry* , **32**, 1393–8.

Larøi, F., Van der Linden, M., & Marczewski, P. (2004). The effects of emotional salience, cognitive effort and meta-cognitive beliefs on a reality monitoring task in hallucination-prone subjects. *Br J Clin Psychol*, **43**, 221–33.

Larøi, F., Van der Linden, M., & Goëb, J.L. (2006). Hallucinations and delusions in children and adolescents. *Curr Psychiatr Rev*, **2**, 473–85.

Lataster, T., van Os, J., Drukker, M., *et al*. (2006). Childhood victimisation and development expression of non-clinical delusional ideation and hallucinatory experiences. *Soc Psychiatry Psychiatr epidemiol*, **41**, 423–8.

Leichsenring, F., & Rabung, S. (2008). Effectiveness of long-term psychodynamic psychotherapy: a meta-analysis. *JAMA*, **300**, 1551–65.

Marra, D., Amoura, Z., Soussan, N., *et al*. (2008). Plasma exchange in patients with stuporous catatonia and systemic lupus erythematosus. *Psychother Psychosom*, **77**, 195–196.

Martin, A., Volkmar, F.R., & Lewis, M. (2007). *Lewis' child and adolescent psychiatry: a comprehensive textbook*. 4th Edn. Philadelphia: Lippincott Williams & Wilkins.

McClellan, J.M., Werry, J., Bernet, W., *et al*. (2001). Practice parameter for the assessment and treatment of children and adolescents with schizophrenia. *J Am Acad Child Adolesc Psychiatry*, **40**(Suppl 7), 4S–23S.

McGee, R., Williams, S., & Poulton, R. (2000). Hallucinations in nonpsychotic children. *J Am Acad Child Adolesc Psychiatry*, **39**, 12–3.

McGorry, P.D., Yung, A.R., Phillips, L.J., *et al*. (2002). Randomized controlled trial of interventions designed to reduce the risk of progression to first-episode psychosis in a clinical sample with subthreshold symptoms. *Arch Gen Psychiatry*, **59**, 921–8.

McQuaid, D. (2001). More on the DICA-IV. *J Am Acad Child Adolesc Psychiatry*, **40**(2), 130–2.

Meltzer, D.W. (1975). *Explorations in Autism: a psychoanalytic study*. Perthshire: Clunie Press.

Morrison, A.P., French, P., Walford, L., *et al*. (2004). Cognitive therapy for the prevention of psychosis in people at ultra-high risk: randomized controlled trial. *Br J Psychiatry*, **185**, 291–7.

Miller, T.J., McGlashan, T.H., Woods, S.W, *et al*. (1999). Symptom assessment in schizophrenic prodromal states. *Psych Q*, **70**, 273–87.

Murray, H.A. (1943). *The Thematic Apperception Test*. Cambridge: Harvard University Press.

Parellada, E. (2006). Clinical experience and management considerations with long-acting risperidone. *Curr Med Res Opin*, **22**(2), 241–55.

Pilling, S., Bebbington, P., Kuippers, E., *et al.* (2002). Psychological treatments in schizophrenia: I. Meta-analysis of family intervention and cognitive behaviour therapy. *Psychol Med*, **32**, 763–82.

Poulton, R., Avshalom, C., Moffitt, T.E., Cannon, M., Murray, R., & Harrington, H. (2000). Children's self-reported psychotic symptoms and adult schizophreniform disorder: A 15-year longitudinal study. *Arch General Psychiatry*, **57**, 1053–8.

Quintana, H. (2005). Transcranial magnetic stimulation in persons younger than the age of 18. *JECT*, **21**, 88–95.

Remschmidt, H., Fleischhaker, C., Hennighausen, K., & Schulz, E. (2000). Management of schizophrenia in children and adolescents. The role of clozapine. *Paediatr Drugs*, **2**, 253–62.

Remschmidt, H., & Theisen, F.M. (2005). Schizophrenia and related disorders in children and adolescents. *J Neural Transm Suppl*, **69**, 121–41.

Rosenberg, D.R., Holttum, J., & Gershon, S. (1994). *Textbook of pharmacotherapy for child and adolescent psychiatric disorders*. New York: Brunner/Mazel Publishers.

Ross, R.G., Heinlein, S., & Tregellas, H. (2006). High rates of comorbidity are found in childhood-onset schizophrenia. *Schizophr Res*, **88**, 90–95 .

Ross, R.G. (2008). New findings on antipsychotic use in children and adolescents with schizophrenia spectrum disorder. *Am J Psychiatry*, **165**, 1369–72.

Schreier, H.A. (1998). Auditory hallucinations in non-psychotic children with affective syndromes and migraines: Report of 13 cases. *J Child Neurol*, **13**, 377–82.

Schreier, H.A. (1999). Hallucinations in nonpsychotic children: more common than we think? *J Am Acad Child Adolesc Psychiatry*, **38**, 623–5.

Schulze, B., Richter-Werling, M., Matschinger, H., & Angermeyer, M.C. (2003). Crazy? So what! Effects of a school project on students' attitudes towards people with schizophrenia. *Acta Psychiatr Scand*, **107**, 142–50.

Sedel, F., Baumann, N., Turpin, J.C, Lyon-Caen, O., Sandubray, J.M., & Cohen, D. (2008). Psychiatric manifestations revealing inborn errors of metabolism in adolescents and adults. *J Inherit Metab Dis* , **30**, 631–41.

Sosland, M.D., & Edelsohn, G.A. (2005). Hallucinations in children and Adolescents. *Curr Psychiatr Reports*, **7**, 180–8.

Sosland, M.D., & Pinninti, N. (2008). Five ways to quiet auditory hallucinations. *Current Psychiatry*, **4**(4), 110.

Tiffin, PA. (2007). Managing Psychotic illness in young people: A practical overview. *Child Adol Ment Health*, **12**, 173–86.

Tordjman, S., Antoine, C., Cohen, D.J., *et al.* (1999). Study of the relationships between self-injurious behavior and pain reactivity in infantile autism. *Encephale*, **25**, 122–34.

Thomas, P., Rascle, C., Mastain, B., Maron, M., & Vaiva, G. (1997). Test for catatonia with zolpidem. *Lancet* ,**349**, 702.

Ulloa, R.E., Birmaher, B., Axelson, D., *et al.* (2000). Psychosis in a pediatric mood and anxiety disorders clinic: phenomenology and correlates. *J Am Acad Child Adolesc Psychiatry*, **39**, 337–45.

van Os J, Hanssen, M., Bijl, R.V., & Ravelli, A. (2000). Strauss (1969) revisited: a psychosis continuum in the normal population ? *Schizophr Res*, **45**, 11–20.

Wamboldt, M.Z., Wamboldt, F.S., Gavin, L., & McTaggart, A.S. (2001). A parent-child relationship scale derived from the child and adolescent psychiatric assessment (CAPA). *J Am Acad Child Adolesc Psychiatry*, **40**(8), 945–53.

Weiner, I.B. (2003). *Principles of the Rorschach interpretation*, 2nd Edn. Odessa: Psychological Assessment Ressources.

White, T., Anjum, A., & Schultz, S.C. (2006). The schizophrenia prodrome. *Am J Psychiatry*, **163**, 376–80.

Wyllie, E. (1993). *The treatment of epilepsy: Principles and practices*. Philedelphia: Lea & Febiger.

Yates, T.T., & Bannard, J.R. (1988). The 'haunted' child: grief, hallucinations, and family dynamics. *J Am Acad Child Adolesc Psychiatry*, **25**, 574–8.

Yoshizumi, T., Murase, S., Honjo, S., Kaneko, H., & Murakami, T. (2004). Hallucinatory experiences in a community sample of Japanese children. *J Am Acad Child Adolesc Psychiatry*, **43**, 1030–6.

Yung, A.R., Yuen, H.P., McGorry, P.D., *et al.* (2005). Mapping the onset of psychosis: the comprehensive assessment of at-risk mental states. *Aust N Z J Psychiatry*, **39**, 964–71.

Zimmerman, G., Favrod, J., Trieu, V.H., & Pomini, V. (2005). The effect of cognitive behavioural treatment on the positive symptoms of schizophrenia spectrum disorders: a meta-analysis. *Schizophr Res*, **77**, 1–9.

Zwijnenburg, P.J., Wennink, J.M., Laman, D.M., & Linssen, W.H. (2002). Alice in wonderland syndrome: a clinical presentation of frontal lobe epilepsy. *Neuropediatrics*, **33**, 53–5.

Chapter 16

Visual hallucinations in Charles Bonnet syndrome

Frank Eperjesi

Introduction

The term Charles Bonnet syndrome (CBS) has been used to describe pseudo-visual hallucinations in the absence of any psychological abnormality (Menon *et al.*, 2003) most often occurring in older persons. Latterly, this term has specifically been used to describe visual hallucinations resulting from visual impairment due to ocular disease (Teunisse *et al.*, 1995; Plummer *et al.*, 2007).

Charles Bonnet syndrome is named after a Swiss philosopher who described the phenomenon in 1769. His 89-year-old grandfather began to experience visual hallucinations of men, women, carriages, and buildings with failing eyesight, but he was aware that they were not actually physically present. Bonnet himself began to experience similar visual hallucinations in his later life (Damas-Mora *et al.*, 1982). It is widely accepted that CBS is an under recognized condition (Teunisse *et al.*, 1996; Menon, 2005), and this has been attributed to sufferers' natural reluctance to admit to their hallucinatory experiences for fear of been diagnosed as mentally unstable (Gittinger *et al.*, 1982; Siatkowski *et al.*, 1990; Scott *et al.*, 2001; Plummer *et al.*, 2007) and to the unfamiliarity of health care practitioners with CBS leading to a tendency to misdiagnose mental illness (Norton-Wilson & Munir, 1987). This chapter is a review of the diagnostic criteria, prevalence, clinical characteristics, pathogenesis, and management of CBS. Increased awareness of this phenomenon amongst eye care and medical practitioners should help improve its recognition and allow sufferers to be directed to appropriate methods of management.

Diagnostic criteria

The following diagnostic criteria are accepted by most authorities (Gold & Rabins, 1989): (1) presence of formed, complex, persistent, or repetitive, stereotyped visual hallucinations, (2) full or partial retention of insight into the unreal nature of the hallucinations, (3) absence of hallucinations in other sensory modalities, and (4) absence of primary or secondary delusions. Menon (2005) adds that insight into the unreal nature of the hallucinations may be delayed, and makes a good case for intact cognition and acquired visual impairment to be added to the list of diagnostic criteria. Others too have stated that impaired visual acuity (VA) and brain dysfunction are required for CBS to develop

(Burgermeister *et al.*, 1965), and there have been several reports of cases where patients experiencing CBS hallucinations have subsequently developed dementia (Brabbins, 1992). It has been claimed that cases of true CBS, that is complex visual hallucinations in the absence of neuropsychiatric disorder and with full insight, are exceedingly rare and most cases described in the literature are CBS plus, that is visual hallucinations in the presence of a neuropsychiatric disorder or with the sufferer totally lacking insight that the halluci-nations are unreal (Howard & Levy, 1994). However, recent work has called this assertion into question, because a large proportion of individuals with age-related macular degen-eration (AMD) with normal mentation experience formed visual hallucinations (Holroyd & Rabins, 1996) and on the basis that some degree of cognitive impairment is universally present in people with CBS (Pfeiffer & Bodis-Wollner, 1996). Furthermore, Gilmour *et al.* (2009) found that 206 from 258 (80%) of CBS subjects knew the images were not real after the first episode; another 20 (8%) after the second episode, while 15 (6%) experienced ten or more episodes before realizing the images were not real.

Prevalence

Various prevalence rates for visual hallucinations have been reported: 57% from a sample of 104 subjects with retinal or neural visual loss (Lepore, 1990); 10–30% in people with 'vision deficits' (Schultz & Melzack, 1991); 15% of 319 patients with acquired vision loss reported 'full fledged' visual hallucinations rising to almost 39% of patients with sight loss when 'questioned in a context they felt safe' (Needham & Taylor, 1992); just under 2% from a group of 434 patients referred for psychogeriatric work up (Norton-Willson & Munir, 1987); almost 53% of 284 consecutive low vision patients experienced photopsias (coloured flickering lights and patterns) (Crane *et al.*, 1994), but these are commonly reported by people with ocular pathology; 11% in partially sighted patients (Teunisse *et al.*, 1995); and 60 from 505 visually handicapped patients (Teunisse *et al.*, 1996). More recently, it has been suggested that one out of seven older patients are likely to have experienced visual hallucinations (Verstraten, 2001). Another study reported a prevalence of 21 of 53 (40%) individuals with bilateral visual impairment due to AMD (Abbott *et al.*, 2007) while Scott *et al.* (2001) found a prevalence of 15.1% of 86 consecutive visually impaired people with retinal disease experienced visual hallucinations. Jackson *et al.* (2007) examined a group of 225 patients referred for low vision rehabilitation and found that 78 (35%) reported CBS hallucinations, while Vukicevic and Fitzmaurice found a prevalence of 35 of 200 (17.5 %) older people with visual impairment of equal to or worse than 6/12 in an Australian older-aged low vision population.

Menon (2005) set out to determine the prevalence of visual hallucinations amongst visually impaired individuals using a 'structured, sensitive and sympathetic history taking approach'. This commenced with non-leading questions about unusual visual symptoms or experiences apart from blurred vision. If a history of visual hallucinations was not forthcoming, patients were advised that some visually impaired individuals experience visual hallucinations, a well-recognized physiological consequence of visual impairment.

Specific and direct inquiry was then made with regard to any complex visual hallucinatory experiences. If hallucinations were admitted to, systematic inquiry was directed toward elucidating the characteristics of the hallucinatory phenomena, namely, image content, movement, triggering and relieving factors, and any associated hallucinations of other sensory modalities. History taking was continued regarding whether the subject had confided in anyone about his or her hallucinations, or had experienced any distress because of the hallucinations. Sympathetic explanation with regard to the benign nature of visual hallucinations in the context of visual impairment was then offered and the patients' reactions recorded. Of 48 consecutive patients with best corrected VA of 6/60 in the better eye due to a range of ocular disease, 30 (63%) experienced hallucinations, unrelated to specific ocular disease. None volunteered the symptoms; two admitted hallucinations on non-leading questions and 28 on direct questioning about experiences of visual hallucinations. More recently Khan *et al.* (2008) found a prevalence of 27% of CBS amongst 360 individuals with end stage AMD, while Gilmour *et al.* (2009) found CBS to be present in 87 of 258 (34%) subjects aged 40 years or more with 6/12 or worse in the better eye or a reduced visual field of 120° or less compared to only 4 of 251 (<1.6%) of a general population with little or no vision loss. The variation in the reported prevalence of CBS is very likely to be due to differences in populations studied, definition of CBS used, history taking technique, and patients' willingness to disclose the symptom perhaps due to concern that this will imply mental incompetence.

Clinical characteristics

Visual impairment

Although visual impairment is present in most cases of CBS, there is, however, no consensus on the role of visual impairment in the development of this condition. Teunisse *et al.* (1994) proposed that although visual impairment is common in CBS, it is not essential for diagnosis. Many investigators, however, recognize a strong relationship between CBS and visual impairment. It has been stated that 'visual hallucinations of the type seen in CBS are associated, almost without exception, with some type of reduction in vision' (Schultz & Melzack, 1991; Scott *et al.*, 2001). Charles Bonnet syndrome rarely occurs in people with decreased vision in only one eye (Fernandes *et al.*, 2000). In one study of CBS sufferers, a mean VA of 6/24 was recorded in the better eye (Teunisse *et al.*, 1996). Abbott *et al.* (2007) found that a group with AMD and CBS had poorer VA (0.20 logMAR) and more extensive visual field loss than a similar group with AMD but not CBS. Some workers have made a point of neither including or excluding visual system pathology as part of their diagnostic criteria for the condition (Fuchs & Lauter, 1992). Bilateral visual impairment has been put forward as a predisposing factor in CBS, but not necessarily its sole cause (Pfeiffer & Bodis-Wollner, 1996). Interestingly, there is a rarity of visual hallucinations in the totally blind and visual hallucinations occur only in the context of acquired visual loss and never in those who are congenitally blind (Ormond, 1925). It is also well recognized that improvement of visual function whether spontaneously or by interventional means often results in cessation of hallucinations (Levine, 1980; Menon, 2005). Some authors suggest that there is no relationship between hallucinatory activity and the degree of visual impairment (Needham & Taylor, 1992), a theory supported by the paradoxical cessation of hallucinatory activity on further visual deterioration (Teuth et al., 1995). Jackson et al. (2007) did not find any association between VA and CBS, but did find that contrast sensitivity in the three poorer quartiles (compared to the best) was strongly associated with the report of hallucinations (OR 4.1, CI 1.1, 15.9; OR 10.5, CI 2.6, 42.1; OR 28.1, CI 5.6, 140.9) after controlling for VA, age, sex, depression, and independence. Khan et al. (2008) found that VA was the most important factor associated with visual hallucinations with an odds ratio (OR) 3.50 and 95% confidence interval (CI) 1.64-7.48, $p = 0.001$ for better eye VA worse than 6/36 and OR 2.26 (95% CI 1.01–5.06), $p = 0.05$) for better eye VA between 6/12 and 6/36. These investigators did not find any association between best VA and the complexity of images, but did note that the incidence of CBS was statistically significantly higher in those with worse VA. Along similar lines, Gilmour et al. (2009) found that CBS symptoms were twice as likely for subjects with a VA of between approximately 6/90 and 6/480.

Ocular disease

Ocular conditions most frequently associated with CBS are AMD, diabetic retinopathy, cataract, glaucoma, and other retinal diseases (Siatkowski et al., 1990; Gilmour et al., 2009), although CBS has been reported in the context of visual impairment secondary to pathology anywhere along the visual pathway from eye to calcarine cortex. A 12% prevalence of CBS among 100 patients with macular choroidal neovascularization has been documented (Brown & Murphy, 1992), while Gilmour et al. (2009) reported that 66 of 194 people with either wet or dry AMD had CBS. Lepore (1990) reported just over 60% of hallucinators had optic nerve dysfunction, 19% post-geniculate loss, 14% with retinal disease, and 6% with optic tract or chiasmal lesions. Visual hallucinations due to CBS have also been linked to undetectable effects of HIV on the brain (Maricle et al., 1995) and have been described in AIDS patients with cytomegalovirus retinitis (Hartmann et al., 1995). It has been argued that it is not uncommon to find visual hallucinatory phenomena of the CBS type in individuals with no sensory deprivation, in fact no impairment of vision at all, while other cases show a long interval (up to 20 years) between impairment of vision and onset of visual phenomena (Morsier, 1967). Since CBS hallucinations have been described in a number of ocular conditions, the emergence of hallucinations may relate more to the degree of visual impairment than to any specific underlying ocular pathology (Teunisse et al., 1995; Scott et al., 2001).

Age

It is thought that CBS occurs mostly, but not exclusively, in the older population. The mean age of onset has been reported as 83.8 years (Norton-Willson & Munir, 1987), 72.0 years (Teunisse et al., 1996), 75.7 years (Batra et al., 1997), 77.7 years (Vukicevic & Fitzmaurice, 2008), and 80 years (Gilmour et al., 2009). In contradiction, one study reported that almost 20% of sufferers were less than 60 years of age (Schultz & Melzack, 1991) and another noted the occurrence of CBS in a subject as young as eight years. Khan *et al.* (2008) did not find an increased risk of CBS with age, while Menon (2005) reported that the emergence of CBS is independent of age, and Abbott *et al.* (2007) found that their AMD group with CBS were younger (median difference four years) than a similar AMD group without CBS. It may be that advanced age is not a cause in itself, and that the higher incidence of CBS in the older population is because visual impairment is more common in old age.

Social and other factors

Pronounced isolation, few social contacts, or experience of loss seem to favour the development of CBS (Schultz & Melzack 1991; Dodd *et al.*, 1999; Vukicevic & Fitzmaurice, 2008). However, counter to this, Khan *et al.* (2008) reported a higher risk of CBS in subjects who were married or living with a partner than those living alone OR 2.22 (95% CI 1.21–4.08, $p = 0.01$). The authors could not explain this finding. Similarly, Abbott *et al.* (2007) found no difference in the proportion of patients who lived alone when a group with AMD and CBS was compared to a similar group with AMD but not CBS. The authors did note that living alone *per se* does not demonstrate the extent of social interaction a person encounters since visits and excursions to and from home are not considered. Gilmour *et al.* (2009) noted that although they did not find that living alone was a risk factor for CBS, 173 of 258 (67%) subjects with CBS reported being alone when experiencing hallucinations.

Other significant risk factors for CBS have been noted as loss of energy, low extroversion, shyness, use of beta-blocking medication and loneliness (Teunisse *et al.*, 1995), and bereavement (Needham & Taylor, 2000), although it has been suggested that bereavement hallucinations differ from true CBS visions in that they are transient, transparent, brief, and situation-specific, and therefore should be classified as illusions since they are distortions and misperceptions of existing objects (Gold & Rabins, 1989).

Properties of visual hallucinations

The onset of visual hallucinations can be before, at the same time, or after the onset of visual impairment (Gold & Rabins, 1989; Teunisse, 1997) and generally occur when the eyes are open (Teunisse *et al.*, 1996). Interestingly, Gilmour *et al.* (2009) found that people diagnosed with an eye condition for more than five years had a 24% greater likelihood of developing CBS. Visual hallucinations due to CBS differ from most other hallucinations in that the observer tends to realize the unreal nature of the hallucinations almost immediately (according to Menon (2005) there may be a delay in some sufferers), that is, they are pseudohallucinations (Gold & Rabins, 1989). Researchers have divided hallucinations into two categories: brief ones lasting a few seconds to a few minutes, which occur when the patient is alert (Needham & Taylor, 1992) and longer ones that occur when the patient is drowsy (White, 1980). Sufferers have very little control over the appearance of the hallucinations or how long they last (Needham & Taylor, 1992). McNamara *et al.* (1982)

proposed that hallucinations associated with CBS differed from those found in people with epilepsy, alcohol withdrawal, and schizophrenia on the basis that CBS sufferers experienced hallucinations continuously rather than episodically, in both visual fields, usually in the context of a visual impairment, are alert, have preserved insight, and have no other signs of cognitive or thought disorders.

Content

The content of hallucinations can be divided into two groups: (1) simple, consisting of coloured shapes, geometric patterns, or white light and (2) complex, involving scenes and groups of people, divine beings, faces, and objects (Plummer et al., 2007; Vukicevic and Fitzmaurice, 2008; Gilmour et al., 2009). Some people begin by having hallucinations of shapes and geometric patterns that progress to full complex scenes while others experience only one type. Hallucinations may also regress from complex to simple before eventually disappearing (Schultz & Melzack, 1991). Eighty-three percent of CBS sufferers reported images of people (Schultz & Melzack, 1991). The images of people can be miniature or dwarfish (Gold & Rabins, 1989), while images of animals such as dogs, cats, birds, and horses are common (e.g., 19% of CBS hallucinations as reported by Gilmour et al., 2009), as well as landscapes and inanimate objects such as furniture and buildings (Schultz & Melzack, 1991). Sufferers typically regard themselves as the onlooker, and it is unusual for them to feel as though they are part of the panorama (Plummer et al., 2007). Abbott et al. (2007) found that CBS sufferers who experienced simple and complex hallucinations had greater visual loss but similar VA and age compared to those who reported only simple or only complex hallucinations. They found no evidence for the hypothesis that increasing visual loss is linked to a progression in the complexity of visual hallucinations experienced. The content of the hallucinations experienced in their study showed a broad variation with 19 subjects experiencing faces (32%), 16 patterns (27%), and ten reported seeing figures (17%). Coloured shapes, objects, scenes, and words were less common.

Menon (2005) reported that of the 48 patients he studied, 14 (30%) observed an adult person, six (13%) of children, four (9%) of faces often with grotesque features, six (13%) of animals such as cats and dogs, and 12 (25%) of inanimate objects. In some cases, individuals remembered hallucinated objects from past experiences, but more often they were not familiar to the patient at all. Menon (2005) reported that patients reported that their visions appeared brilliantly clear and detailed in contrast to their usual blurred images of the real world.

In a recent study of 360 subjects with end stage AMD, Khan et al. (2008) found 97 cases of CBS. The images tended to be coloured (72.2%), straight ahead and within the central scotoma (84.5%), occurring once a day (34%), at any time of the day (53.6%), and having moving parts (62.9%). The single most common type was of people (19.6% of images) followed by geometric patterns (15.8% of images). There is a suggestion that coloured images are more common when visual impairment is due to AMD (Santhouse et al., 2000; Khan et al., 2008). Interestingly, Abbott et al. (2007) found that for a group of 21 subjects with bilateral AMD and CBS that the hallucinations were rarely restricted to the area corresponding to the visual field loss.

Functional MRI investigations have shown that coloured hallucinations are accompanied by increased activity in cortex specialized for colour; face hallucinations, increased activity in cortex specialized for faces; and object hallucinations, increased activity in cortex specialized for objects. Also the pathophysiology of the hallucinations involved a localized increase in cerebral activity (Ffytche et al., 1998).

Frequency and temporal factors

The frequency of hallucinations ranges from one episode a year to several daily (Teunisse et al., 1996). It can increase or decrease with time and these changes may be associated with progressive visual loss (White, 1980). The hallucinations can last from a few seconds (Gilmour et al., 2009) to several hours (Schultz & Melzack, 1991). The period of time over which a sufferer has hallucinations varies considerably. Some may be continuous whilst others have remission phases with periods without hallucinations. Hallucinations may begin again spontaneously or be triggered by a systemic health problem; these are called periodic. Hallucinations may also be episodic lasting from 3 to 90 days (Batra et al., 1997). Interestingly, Vukicevic and Fitzmaurice (2008) found that if the onset of hallucinations was more than six months prior to involvement in their study, then the person was likely to hallucinate less frequently than one who had only just begun to experience visual hallucinations.

Appearance

Hallucinations can be in black and white or in colour, and can be clearer, equally clear or less clear than reality. Hallucinated objects have been reported as floating, projected on a wall or on the ceiling. However, the objects may also appear to fit well into the observer's surroundings (Teunisse et al., 1996). Hallucinatory images may be motionless (static), have intrinsic movement (dynamic), or move as a whole in an individual's visual field (moving). Menon (2005) noted that for 6 of the 48 subjects in his study, images remained motionless, manifested en bloc movement (movement of the whole image without relative movement of its constituent parts) for five subjects, with intrinsic movement (internal movement of the various parts of an image, e.g., hands and feet) for 17 subjects, and en bloc as well as intrinsic movement for one subject.

Emotional reaction

In one study, it was noted that although fearful emotional responses tended to occur with continuous visions or distorted characters, the predominant reaction was one of enjoyment, curiosity, and delight (Holroyd et al., 1992). When experiencing a hallucinatory episode for the first time, some observers may react negatively as they are unaware of the cause of their hallucinations. Patients might react with anxiety until they know more about the underlying process (Gold & Rabins, 1989). Once individuals begin to understand the cause of their hallucinations, they are usually no longer anxious, and in some cases begin to enjoy the hallucinations (Gittinger *et al.*, 1982). When 47 hallucinating subjects were interviewed, eight (17%) reported negative emotions of anger, anxiety, and fear, and nine (20%) reported pleasant emotions. Interestingly, the remaining 30 (63%) of hallucinators had a neutral emotional response to their hallucinations (Fuchs & Lauter, 1992). Pleasant emotional reactions can be associated with well-defined and proportioned figures, whereas reactions of fear and anxiety usually occur with distorted and ill-formed faces and figures (Gold & Rabins, 1989). Of 97 subjects with CBS studied by Khan *et al.* (2008), 71.1% felt impartial towards the experience; 24% described the experience as unpleasant, a figure similar to the 23% reported by Menon (2005); only 5.2% described the experience as pleasant. In another study, 10 of 35 (29%) CBS sufferers reported experiencing severe stress and 17 reported mild stress. The stress was due to worry about the cause rather than the content of the hallucinations (Vukicevic & Fitzmaurice, 2008).

Sixteen (94%) of 17 concerned patients admitted to deriving emotional and psychological comfort from sympathetic explanation that their hallucinations represented a release phenomenon in the context of visual impairment analogous to that of the phantom limb syndrome and represented neither sinister pathology nor imminent insanity (Menon, 2005). Gilmour *et al.* (2009) found that emotional responses changed from 63% neutral, 34% negative, and 6% positive with the initial episode to 71% neutral, 18% negative, and 6% positive by the last episode. These authors also noted that 14% felt psychotic after the first episode.

Theories of pathogenesis

The visual hallucinations in CBS are widely considered to represent a release phenomenon (Cogan, 1973) secondary to deafferentation or denervation (silencing of main afferents) of the visual association areas of the cerebral cortex (Berrios & Brook, 1982), analogous to that seen in the phantom limb syndrome (Schultz & Melzack, 1991). This could lead to the hyperexcitability of the affected neurons. Complex visual hallucinations are believed to originate in the visual association areas of the cerebral cortex (Lance, 1976), notably the lateral temporal cortex, corpus striatum, and thalamus (Adachi *et al.*, 2000). Neuroimaging studies suggest that activation of different areas of visual association cortex may result in different specific hallucinatory images (Ffytche *et al.*, 1998). These investigators also suggest that CBS is an example of positive visual phenomena in which there is increased function in specific pathways (Ffytche *et al.*, 1998). However, some researchers have considered the episodic nature of the hallucinations typical of CBS and have promoted an irritative theory to explain this phenomenon. Theories that have been proposed to explain the cause of CBS hallucinations are further described in the next section.

Irritative theory

An imitative theory for CBS visual hallucinations was put forward by Cogan (1973) who divided the hallucinations into two distinct categories by aetiology: ictal (that is irritative) phenomena and release phenomena. Ictal visual hallucinations, resulting from epileptic discharges, are intermittent and usually stereotyped. They may be simple and unformed, such as circles of colour, or may consist of complex identifiable figures such as animals or people. Other research has suggested that the complex visual hallucinations experienced in people with CBS are often episodic rather than continuous (Berrios & Brook, 1982) and the fact that cells of the visual cortex are more likely to discharge spontaneously when sensory deprivation leads to the reduction of normal afferent input as in CBS (Rosenbaum *et al.*, 1987) reinforced the possibility that CBS hallucinations are an irritative phenomenon. However, other studies on people with visual hallucinations have shown an absence of abnormal brain activity (Bartlett, 1951; Pliskin *et al.*, 1996), and in addition to this, an irritative focus within the brain has not yet been found. Despite the lack of evidence for an irritative aetiology for CBS, some sufferers have been treated successfully with antiepileptic drugs (Bhatia *et al.*, 1992; Chen *et al.*, 1996), but Berrios and Brook (1982) found neuroleptics to be of little benefit, and Miller *et al.* (1987) suggested that these agents may lower the seizure threshold and intensify visual hallucinations in some cases.

Release/deafferentation theory

The release theory was originally proposed by West (1962) and later added to by others (Cogan, 1973; Olbrich *et al.*, 1987; Siatkowski *et al.*, 1990). West (1962) postulated that the brain is constantly bombarded by a surfeit of sensory stimuli, which are normally excluded from consciousness that selectively acts to keep out everything that is unwanted or unneeded. When the usual information input level no longer suffices to inhibit this emergence the precepts, or memory traces (sometimes referred to as engrams) may be released as hallucinations (Gittinger *et al.*, 1982). In other words, sensory deprivation (such as reduced vision due to peripheral or central leisons) creates hallucinations by a 'release' mechanism resulting from a decrease in afferent input and the underlying behaviour of neural tissue may then become evident. More specifically, this theory suggests that a mechanism exists in all individuals, which screens input from sensory pathways in order to filter out unimportant information and scans the input for important information. This mechanism also generally arouses the reticular activating system and therefore supports normal awareness. When sensory input is decreased, the scanning and screening processes are usually disrupted and awareness is reduced. However, in some cases, when sensory input is decreased, the arousal of the reticular activating system may be at a sufficient level to support awareness, but the scanning and screening processes fail to inhibit perceptual traces. These perceptual traces are therefore released and may be experienced by the individual as visual hallucinations. Cortical input from other areas of the brain such as the memory association areas, which are closely involved with the occipital lobes are thought to fill in for the sensory deficit and to produce the hallucinogenic effect (Dodd *et al.*, 1999). Many of these affects seem to occur when the person is quite inactive with reduced external stimuli; for example, when sitting in a chair with no radio or television, or just before retiring for the evening. This additional loss of sensory input would seem to further cause disinhibition of those neural circuits, which ordinarily prevent hallucinations from entering awareness (Gittinger *et al.*, 1982). Cogan (1973) also believes that aging contributes to the disinhibition of higher centres.

The release theory is supported by deafferentation theory (Berrios & Brook 1982; Needham & Taylor, 1992) by which it has been proposed that reduced vision and/or hearing are responsible for the creation of hallucinations, in that the reduction stimulates private perceptual mechanisms to create or fill in the absent or incomplete stimuli, as in the 'phantom limb' syndrome described by Bromage and Melzack (1974). Support for this can be found in the findings of a study by Scott *et al.* (2001) who reported that subjects with bilateral visual impairment and those with worse VA were at increased risk of developing visual hallucinations and Vukicevic and Fitzmaurice (2008) who found that people with visual and hearing impairment were more likely to suffer with CBS than those with just visual impairment. Along these lines, it has been postulated that in AMD cone photoreceptor loss and subsequent, retino-thalmic deafferentation might lead to a functional deafferentation in the visual cortex with the subsequent manifestation of coloured 'positive' visual hallucinations (Santhouse *et al.*, 2000).

While the release/deafferentation theory has received much support (Abbott *et al.*, 2007), Gittinger *et al.* (1982) have suggested that the release theory rests on the assumption that life's experiences affect the brain so as to leave permanent neural traces, imprints, or ingrams and that the brain is a vast store house of previous experiences, while McNamara *et al.* (1982) have questioned the release phenomenon and asked if hallucinations are due to the release phenomenon then why aren't they experienced by every person with a visual impairment. Furthermore, in some cases, individuals remembered hallucinated objects from past experiences, but more often they were not familiar to the patient at all (Menon, 2005).

Neuromatrix theory

Some authors challenge the theory of perceptual release and refer to the neuromatrix theory. Melzack (1989, 1990) has likened the visual hallucinations associated with CBS to the experience of phantom limbs experienced by some amputees. This phenomenon may occur as a result of nerve impulse patterns flowing through a widely distributed series of neural networks, and this has been termed the neuromatrix. In the absence of sensory input, the neuromatrix acts as a substrate for somatic experience. Similarly, CBS hallucinations could be generated by nerve impulse patterns flowing through the neuromatrix in those areas of the brain involved with vision. It is thought that the nerve impulse patterns may be initiated by non-specific input of the ascending reticular formation, the activity of intact visual receptors, or the hyperactivity of cells central to damaged visual areas. These authors argue that sensory changes to sensory input may trigger or modulate the output of this neuromatix but do not dictate the qualities of the experience (Menon *et al.*, 2003). In other words, the existence of an inherited, although modifiable neural network of the 'bodyself' that generates sensory phantoms. This model is supported by clinical and laboratory research (Needham & Taylor, 1992).

CBS and pupil size

Pankow *et al.* (1997) suggested that there was case study evidence from their own research and also in the literature for some association between changes in lighting and hallucination occurrence (Vukicevic & Fitzmaurice, 2008). They went onto postulate that there might be a link between changes in pupil size and neurological impulses creating hallucinations. It has also been reported that closing the eyes tends to eliminate hallucinations (Tenuisse *et al.*, 1994). Pankow *et al.* (1997) went on to suggest that the lack of sensory input due to visual impairment may affect the parasympsthetic papillary innervations at any one of a number of areas in the brain and that more than one may be affected. These authors do acknowledge that there is very little evidence to substantiate their theory that pupil size changes result in CBS hallucinations.

CBS and dementia

Most studies show CBS and dementia to be unrelated (Norton-Willson & Munir, 1987; Needham & Taylor, 1992). The criteria of Gold and Rabins (1989) suggest that 'the retention of insight and absence of delusions are of critical importance to discriminate CBS from true psychotic syndromes, including those in patients with dementia' and that 'as yet there is no reliable evidence that classic CBS patients are more at risk for dementia'. However, in one study, 15 subjects with CBS were compared with 11 controls and impairment of neuropsychological function was found to be associated with CBS. It was suggested that isolated visual hallucinations in older adults with visual impairment are actually an indication of the early stages of dementia (Pliskin *et al.*, 1996). All of the 48 subjects with CBS studied by Menon (2005) manifested insight into the unreality of their hallucinations; however, 18 (60%) attained such insight only after an initial phase of deception, especially when the hallucinations were realistic and appeared consistent with the surroundings. In the same study, 17 (57%) subjects expressed concern about their hallucinations and seven (23%) had experienced disturbing or frightening images. Nineteen (63%) feared being labelled as insane were they to admit to their hallucinations, while ten (33%) were fearful that they were becoming insane or senile. Ten subjects (33%) had previously admitted the existence of their hallucinations, seven of these to family members. Three of these seven were already aware of CBS, while four had been experiencing disturbing images. Interestingly, only 2 of 13 sufferers had informed their physician in a study conducted by Scott *et al.* (2001) and only 36% of the 97 cases of CBS assessed by Khan *et al.* (2008) had discussed their visual hallucinations with a general practitioner or their ophthalmologist. Furthermore, using a modified Mini-Mental State Examination (with two tasks that required good visual function removed). Menon (2005) demonstrated intact cognition among patients with CBS and made the excellent point that a good performance by a CBS sufferer on a formal test of cognition lends credibility to any reassurance provided by a health care practitioner because patients frequently harbour fears of impending dementia (Teunisse *et al.*, 1996; Gilmour *et al.*, 2009). However, Plummer *et al.* (2007) have warned that the Mini-Mental State Examination score, used as evidence against dementia in many CBS studies may not detect higher order cognitive deficits.

Management

Visual

Even though the phenomenology of CBS hallucinations does not appear to correlate with underlying ocular disease, significant bilateral loss of VA appears to be a primary trigger (Scott *et al.*, 2001; Abbott *et al.*, 2007) and several studies have reported that hallucinations attributed to CBS may disappear after treatment of the underlying cause of visual impairment. For example, an 82-year-old female with bilateral cataracts who had experienced visual hallucinations reported VA improvement and cessation of hallucinations following removal of one cataract (Rosenbaum *et al.*, 1987). Similarly, hallucinations ceased for a 39-year male patient with proliferative diabetic retinopathy after VA had been improved from counting fingers at 1.6 m to 6/60 following surgical intervention (Teuth *et al.*, 1995). A reduction in hallucinations has also been noted after treatment of a sub-retinal haemorrhage with laser photocoagulation (Siatkowski *et al.*, 1990), and in another case when temporal arteritis was treated with prednisolone (Sonnenblick *et al.*, 1995). Optical management has included trial with Fresnel prisms displacing what appeared in the left visual field to midline for a patient with left hemianopia, later replaced with ground prism; a 2.8× monocular telescope, combined with a patch over the other eye, for TV viewing for a person that saw hallucinations while watching TV; and increased localized illumination during night-time reading for a patient who experienced hallucinations on waking. For another patient, with peripheral field loss due to glaucoma and central field loss due to scarred corneas and no cognitive loss, hallucinations disappeared over a sustained period of nine months using a combination of full-time spectacle wear, tinted over-shields when in bright environments and night lights for bedroom and bathroom (Pankow & Luchins, 1997). Interestingly, Abbott *et al.* (2007) found that the extent of visual loss did not predict which people would experience hallucinations or the complexity of reported hallucinations.

It is likely that relief from CBS symptoms is more likely with provision of clear retinal images through a combination of maximizing remaining vision and removing or reducing the effects of adverse factors such as blur, glare, and visual field loss. It is unlikely that resolution occurred spontaneously in the cases described here, as hallucinations were noted to return when the interventions were halted.

In summary, visual interventions ranging from the simple such as optimum spectacles and night lights to the more complex such as telescopes and prisms can be very effective at reducing the frequency and even totally halting the occurrence of CBS associated visual hallucinations. Therefore, it would seem sensible for a person with CBS to consult an eye care practitioner if they have not done so recently.

Social

Several groups have purported that the best form of rehabilitation for CBS is reassurance, counselling, and an explanation of the underlying causes using the phantom limb analogy (Needham & Taylor, 1992; Crane *et al.*, 1994; Teunisse *et al.*, 1996; Verstraten 2001;

Menon, 2005; Gilmour *et al.*, 2009). Reassurance of the benign nature of the hallucinations has been reported to have a great therapeutic effect (Needham & Taylor, 1992; Crane *et al.*, 1994), and individuals may learn to coexist with visual hallucinations with relative ease. Also, patients are more likely to admit to experiencing visual hallucinations when a non-judgemental, open-ended 'third party' interview technique is used (Crane *et al.*, 1994). The possibility of hallucinations should also be discussed with those people who have not acknowledged their presence or who have not yet have experienced them (Needham & Taylor, 1992).

Abbott *et al.* (2007) found that 15 (71%) patients had no prior knowledge of CBS and did not know that visual hallucinations could be a feature of visual impairment. In another study, it was found that proper diagnosis had only been made in one of 16 patients who had consulted a general medical practitioner about the hallucinations they were experiencing (Teunisse *et al.*, 1996). Only 8 of 87 CBS subjects sought medical advice, 4 visited an ophthalmologist and 4 saw a general practitioner; only 4 or those that did seek medical advice received an explanation of CBS.

Verstraten (2001) advocated the referral of patients with visual hallucinations (apart from those obviously due to true CBS and who are not distressed) to a psychologist for a structured interview and psychological testing. Cases where the diagnosis is likely to be something other than CBS can then be further referred to other specialists. Misdiagnosis is less likely to occur using this strategy. Cases that can be definitely diagnosed as true CBS could be given the opportunity to join a 'self-help group' (without having to undergo psychological testing) where sufferers could be encouraged to meet, obtain reassurance, and be supplied information and advice on specific techniques for reducing the duration of hallucinations.

Pharmacological

There are many reports in the literature on the use of pharmacological agents in the management of CBS; however, there have been no controlled clinical trials published. Three subjects, treated with between 25 and 100 mg of melperone (an atypical, low-potential neuroleptic agent with minimal side effects makes melperone especially tolerable for older patients), experienced a reduction or total cessation of hallucinations. In one case, the treatment was interrupted for a period of 15 days, after which the patient reported the recurrence of visual hallucinations. When pharmacological treatment was resumed, symptoms again quickly reduced (Batra *et al.*, 1997). Haloperidol has also been reported to have had limited success in treating CBS (Chen *et al.*, 1996; Fernandez *et al.*, 1996), although others found it to be of no use (Miller *et al.*, 1987; Casy & Wandziak, 1988, Bhatia *et al.*, 1992). Neuroleptic agents did not have any effect on CBS hallucinations for eight subjects described by Teunisse and colleagues (1999).

One older patient, who had been experiencing visual hallucinations associated with CBS for 18 months, was successfully treated with 200 mg carbamazepine (an anti-seizure drug) daily (Hosty, 1990). Another case report, describing the cessation of visual hallucinations with 300 mg carbamazepine daily is interesting in that the patient was 38 years old and did not have any visual impairment (Bhatia *et al.*, 1992). A combination of car-bamazepine and clonazepam has been found to be successful (Terao, 1998) as has 400–800 mg per day of valproate, which has fewer potential side effects than carbamazepine (Hori *et al.*, 2000).

One reported case of CBS was successfully treated with ondansetron, a serotonin antag-onist that has limited side effects and is frequently used as an antiemetic for cancer patients receiving cytotoxic drugs (Nevins, 1997). When treatment was stopped, halluci-nations promptly recurred and when treatment was resumed, the hallucinations ceased again. Cisapride, a drug that shares some pharmacologic properties with ondansetron, has been proposed as an alternative and two cases (30–40 mg per day) describing cessa-tion of hallucinations associated with CBS have been reported (Ranen *et al.*, 1999).

Other successful pharmacological treatments include risperidone, a drug used in the treatment of hallucinations associated with dementia, which was successful in reducing symptoms in one case of CBS plus when prescribed twice daily in a 0.5 mg dose (Howard *et al.*, 1994). Diazepam prescribed twice daily in 2 mg doses was found to diminish visual hallucinations in one case of true CBS (Raschka & Sclager, 1982). Pliskin *et al.* (1996) treated nine people with CBS using various psychiatric medications, all of which were found to be ineffective in alleviating the hallucinations.

In summary, the literature indicates mixed success with the use of pharmacological agents in the management of CBS. No specific medications have been shown to treat all CBS visual hallucinations although some anticonvulsants may be helpful in some specific cases. There is an important ethical issue to consider here and that is the use of antipsychotic drugs developed for psychotic patients (where both the hallucinations and underlying neuroreceptor mechanisms are different) by CBS sufferers who by definition are not psychotic. There are also issues associated with polydrug use in that the greater the number of drugs a person uses the more side effects they are likely to experience. It would seem sensible to try and reduce CBS visual hallucinations through less aggressive and invasive means such as through the improvement of visual function (optimum spectacles, prisms telescopes, night lights) along with the improvement of the sufferers social situation and use pharmacological agents only in those cases where the person is disturbed by visual hallucinations and no other form of management has been successful.

Triggers and stoppers

Abbott *et al.* (2007) noted that in a group of individuals with AMD and CBS, visual hal-lucinations appeared suddenly and patients were unable to control what subsequently happened to the image. In this group, common triggers included relaxation, solitary conditions, and evening periods, and the investigators went on to suggest that in these situations, a person would be in a state of reduced sensory stimulation and could be con-sidered to be in 'stand-by mode' and may employ cognitive constructs to interpret the visual scene. As these investigators were unable to predict which of 53 subjects with AMD were likely to report CBS hallucinations despite differences in VA and central field losses, they proposed that cognitive factors such as state of arousal, play a central role in the appearance of the visual hallucinations once the visual loss has reached a threshold level. No common stoppers were evident in this study. It has been reported that closing (Khan *et al.*, 2008; Vukicevic & Fitzmaurice, 2008) or opening the eyes, blinking or putting on a light, concentrating on something else/looking for distraction, hitting the hallucination, or shouting at the hallucination may reduce the length of the hallucinatory period (Alroe & McIntyre, 1983; Teunisse *et al.*, 1996).

Future therapies

A universally effective remedy for CBS remains elusive. Some of the techniques used in psychological therapy for phantom limb pain such as hypnosis, distraction techniques, cognitive restructuring, and relaxation training can be used to minimize the effects of intrusive visual hallucinations (Needham & Taylor, 1992), but the mainstay of treatment of CBS remains sensitive reassurance as sympathetic explanation of the benign nature of such hallucinatory experiences affords significant emotional relief (Menon, 2005). This form of treatment should be aimed at the sufferer and immediate carers and/or relatives. The clinician also needs to bear in mind before treating a CBS sufferer that some people with CBS do enjoy and welcome their hallucinations and may not want to lose them. Furthermore, it would be sensible to advise all visually impaired people, even those who do not admit hallucinatory experiences, of the possible future occurrence of hallucinations to render them better prepared to deal with such experiences should they arise (Menon, 2005; Gilmour *et al.*, 2009).

Functional magnetic resonance imaging (Ffytche *et al.*, 1998), computed tomography, and single photon emission computed tomography (Adachi *et al.*, 1994) show promise as alternative investigative techniques in the search for the aetiology of CBS. Future treatment may involve improvement of sensory input in addition to correction of the primary lesion or simply the provision of education and reassurance. Psychosocial intervention may also be helpful.

Fernandez *et al.* (1996) comment that work remains in organizing and understanding CBS. They suggest that hallucinations should be defined systematically (onset, content, duration, frequency, and comorbidity) and that cognitive, visual impairment, and level of arousal need to be quantified along with the prevalence of hallucinations in cognitive or visually impaired elderly and risk factors for CBS. They go onto say that treatment trials should include increasing sensory stimulation and level of arousal with such tools as improved vision, relocation, and psychostimulants.

Conclusions

Although CBS was first described in 1769, there is still much to be learned about the condition. Accurate diagnosis is critical in order to avoid misdiagnosis and inappropriate intervention (McNamara *et al.*, 1982; Abbott *et al.*, 2007) and although awareness is growing, many medical professionals know little about the condition.

It has been suggested that the typical CBS hallucination occurring in association with AMD (the most common eye condition causing visual impairment) is that of a person, in colour, within the central scotoma, occurring any time of the day, on most days, lasting a few seconds and not generally associated with pleasant or unpleasant feelings and possibly resolving on closing the eyes. Studies show that many people do not report their hallucinations to doctors or optometrists because they believe that they may be thought of as mentally ill. Sufferers invariably do not admit to their hallucinations unless specifically asked. It is therefore important for clinicians to inform those who are susceptible to CBS about the condition, and also to ask direct questions about the appearance of hallucinations if CBS is suspected during a sensitive and sympathetic history taking. Early reassurance is important in patient care, with sympathetic understanding and explanation providing emotional relief. Sympathetic explanation of the benign nature of such hallucinatory experiences is a source of considerable emotional relief. It is sensible to advise all visually impaired people, even those who do not admit hallucinatory experiences, of the possible future occurrence of hallucinations to render them better prepared to deal with such experiences should they arise.

Pharmacotherapy is disappointing as demonstrated by the diverse range of therapeutic agents advocated in this condition (Menon, 2005). A trial of pharmacotherapy may be justified under the guidance of an expert physician or psychiatrist in the context of persistent disturbing hallucinations in a subject refractory to reassurance (Menon, 2005).

It is my view that primary health care practitioners such as optometrists and general medical practitioners should ask about the occurrence of visual hallucinations or warn about their possible onset when they encounter patients who are old and have an eye disease (Melzack, 1989) (particularly AMD as it is a common eye disease in older people) that causes the VA to be reduced to a level where it is 6/24 in the better eye. Those with suspected CBS should initially be referred to a low vision specialist who may be able to reduce or alleviate hallucinatory activity by optimizing visual function, providing reassurance and information, and recommending methods that can help reduce the duration of hallucinatory periods. At the same time, if there is a self-help group in the locality, the patient should be given the opportunity of attending. If this approach fails to have a satisfactory impact on hallucinatory activity then, in those cases where there is an operable ocular condition such as cataract, the patient could be considered for surgery. When optical or surgical intervention is not an appropriate option, then a referral to a specialist for pharmacological therapy can be instigated. Finally, greater awareness of CBS is necessary to avoid inappropriate labelling and treatment for non-existent psychosis.

Resources

Further information on CBS and support in dealing with this condition can be obtained from the following self-help groups.

In the UK: the Macular Disease Society www.maculardisease.org and the Royal Natinal Institute for the Blind www.rnib.org.uk.

In the USA: The American Foundation for the Blind www.afb.org

References

Abbott, E.J., Connor, G.B., Artes, P.H., & Abadi, R.V. (2007). Visual loss and visual hallucinations in patients with age-related macular degeneration (Charles Bonnet syndrome). *Investigative Ophthalmology and Visual Science*, **48**, 1416–1423.

Adachi, N., Nagayama, M., Anami, K., Arima, K., & Matsuda, H. (1994). Assymetrical blood flow in the temporal lobe in the Charles Bonnet syndrome: serial neuroimaging study. *Behav Neurol*, **7**, 97–99.

Alroe, J., & McIntyre, J.M. (1983). Visual hallucinations the Charles Bonnet syndrome and bereavement. *Med J Aust*, **2**, 674–675.

Bartlett, J.E. (1951). A case of organized visual hallucinations in an old man with cataract, and their relation to the phenomena of the phantom limb. *Brain*, **74**, 363–373.

Batra, A., Bartels, M., & Wormstall, H. (1997). Therapeutic options in Charles Bonnet syndrome. *Acta Psychiatr Scand*, **96**, 129–133.

Berrios, G.E., & Brook, P. (1982). The Charles Bonnet syndrome and the problem of visual perceptual disorders in the elderly. *Age Ageing*, **11**, 17–23.

Bhatia, M.S., Khastgir, U., & Malik, S.C. (1992). Charles Bonnet Syndrome. *Br J Psychiatry*, **161**, 409–410.

Brabbins, C.J. (1992). Dementia presenting with complex visual hallucinations. *Int J Geriatr Psychiatry*, **7**, 455–460.

Bromage, P.R., & Melzack, R. (1974). Phatom limb abd the body schema. *Canadian Anaesthetists' Society Journal*, **21**, 267–274.

Brown, C.G., & Murphy, P.R. (1992). Visual symptoms associated with choroidal neovascularisation: photopsias and the Charles Bonnet syndrome. *Arch Ophthalmol*, **110**, 1251–1256.

Burgermeister, R., Tissot, R., & de Ajuriaguerra, J. (1965). Les hallucinations visualles des ophthalmopathes. *Neuropsychologia*, **3**, 9–38.

Casy, D.A., & Wandziak, T. (1988). Senile macular degeneration and psychosis. *J Geriatr Psychiatry Neurol*, **1**, 108–109.

Chen, J., Gomez, M., Veit, S., & O'Dowd, M.A. (1996). Visual hallucinations in a blind elderly woman: Charles Bonnet syndrome, an under recognised clinical condition. *Gen Hosp Psychiatry*, **18**, 453–455.

Cogan, D.G. (1973). Visual hallucinations as a release phenomena. *Graefes Archives of Clinical and Experimental Ophthalmology*, **188**, 139–150.

Crane, W.G., Fletcher, D.C., & Schuchard, R.A. (1994). Prevalence of photopsias and Charles Bonnet Syndrome in a low vision population. *Ophthalmol Clin North Am*, **7**, 143–149.

Damas-Mora, J., Skelton-Robinson, M., & Jenner, F.A. (1982). The Charles Bonnet syndrome in perspective. *Psychol Med*, **12**, 251–261.

Dodd, J., Heffernan, A., & Blake, J. (1999). Visual hallucinations associated with Charles Bonnet syndrome—an ever increasing diagnosis. *Ir Med J*, **92**, 344–345.

Fernandes, L.H., Scassellati-Sforzolini, B., & Spaide, R.F. (2000). Estrogen and visual hallucinations in a patient with Charles Bonnet syndrome. *Am J Ophthalmol*, **129**, 407.

Fernandez, A., Lichtshein, G., Vieweg, W.V.R., *et al.* (1996). Charles Bonnet syndrome with peripheral and central findings. *Int J Geriatr Psychiatry*, **11**, 773–778.

Fuchs, T., & Lauter, H. (1992). Charles Bonnet syndrome and musical hallucinations in the elderly: functional disorders. In Katona, C. and Levy, R. (ed.) *Delusions and Hallucinations in Old Age*, pp.187–198, London: Gaskill.

Ffytche, D.H., Howard, R.J., Brammer, M.J., David, A., Woodruff, P., & Williams, S. (1998). The anatomy of conscious vision: an fMRI study of visual hallucinations. *Nat Neurosci*, **1**, 738–742.

Gilmour, G., Schreiber, C., & Ewing, C. (2009). An examination of the relationship between low vision and Charles Bonnet syndrome. *Can J Ophthalmol*, **44**, 49–52.

Gittinger, J.W. Jr, Miller, N.R., Keltner, J.L., & Burde, R.M. (1982). Sugarplum fairies. Visual hallucinations. *Surv Ophthalmol*, **27**, 42–48.

Gold, K., & Rabins, P.V. (1989). Isolated visual hallucinations and the Charles Bonnet syndrome: a review of the literature and presentation of six cases. *Compr Psychiatry*, **30**, 90–98.

Hartmann, P.M., Kosko, D.A., & Cohn, J.A. (1995). The Charles Bonnet syndrome in an AIDS patient with cytomeglovirus retinitis. *J Nerv Ment Dis*, **183**, 540–549.

Holroyd, S., Rabins, P.V., Finkelstein, D., Nicholson, M.C., Chase, G.A., & Wisniewski, S.C. (1992). Visual hallucinations in patients with macular degeneration. *Am J Psychiatry*, **149**, 1701–1706.

Holroyd, S., & Rabins, P.V. (1996). A three-year follow-up study of visual hallucinations in patients with macular degeneration. *J Nerv Ment Dis*, **184**, 188–189.

Hori, H., Terao, T., Shiraishi, Y., & Nakamura, J. (2000). Treatment of Charles Bonnet syndrome with valporate. *Int Clin Psychopharmacol*, **15**, 117–119.

Hosty, G. (1990). Charles Bonnet syndrome: a description of two cases. *Acta Psychiatr Scand*, **82**, 316–317.

Howard, R., & Levy, R. (1994). Charles Bonnet syndrome plus: complex visual hallucinations of Charles Bonnet syndrome type in late paraphrenia. *Int J Geriatr Psychiatry*, **9**, 399–404.

Howard, R., Meehan, O., Powell, R., *et al.* (1994). Successful treatment of Charles Bonnet syndrome type visual hallucinosis with low dose risperidone. *Int J Geriatr Psychiatry*, **9**, 677–678.

Jackson, M.L., Bassett, K., Nirmalan, P.V., & Sayre, E.C. (2007). Contrast sensitivity and visual hallucinations in patients referred to a low vision rehabilitation clinic. *Br J Ophthalmol*, **91**, 296–298.

Khan, J.C., Shahid, H., Thurlby, D.A., Yates, J.R., & Moore, A.T. (2008). Charles Bonnet syndrome in age-related macular degeneration: the nature and frequency of images in subjects with end-stage disease. *Ophthalmic Epidemiol*, **15**, 202–208.

Lance, J.W. (1976). Simple formed hallucinations confined to the area of specific visual field. *Brain*, **99**, 719–734.

Lepore, F.E. (1990). Spontaneous visual phenomena with visual loss: 104 patients with lesions of retinal neural afferent pathways. *Neurology*, **40**, 444–447.

Levine, A.M. (1980). Visual hallucinations & cataracts. *Ophthalmic Surg*, **11**, 95–98.

Maricle, R.A., Lance, D.T., & Lehman, K.D. (1995). The Charles Bonnet syndrome: a brief review and case report. *Psychiatr Serv*, **6**, 289–291.

McNamara, M.E., Heros, R.C., & Boller, F. (1982). Visual hallucinations in blindness: the Charles Bonnet syndrome. *Int J Neurosci*, **17**, 13–15.

Melzack, R. (1989). Phantom limbs, the self and the brain. *Can Psychol*, **30**, 1–16.

Melzack, R. (1990). Phantom limbs and the concept of a neuromatrix. *Trends Neurosci*, **13**, 88–92.

Menon, G.J., Rahman, I., Menon, S.J., & Dutton, G.N. (2003). Complex visual hallucinations in the visually impaired: the Charles Bonnet Syndrome. *Surv Ophthalmol*, **48**, 58–72.

Menon, G.J. (2005). Complex visual hallucinations in the visually impaired: a structured history-taking approach. *Arch Ophthalmol*, **123**, 349–355.

Miller, F., Magee, J., & Jacobs, R. (1987). Formed visual hallucinations in an elderly patient. *Hospital Community Psychiatry*, **38**, 527–529.

Morsier, G. de. (1967). Les syndrome de Charles Bonnet: hallucinations visuelles de vieillards san deficience mentale. *Annales Médico-Psychologiques*, **125**, 677–702.

Needham, W.E., & Taylor, R.E. (1992). Benign visual hallucinations, or 'phantom vision' in visually impaired and blind persons. *Journal Visual Impairment and Blindness*, **86**, 245–248.

Needham, W.E., & Taylor, R.E. (2000). Atypical Charles Bonnet hallucinations: an elf in the woodshed, a spirit of evil, and the cowboy malefactors. *J Nerv Ment Dis*, **188**, 108–115.

Nevins, M. (1997). Charles Bonnet syndrome. *Journal of the American Geriatic Society*, **45**, 894–895.

Norton-Willson, L., & Munir, M. (1987). Visual perceptual disorders resembling the Charles Bonnet syndrome. A study of 434 consecutive patients referred to a psychogeriatric unit. *Fam Pract*, **4**, 27–31.

Ormond, A.W. (1925). Visual hallucinations in sane people. *Br Med J*, **2**, 376–377.

Pankow, L., & Luchins, D. (1997). An optical intervention for visual hallucinations associated with visual impairment in an elderly patient. *Optometry Vision Science*, **74**, 138–143.

Pfeiffer, R.F., & Bodis-Wollner, I. (1996). Charles Bonnet syndrome. *Journal of American Geriatric Society*, **44**, 1128–1129.

Pliskin, N.H., Kiolbasa, T.A., Towle, V.L., *et al.* (1996). Charles Bonnet syndrome: an early marker for dementia? *Journal of American Geriatric Society*, **44**, 1055–1061.

Plummer, C., Kleinitz, A., Vroomen, P., & Watts, R. (2007). Of Roman chariots and goats in overcoats: the syndrome of Charles Bonnet. *J Clin Neurosci*, **14**, 709–714.

Ranen, N.G., Pasternak, R.E., & Rovner, B.W. (1999). Cisapride in the treatment of visual hallucinations caused by visual loss: the Charles Bonnet syndrome. *Am J Geriatr Psychiatry*, **7**, 264–266.

Raschka, L.B., & Sclager, F.M. (1982). On the diversity of visual hallucinations. *Can J Psychiatry*, **27**, 48–51.

Rosenbaum, F., Harati, Y., Rolak, L., & Freedman, M. (1987). Visual hallucinations in sane people: Charles Bonnet syndrome. *Journal of American Geriatric Society*, **35**, 66–68.

Santhouse, A.M., Howard, R.J., & Ffytche, D.H. (2000). Visual hallucinatory syndromes and the anatomy of the visual brain. *Brain*, **123**, 2055–2064.

Schultz, G., & Melzack, R. (1991). The Charles Bonnet syndrome: 'phantom visual images'. *Perception*, **20**, 809–825.

Scott, I.U., Schein, O.D., Feuer, W.J., & Folstein, M.F. (2001). Visual hallucinations in patients with retinal disease. *Am J Ophthalmol*, **131**(5), 590–8.

Siatkowski, R.M., Zimmer, B., & Rosenburg, P.R. (1990). The Charles Bonnet syndrome: Visual perceptive dysfunction in sensory deprivation. *J Clin Neuroophthalmol*, **10**, 215–218.

Sonnenblick, M., Nesher, R., Rozenman, Y., & Nesher, G. (1995). Charles Bonnet syndrome in temporal arteritis. *J Rheumatol*, **22**, 1596–1597.

Terao, T. (1998). Effect of carbamazepine and clonazepam combination on Charles Bonnet syndrome: a case report. *Human Psychopharmacology: Clinical and Experimental*, **13**, 451–453.

Teunisse, R.J., Zitman, F.G., & Raes, D.C. (1994). Clinical evaluation of 14 patients with the Charles Bonnet syndrome (isolated visual hallucinations). *Compr Psychiatry*, **35**, 70–75.

Teunisse, R.J., Cruysberg, J.R., Verbeek, A., & Zitman, F.G. (1995). The Charles Bonnet syndrome: a large prospective study in the Netherlands. *Br J Psychiatry*, **166**, 254–257.

Teunisse, R.J., Cruysberg, J.R., Hoefnagels, W.H., Verbeek, A.L., & Zitman, F.G. (1996). Visual hallucinations in psychologically normal people: Charles Bonnet's syndrome. *Lancet*, **347**, 794–797.

Teunisse, R.J. (1997). Charles Bonnet syndrome, insight and cognitive impairment. *Journal of the American Geriatric Society*, **45**, 892.

Teunisse, R.J., Cruysberg, J.R., Hoefnagels, W.H., Kuin, Y., Verbeek, A.L., & Zitman, F.G. (1999). Social and psychological characteristics of elderly visually handicapped patients with the Charles Bonnet syndrome. *Compr Psychiatry*, **40**, 315–319.

Teuth, M.J., Cheong, J.A., & Samander, J. (1995). The Charles Bonnet syndrome: a type of organic visual hallucinosis. *J Geriatr Psychiatry Neurol*, **8**, 1–3.

Verstraten, P. (2001). Experiences with a protocol for the Charles Bonnet syndrome. In Whal, H.W. and Schulze, H.E. (ed.) *On the special needs of blind and low vision seniors: research and practice concepts*, pp.209–213. Amsterdam: IOS Press.

Vukicevic, M., & Fitzmaurice, K. (2008). Butterflies and black lacy patterns: the prevalence and characteristics of Charles Bonnet hallucinations in an Australian population. *Clinical and Experimental Ophthalmology*, **36**, 659–665.

West, L.J. (1962). A general theory of hallucinations and dreams. In West, L.J. (ed.) *Hallucinations*, pp. 275–291, New York: Grune and Stratton.

White, N.J. (1980). Complex visual hallucinations in partial blindness due to eye disease. *Br J Psychiatry*, **136**, 284–286.

Chapter 17

Hallucinations in the context of dementing illnesses

Urs Peter Mosimann and Daniel Collerton

Dementia and hallucinations

In this chapter, we will review the current epidemiological, clinical, and biological evidence on the relationships between hallucinations and dementing illnesses, particularly Lewy Body Dementia (LBD) and Parkinson's disease dementia (PDD) where visual hallucinations are common (see also Fénelon, this volume). We will compare dementia-specific models for their genesis with models derived in other disorders. We will then evaluate assessment, treatment, and support options, and finally, look to unresolved issues and the potential for further developments.

Dementia can be neatly defined as an acquired, generally progressive global impairment of cognition in the absence of impaired consciousness. As with all neat definitions, its simplicity is clinically useful but may also be misleading. In most cases, impairments are not equal in all cognitive areas (the exact nature of cognitive change varies by the stage and type of dementing illness), and consciousness may be variably affected. The focus on cognition alone distracts attention from the non-cognitive effects of dementia—emotional, behavioural, psychological, and psychiatric—including hallucinations. There is only a difference of degree between cognitive impairments which are, or are not, severe enough to be classed as dementia. It may be more helpful to think of a dementing process, rather than a state of dementia. The reader with a special interest in the assessment and management of dementia may find more detailed information in specific textbooks or in up-to-date assessment guidelines, for example, the European Federation of Neurological Societies Guidelines (Waldemar *et al.*, 2007).

The overall prevalence of dementia in Western Europe is about 5.4% for those over the age of 60 years, and the estimated annual incidence is 8.8 per 1,000 inhabitants. The prevalence increases exponentially with age: 1% (60–64 years), 1.5 % (65–69 years), 3.6% (70–74 years), 6% (75–79 years), 12.2% (80–84 years), and 24.8% (≥85 years). Global prevalence rates will double in the next 20 years, mainly due to an increased life expectancy in the third world (Ferri *et al.*, 2005). The economical cost of dementia in Europe exceeds 55 billion Euros per year with the major costs emerging in institutional care (Johnson *et al.*, 2005). If the unpaid work of family and other carers is included, the costs rise threefold.

The associations between dementia, hallucinations, disability, and carer burden

Dementia and hallucinations commonly coexist, particularly in later life. We have previously estimated that amongst the total population of people with complex visual hallucinations, cases of dementia are as frequent as psychosis and eye disease, and a third of the frequency of the most common association, delirium (Collerton *et al.*, 2005).

Visual hallucinations are found in a third of patients with dementia, with auditory hallucinations in a third of that number (Ballard *et al.*, 1995). They are closely associated with LBD (McKeith *et al.*, 2005) and are also a core diagnostic feature for PDD (Emre *et al.*, 2007a) and an exclusion criterion for progressive supranuclear palsy (Litvan, 1997). Since recurrent visual hallucinations are rare features in vascular dementia, frontotemporal dementia, and early Alzheimer's disease, the main focus of this chapter will be on LBD and PDD.

Dementia is not a one person disease (Brodaty, 2007). It affects caregivers with a major contributor to their burden being neuropsychiatric features, in particular hallucinations, delusions, and sleep disturbances (de Vugt *et al.*, 2006, Sink *et al.*, 2006). In people with dementia, hallucinations are associated with increased distress and disability and lead to earlier institutionalization (Craig *et al.*, 2005; Ropacki & Jeste, 2005; Scarmeas *et al.*, 2005; Allegri *et al.*, 2006; Aarsland *et al.*, 2007; Capitani *et al.*, 2007; Fujishiro *et al.*, 2007).

The assessment and management of dementing illnesses

It is helpful to distinguish between *dementia*, the variable clinical syndrome, and its causes that are a number of *dementing illnesses* (Fig. 17.1). Identification of the dementing illness is more helpful than the label of dementia in that it allows the patient to be given a more accurate prognosis and more specific treatment.

In the context of hallucinations, the key task is to assess whether a dementing illness is the more likely cause than the other common aetiologies in this age group: delirium, sensory impairment, or psychosis. Dementia is generally characterized by chronic, progressive cognitive decline over more than 6 months, associated with impairments in activities of daily living (WHO, 2003). Common complaints of patients and informants include poor memory, disorientation, getting lost in a familiar environment, lack of recognition of relatives, lack of insight or judgement, impaired comprehension, and word finding difficulties. Abrupt onset is not common. The early stages of dementing illnesses may present as a mild cognitive impairment, which is difficult to distinguish from normal ageing, depression, or the effects of ill health (WHO, 2003).

Dementing illnesses

The classification of dementing illnesses has developed historically and is not entirely consistent. Disorders are either based on the presumed neuropathology (e.g., LBD, Alzheimer's disease, vascular dementia) or on the dysfunction of focal brain areas, e.g.,

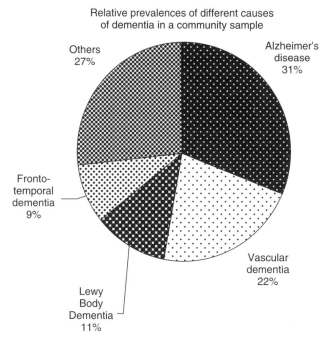

Fig. 17.1 Causes of dementia in later life (Stevens *et al.*, 2002).

fronto-temporal degeneration. The most common dementing illnesses of later life are described in Table 17.1. Heterogenous and mixed pathology is common in old age, but there are currently no clinical diagnostic criteria for mixed dementia. The pathological features of dementing illnesses (plaques, tangles, vascular damage, and Lewy bodies) are common in old age and the pathological separation between normal ageing and dementia is often one of threshold or density of neuropathology in a specific brain area rather than the simple presence of the pathology itself. The boundaries between the different causes of dementia, and even dementia and normal ageing, are therefore not clear.

The clinical assessment and diagnosis of dementia

The clinical classification of dementing illnesses is based upon pattern recognition. Clinical symptoms need to be related to the severity of dementia to be helpful for the differential diagnosis. For example, slowly progressive memory impairment at onset of the disease supports the diagnosis of Alzheimer's disease; however, it loses diagnostic specificity when found in later disease stages (Metzler-Baddeley, 2007). Recurrent visual hallucinations and visuo-perceptual impairments at the initial disease presentation are often followed by Lewy body pathology at autopsy (Tiraboschi *et al.*, 2006). Hallucinations in moderate to severe dementia have less diagnostic specificity. They are more often a symptom of co-morbidity such as delirium, psychosis, or visual impairment.

The identification of dementia is based on a detailed history of the initial symptoms of cognitive decline and the progression of the disease, which includes an informant report.

Table 17.1 Characteristics of the most common dementing illnesses

Type	Core clinical features	Diagnostic criteria
Alzheimer's disease	Established dementia (APA, 1994, WHO, 2003) with progressive impairment of episodic memory and other cognitive deficits; the absence of disturbed consciousness and other disorders, which themselves could account for progressive cognitive impairments. The diagnosis is supported by impaired activities in daily living, a positive family history of dementia, normal lumbar puncture, and evidence of cerebral atrophy on CT or MRI. Features that make the diagnosis uncertain include sudden onset of cognitive impairment, focal neurological findings, seizures or gait disturbance at presentation (Allan et al., 2005).	National Institute of Neurological Disorders and Stroke-Alzheimer's Disease and related disorders (McKhann et al., 1984), revised research criteria (Dubois et al., 2007).
Vascular dementia	*Vascular cognitive disorders* have been suggested as an umbrella term (Roman et al., 2004) including *vascular dementia* (Roman et al., 2004) and *vascular cognitive impairment* (O'Brien, 2006). The diagnosis vascular dementia requires (a) dementia and (b) cerebrovascular disease, which manifests by the presence of focal neurological signs and cerebrovascular disease in CT or MRI. To fulfill diagnostic criteria a relationship between (a) and (b) is needed; either abrupt start with stepwise progression or dementia following a stroke within a couple of months. Early presence of gait disturbance, history of falls, early change in urinary frequency, pseudobulbar palsy, and personality changes are consistent with this diagnosis. Subtypes of vascular dementia are cortical vascular dementia (multi-infarct dementia), subcortical vascular dementia (small vessel dementia or Binswanger disease), strategic infarct dementia, hypoperfusion dementia, hemorraghic dementia, and hereditary vascular dementia (Grand et al., 1988).	National Institute of Neurological Disorders and Stroke and Association Internationale pour la Recherche et l'Enseignement en Neurosciences Guidelines (Roman et al., 1993).
Lewy body dementias	LBD is defined as a distinct clinical syndrome with progressive cognitive impairment, usually prominent executive and visuo-constructional impairments. The three core features supporting this diagnosis are parkinsonism, recurrent visual hallucinations, and fluctuation of cognition (McKeith et al., 2005). Suggestive features are REM-sleep behaviour disorder, severe neuroleptic sensitivity, and reduced striatal dopamine activity. A diagnosis of probable LBD is recommended if one or more suggestive features are present in conjunction with at least one of the core features. A diagnosis of possible LBD is recommended when the central feature—progressive cognitive decline—co-exists with at least one suggestive feature. Stroke disease and other physical or neurological conditions sufficient to account for the clinical picture are exclusion criteria.

PDD has a similar clinical and pathological profile, but disease progression is different. Patients are classified as having PDD if Parkinson's disease predates dementia. In LBD parkinsonism develops simultaneously or after cognitive impairment. | Lewy body dementias include Lewy Body Dementia (LBD) (McKeith et al., 2005) and Parkinson's disease dementia (PDD) (Emre, 2007a). |
| Fronto-temporal dementia | Three clinical syndromes have been defined: frontotemporal dementia, progressive nonfluent aphasia, and semantic dementia. Initial symptoms are often personality change and impaired executive function before cognitive impairment (often language impairment) evolves (Neary et al., 1998, McKhann et al., 2001). | Consensus diagnostic criteria (Neary et al., 1998, McKhann et al., 2001). |

Formal assessment of cognition involves neuropsychological testing, which includes a cognitive screening test (e.g., Mini Mental State Examination (MMSE)) (Folstein *et al.*, 1975), which may then be followed by a more comprehensive cognitive test battery, e.g., Cambridge Cognitive Assessment (CAMCOG) (O'Connor, 1990). Given that dementia is not merely a cognitive disorder, scales to measure disability, e.g., Clinical Dementia Rating (CDR) (Morris, 1993) or behavioural and psychological symptoms, e.g., Neuropsychiatric Inventory (NPI) (Cummings *et al.*, 1994) are commonly included in the assessment process as well.

A major focus of the medical assessment of suspected dementia is on the exclusion of potentially treatable causes. A blood sample helps to exclude metabolic (e.g., hypothyroidisms, vitamin B12 and folic acid deficiency) or inflammatory co-morbidities (e.g., neurosyphilis) causing or contributing to cognitive impairments. A physical assessment may give other diagnostic pointers, e.g., extrapyramidal motor symptoms for LBD and PDD, or focal neurological symptoms for vascular dementia. Structural (e.g., computerized tomography (CT) or magnetic resonance imaging (MRI)) or functional neuroimaging (e.g., single photon computer tomography (SPECT) and positron emission tomography (PET)) are other helpful tools to establish the illness underlying dementia and to exclude treatable causes. In an elderly patient with newly occurring recurrent complex visual hallucinations without visual impairment, a CT or MRI scan may identify structural abnormalities within the visual system, for example, a cerebrovascular lesion in the occipital cortex. Early diagnosis is important to exclude treatable causes of cognitive impairment and will become even more important in the future once biomarkers and disease modifying treatments will become available (Mollenhauer *et al.*, 2007). The highest accuracy for the clinical diagnosis is *possible* or *probable* disease. Autopsy is required to establish the *definite* cause of dementia.

> Mrs B had an 18 month history of hallucinations of 'waterfalls of rain' occurring almost continually. She had a mild cognitive impairment (MMSE 28/30) of uncertain aetiology. A CT scan showed atrophy consistent with her age but she had significant visual loss due to cataracts. There was no evidence of other neurological symptoms. A diagnosis of hallucinations associated predominantly with eye disease was made with her mild cognitive impairment being a minor contributory factor. Treatment of her cataracts reduced, but did not abolish her hallucinations.

Identifying and assessing hallucinations in the context of cognitive impairment

Hallucinations are, by nature, internal experiences that are not directly accessible to others. This poses particular challenges when assessing hallucinations in people with cognitive impairment who may not volunteer or be able to describe their experiences. The co-existence of other types of sensory dysfunctions, including illusions, misperceptions, and a range of perceptually influenced delusions, can make it exceptionally difficult to be confident whether a person is truly hallucinating or merely reporting a perceptual disturbance. For instance, faces may appear from patterned carpets or curtains. The boundary between a distortion and a hallucination cannot be objectively drawn. Further questioning in these circumstances is rarely productive. Experience of the full range of perceptual disturbances in dementia can make differential classification easier but not always easy.

Until lately, there was a lack of instruments for quantifying hallucinations in people with significant cognitive impairment, though there are several new measures for other populations, particularly Parkinson's disease and visual impairment (Wada-Isoe et al., 2008). We recently developed a new screening tool to assess the presence of visual hallucinations in elderly patients regardless of the presence of cognitive or visual impairments (North East Visual Hallucinations Interview—NEVHI) (Mosimann et al., 2008). The first section of NEVHI establishes the presence or absence of visual hallucinations, visual misperceptions, or a sense of presence. This first section has good internal consistency (Cronbach alpha: 0.71) and inter-rater reliability (Kappa: 0.72–0.83). In screening for hallucinations, we found that it is best to avoid the term hallucinations in initial questions because a proportion of patients do not refer to them as such. The questions 'Do your eyes ever play tricks on you?' or 'Have you ever seen something, which other people could not see? are more likely to facilitate the disclosure of hallucinations than questions directly referring to them. The second section of the NEVHI documents visual hallucinations experienced in the month prior to the assessment and establishes their frequency together with any associated emotions (e.g., anxiety), cognitions (e.g., fear of suffering from a mental illness), or behaviours (e.g., acting upon hallucinations).

An informant version of NEVHI has also been developed. We have shown that patients with mild to moderate dementia (MMSE down to 13) are well able to provide details about the phenomenology of hallucinations (Mosimann et al., 2006). Informants provide more reliable information about the frequency of complex visual hallucinations in patients with moderate dementia (MMSE below 20), but they under-report the presence of hallucinations in the cognitively less impaired (Mosimann et al., 2008). A comprehensive hallucination assessment for patients with cognitive impairment or dementia should therefore include patient's and informant's views. Contradictory reports need to be resolved on a case-by-case basis. Hallucinations in the most severely demented may have to be inferred from behaviour, though this is difficult to do reliably. Some patients, for example, may appear to be conversing with invisible companions, or picking at invisible objects, but whether this is in response to hallucinations is impossible to say for certain.

As well as assessing hallucination phenomenology, it is crucial to bear in mind that potential targets for the treatment of hallucinations are not only frequency, but also their consequences including emotions (e.g., fear), cognitions (e.g., the interpretation of a figure as a visitor), and the behaviour associated with them (e.g., shouting at supposed burglars). Frequency, emotions, cognitions, and behaviours are potential outcome variables for the treatment of hallucinations. We have seen numerous patients with hallucinations whose suffering was related to the belief resulting from their hallucinations—e.g., the fear of suffering from an additional mental illness—and not the hallucination *per se*. In these situations, psychoeducation of patient and informant is often sufficient to alleviate distress. Other patients find their visual hallucinations amusing and entertaining, and the stress caused is mainly on the caregiver side. It is therefore essential to explore emotions, cognitions, and behaviours associated with hallucinations in order to plan the most efficient treatment strategy.

Mrs A lived alone. She had a 6 month history of hallucinating figures of three men appearing in her kitchen in the early evening. She had a moderately severe cognitive impairment (MMSE 19/30) with a retrograde amnesia dating back several decades and little day-to-day learning. She interpreted her hallucinations as visiting workmen. She was not distressed but tried to feed them, reasoning that they must be coming at teatime for a meal. She could not be persuaded otherwise. The main problems were of wasted food and the worries of her family. The former was dealt with by providing non-perishable food that could be reused, and the latter by education. On follow up over 6 months, the hallucinations had resolved.

Modality and phenomenology

Across dementia as a whole, complex visual hallucinations (formed hallucinations of people, body parts, animals, pictures, furniture, and plants) (Mosimann *et al.*, 2008) are reported more frequently than simple hallucinations (lights, circles, rings, wheels, stars, spots, shapes, and shadows) (Weinberger, 1940), though this may be a reflection of salience in the minds of the patient and the examiner rather than a true reflection of prevalence. When they are associated with hallucinations of other modalities, the most common association is with auditory. Visuo-tactile or visuo-gustatory hallucinations are much rarer. Some patients may have hallucinations in more than one modality but these may not be synchronized, e.g., talking visual hallucinations are rarely encountered. This may irritate patients when they fail to get an answer when questioning what they believe to be an intruder or guest. Common neuropsychiatric features associated with visual hallucinations are apathy and delusions. Isolated auditory or musical hallucinations are relative uncommon, but where they do occur, they tend to lack the personal reference of psychotic experiences.

Chronicity, duration, and frequency

Prevalence of hallucinations rises through early dementia but then remains constant (Awata *et al.*, 2005, Hamuro *et al.*, 2007). There is an apparent drop in the most severe dementia, which may reflect difficulties in ascertainment. Hallucinations in most people with dementia usually span a number of weeks or months, with persistence over years being relatively rare, though patients with LBD tend to have hallucinatory periods for longer parts of their disease. Hallucinations generally last for minutes, or at most a few hours. Fleeting hallucinations (seeing something out of the corner of the eye) are less common in patients with dementia. In a hallucinatory period, daily hallucinations are not uncommon. Timing may be consistent within an individual patient with transitions from sleep to waking, or times of reduced alertness triggering hallucinations.

Variations of hallucinations with type of dementing illness

As Figure 17.2 shows, there is a distinct variation in levels of reported hallucinations across disorders. Gender and other factors are also important (Steinberg *et al.*, 2006). However, studies have used a variety of designs and instruments, so it may be that the actual differences are less or more striking.

A comparison of the phenomenology of hallucinations across dementing illnesses is fraught with difficulty. The lack, until recently, of measures validated across clinical groups, and intrinsic differences between the reporting capabilities of people with dementia, means that conclusions are unreliable at present. There is even more difficulty in comparing hallucinations between dementing illnesses and other disorders with high rates of hallucinations, for instance, psychosis and eye disease. From the somewhat unreliable data currently available, it does not seem that the basic phenomenology of hallucinations is definitively different across disorders, though associated factors may differ.

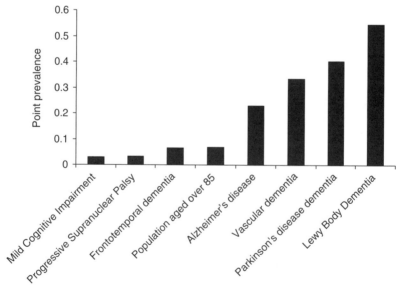

Fig. 17.2 Variation of prevalence of complex visual hallucinations by disorder (Collerton *et al.*, 2005). Reproduced with permission.

The great distress seen in psychotic disorders is uncommon for example in people with dementia, while bizarre distortions are possibly more specific for eye disease.

Causes of hallucinations in dementia

Coincidental other disorders

Eye disease is no less frequent in people with dementia than it is in the general older population. Though Charles Bonnet syndrome can be defined to exclude people with dementia, cognitive impairment is a risk factor for hallucinations in eye disease (Graham *et al.*, in press), and poor vision is a risk factor for visual hallucinations in dementia (Chapman *et al.*, 1999). Similarly, poor hearing is a risk factor for auditory hallucinations and dual sensory impairment contributes to both. People with dementia are particularly prone to develop delirium in response to ill health with an associated multi-modal hallucinatory episode. A *de novo* coincidental psychosis is rare in dementia, though hallucinations, illusions, and misinterpretations with the character of delusions may be misleading. Occasionally, people with a chronic psychosis may develop dementia in later life, though generally, by that stage, active hallucinations have disappeared. Particularly in people with a liability to hallucinations, multiple medications, especially drugs with anticholinergic effects or side effects, contribute to the experience of hallucinations. It is therefore likely that, in most patients, hallucinations have multiple causes.

Mr B has a 6 year history of dementia, probably due to Alzheimer's disease. He developed a severe infection leading to hospital admission. He was placed in a single room facing a blank wall. He soon became greatly distressed by hallucinations of distorted faces appearing from the wall and the curtains around his bed. He was confused with poor attention. A diagnosis of delirium was made. He was moved into a more stimulating environment, and his infection responded to treatment. His hallucinations stopped over a 48-hour period and have not recurred.

As we noted above, the relative rareness of hallucinations in disorders other than LBD, strongly suggests that co-morbidities (e.g., delirium, visual impairment) or medication (e.g., drugs with anticholinergic properties) contribute to the experience of hallucinations in Alzheimer's disease, vascular dementia, and frontotemporal degeneration.

Dementia-specific factors

Cognitive impairment

Several groups have now reported an association between impaired attentional and executive performance and liability to visual hallucinations (Collerton *et al.*, 2005). However, it is not clear which specific aspects of attention or executive function need to be impaired, given the tendency for people with dementia to be impaired in most cognitive domains. As with attentional factors, failures in visual perceptual processing are associated with visual hallucinations, though again since dementia causes impairments at many stages of the visual system, it is not known whether a single specific impairment in each cognitive area is sufficient, or whether multiple, cumulative dysfunctions are needed.

Neuropathology of hallucinations in dementia

Visual hallucinations have a close relationship with Lewy body pathology within visual pathways. Tiraboshi *et al.* reviewed clinical symptoms at the first presentation of dementia in patients with LBD and Alzheimer's disease (Tiraboschi *et al.*, 2006). As would be expected from diagnostic criteria, visual hallucinations were more common in clinically diagnosed LBD than in Alzheimer's disease. However, pathological follow-up confirmed that patients with visual hallucinations or visuo-constructional impairment at initial presentation usually had Lewy body pathology at autopsy. Johnson *et al.* compared clinical features of patients with either pure LBD, mixed LBD/Alzheimer's disease or pure Alzheimer's disease (Johnson *et al.*, 2005). They found that patients with Lewy body pathology performed poorly in visuo-spatial tasks, whereas patients with Alzheimer's disease pathology did worse in memory tasks. Combined pathology affected visuo-spatial but not memory performance. Furthermore, Alzheimer's disease neuro-fibrillary pathology modifies the presence of hallucinations. LBD patients with low tangle pathology have more hallucinations than those with many tangles (Braak stages 3–6) (Merdes *et al.*, 2003). Ballard *et al.* confirmed an association between persistent visual hallucinations and Lewy body pathology and an inverse relationship between hallucinations and tangle pathology in LBD (Ballard *et al.*, 2004). These findings suggest that Lewy body pathology is essential for visuo-perceptual impairment independent of associated Alzheimer's disease pathology (Gomez-Isla *et al.*, 1999).

Lewy body pathology is usually found throughout the brainstem and anterior portions of the ventral visual pathway amongst others (Merdes *et al.*, 2003, Williams & Lees, 2005, Tiraboschi *et al.*, 2006) with primary sensory areas being relatively spared (Harding *et al.*, 2002). Early onset of hallucinations was associated with higher Lewy body densities in the parahippocampal and the inferior temporal cortices in LBD. A similar association was found in patients with PDD (Liang *et al.*, 2005).

Neurochemical changes and hallucinations

Numerous neurochemical changes occur in dementing illnesses. Investigations to date have focused on cholinergic and dopaminergic losses. Both are noticeably more pronounced in LBD than in Alzheimer's disease (Perry *et al.*, 1985, Tiraboschi *et al.*, 2002). Both deficits may contribute to the generation of visual symptoms with cholinergic function having a primary and dopaminergic function a secondary role (Collerton *et al.*, 2005). Striatal dopaminergic loss likely interferes with information selection, because the basal ganglia are vital to direct the eyes to objects of interest (Hikosaka *et al.*, 2000). Furthermore, dopamine is crucial for retinal visual processing (Witkovsky, 2004), namely for light adaptation (Iuvone *et al.*, 1978), colour, and contrast perception (Djamgoz *et al.*, 1997). It is released when light increases and is involved in the switching from cone perception to light-sensitive rod perception (Wink & Harris, 2000). The lack of retinal dopamine in patients with Parkinson's disease is associated with impaired light adaptation and contrast vision (Harnois & Di Paolo, 1990, Harris *et al.*, 1992).

The cholinergic system plays an essential role in visual information processing (Kimura, 2000), because it is crucial for visual perception and saccade control (Kitagawa *et al.*, 1994, Kobayashi *et al.*, 2001). Experimental work suggested that acetylcholine contributes to the switch from top–down visual processing to bottom–up processing (Kobayashi & Isa, 2002). The cholinergic deficits are associated with visual hallucinations (Court *et al.*, 2001), particularly in Lewy body disease with profound cholinergic deficits in the temporal and parietal lobes (Perry *et al.*, 1995, Ballard *et al.*, 2004). In contrast to the dopaminergic hypotheses, the cholinergic hypothesis is supported by recent treatment studies, showing that hallucinations may well improve when treated with cholinesterase inhibitors (Aarsland *et al.*, 2004, McKeith & Mosimann, 2004).

Neuroimaging of hallucinations in dementia

The relationship of perception, hallucinations, and imaging findings is complex and not yet clear. Functional imaging studies assessing cortical perfusion or glucose metabolism in LBD showed extensive changes in visual association areas. Most studies reported more occipital or occipito-parietal hypoactivity in LBD compared to Alzheimer's disease (Donnemiller *et al.*, 1997, Ishii *et al.*, 1998, Higuchi *et al.*, 2000, Imamura *et al.*, 2001, Lobotesis *et al.*, 2001, Minoshima *et al.*, 2001, Pasquier *et al.*, 2002, Firbank *et al.*, 2003). A recent diffusion tensor imaging study (Bozzali *et al.*, 2005), a technique helpful to assess the integrity of the white matter, showed different white matter disintegration in the occipito-parietal compared to the occipito-temporal region in LBD. Sauer *et al.* (Sauer *et al.*, 2006) found more activation in the superior temporal sulcus during motion perception in LBD when compared to Alzheimer's disease or controls. Taken together, these studies suggest disease specific activation changes in the visual system in LBD, which are present at rest or when perceiving a visual stimulus.

Other researchers have compared patients with and without visual hallucinations. A ^{18}F-fluorodeoxyglucose PET study revealed that patients with LBD and visual hallucinations have less hypometabolism in the right temporo-parietal and lateral occipital areas compared to those without them (Imamura *et al.*, 1999). Whether occipital hypoperfusion differs in patients with and without hallucinations is not clear (Lobotesis *et al.*, 2001, Pasquier *et al.*, 2002). An exceptional fMRI single case study (Howard *et al.*, 1997) assessed visual information processing in a patient with LBD whilst he was experiencing visual hallucinations. Photic stimulation during hallucination induced very limited activation of the striatal cortex. The same stimulation in the absence of hallucinations was followed by normal bilateral activation. If replicated and confirmed in a larger sample this may well suggest state dependent, bottom–up perceptual changes whilst experiencing hallucinations.

Models of the generation of hallucinations in dementia

We have previously suggested the requirements for a good model of visual hallucinations (Collerton *et al.*, 2005). It should account for who hallucinates, what they see, and when and where they see it. It has to explain the associations within disorders with poor vision, disturbed alertness, and intellectual impairment. Finally, it needs to account for the phenomenology of recurrent complex visual hallucinations; for the frequency of hallucinations of people and animals; for their abrupt onset and offset, and their movement; for temporal and situational regularities where they exist; and last, for their extinction with eye closure.

Dementia-specific models

Drawing on the character of LBD, we have proposed the Perception and Attention Deficit (PAD) model of the genesis of visual hallucinations (Collerton *et al.*, 2005). We were guided by the cognitive and pathological characteristics of the disorder with the most consistent evidence for the highest levels of visual hallucinations in LBD. Coupling this with the phenomenological character of hallucinations (their occurrence at the focus of visual attention in an otherwise unchanged scene) led us to propose that most cases of visual hallucinations are a result of combined attentional and visual perceptual impairments interacting with scene representations to produce the activation of an incorrect, but environmentally expected, perceptual proto-object. This model is consistent with data on the character of hallucinations and variations in frequency across the major dementing disorders and can, we have argued, also account for hallucinations in other disorders as well (Fig. 17.3).

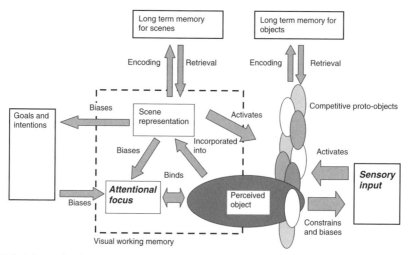

Fig. 17.3 Schematic of PAD model reproduced from Collerton *et al.* (2005). (Italics indicate areas of impairment). Reproduced with permission.

However, PAD is far from the only model. A large number of models, reviewed in this volume and Collerton *et al.* (2005), have been developed within specific disorders such as eye disease and psychosis.

Some models have potential application to dementing illnesses. Horowitz's perceptual nidus theory (Horowitz, 1975) suggests that the primary pathology lies in the generation of images rather than their tagging as internal or external. He suggests that hallucinations occur when there is a combination of an ambiguous relationship between an internal image and reality (the perceptual nidus), in combination with a template of expectancy (derived from psychoanalytic drives and other wishes) and an active memory or fantasy image. This shares several central features with our PAD model.

Recent biological models of psychosis have focused on the role of the thalamus in coordinating the multiple brain areas that subserve attention and perception (e.g., Pelaez, 2000, Lee *et al.*, 2003, Behrendt, 2004). They suggest that thalamic dysfunction creates a stable perception that incorporates incorrect elements. Though attractive in that they can reconcile the need for multiple factors interacting, these models are at odds with the lack of relationship between thalamic dysfunction and rates of recurrent complex visual hallucinations across different disorders (Collerton *et al.*, 2005).

Diederich *et al.* (2004) and Aleman and Larøi (2008) have also proposed novel models, which propose modulated interactions between top–down and bottom–up attentional processes to account for hallucinations, which are shared factors to the PAD model. At present, no model is sufficiently specified to allow unique predictions that might be used to test their respective utility.

Models of the consequences of hallucinations

Emotional reactions to visual hallucinations in dementia

The content of visual hallucinations in people with dementia is generally prosaic compared to the violent or disturbing images seen in other disorders (Zarroug, 1975, Pliskin *et al.*, 1996). Most people see unfamiliar figures or animals. Only half of patients with dementia are distressed by their hallucinations, though their association with carer distress may mean that the patient may be treated to reduce the burden on a carer to prevent caring breaking down altogether. In these cases, careful consideration needs to be given to the patient's best interest before initiating treatment.

> Mr T lives in a nursing home. He has severe dementia with a diagnosis of LBD. He has frequent hallucinations of a black dog who reminds him of a long dead pet of his own. He takes pleasure in the dog's company. Staff support the hallucination.

Collerton and Dudley (Collerton & Dudley, 2004) (Fig. 17.4) have suggested a cognitive behavioural framework for understanding distressed reactions to visual hallucinations. In analogy with psychological treatments for auditory hallucinations in

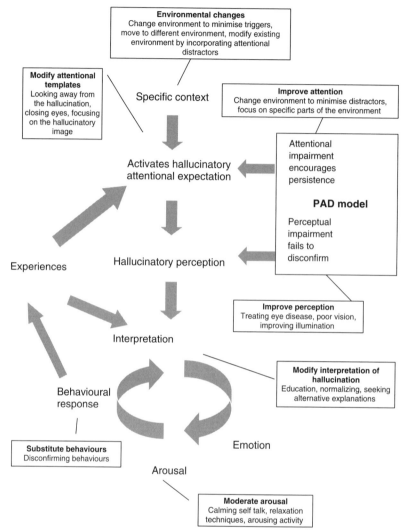

Fig. 17.4 Model of emotional distress associated with visual hallucinations with potential treatment options reproduced from Collerton & Dudley (2004). Reproduced with permission.

people with psychosis, they suggest that modifying the interpretation of the hallucination may be of significant benefit (Smith *et al.*, Johns & Wykes, both this volume). In common with cognitive behavioural models of distressing auditory hallucinations (Chadwick & Birchwood, 1994, Morrison, 1998) (Trower *et al.*, this volume) and of obsessional concerns, this framework proposes that the emotional reaction to a hallucination is an understandable consequence of the cognitive appraisal of unusual experiences, in this case the hallucinated image. It is therefore not the content of the hallucination *per se* but the appraisal of it that leads to distress.

The role of cognitive impairment in modifying reactions to hallucinations

Insight into hallucinations in people with dementia is variable. Severity of dementia may be a factor in whether people believe hallucinations to be true experiences, but there is no systematic evidence to support this and we have seen people in all stages of dementia who act as if their hallucinations are real. Partial or fluctuating insight is common. Understanding may develop over time, especially in response to education, but may not, especially in severe dementia or if delusions are present.

People with dementia tend to react to their immediate understanding of what they are experiencing. Thus, common interpretations of hallucinated figures as visitors or intruders produce understandably different emotional impacts. Behavioural responses are usually consistent with the patient's explanation of what they are experiencing: hospitality for visitors (we have had patients who regularly cook a meal) and hostility for intruders (others have attacked their visions with the poker). Regardless of the interpretation, the lack of response of the hallucination often leads to irritation. In contrast to other patient groups, concerns around the meaning of experiencing hallucinations (as a sign of mental breakdown, for example) are rare.

As an aside, it is important to note that visual hallucinations may also be incorporated into existing delusional beliefs or even lead to such beliefs (Maher, 1974; 2005), though there is little evidence that in themselves they necessarily lead to delusional explanations (Holroyd *et al.*, 2001).

> Mrs B incorporated her hallucinations into a belief that her neighbours thought that her husband was a child abuser. Over time, her hallucinations changed into people carrying placards with that message. As with hallucinations themselves, delusions merge imperceptivity into the misunderstandings and misinterpretations common in dementia.

In common with existing cognitive behavioural treatment models of psychosis, once an appraisal has been made, reinforcing loops, behavioural, physiological, attentional, and environmental, may act to maintain and strengthen this cycle. The more often a hallucination occurs, the more it becomes an expected part of that specific environment, and hence the more frequently it recurs. As a consequence, hallucinations may tend to occur in a specific location at specific times, and have a recurring theme.

Interactions with the environment are not uncommon (Heron *et al.*, 1956, Flynn, 1962). An isolated person with dementia may have low emotional arousal and sensory deprivation from impoverished visual environments. It is not uncommon for patients to spend many hours staring at blank or highly patterned walls with little to occupy them. Conversely, periods of high arousal on busy wards or nursing homes are also associated with increased experiences of verbal and visual hallucinations (Manford & Andermann, 1998) especially in periods of acute stress and prolonged arousal.

> Mrs W hallucinated water on the floor of his room from waking till he went for break-fast. This was a time of low activity and arousal, and encouraging her to be more active reduced the incidence of hallucinations.

Management considerations in patients with dementia

As we suggested earlier, assessment of hallucinations needs to focus not only on the hal-lucination itself but also on the consequences for the person and their carers. As a general principle, cognitive impairment in itself does not affect response to treatments until it reaches moderate to severe disease stages.

Selecting treatment targets

There is little specific evidence that there are treatments that can abolish hallucinations in dementia. Studies have generally included hallucinations in an overall measure of behav-ioural and psychological disturbance, so the specific response of hallucinations to even generally effective treatments is not known. Residual symptoms are common. Management therefore aims first at reducing the risk factors for hallucinations, then at reducing the distress, which may be associated with hallucinatory experiences.

Hallucinations can be caused by co-morbidity, e.g., auditory impairment due to ear disease or delirium in addition to dementia. A consequence of the poly-morbidity com-mon in later life is poly-pharmacy and drug interactions or anticholinergic side effects commonly contribute to hallucinations or psychosis.

Accurate ascertainment of delirium in the context of dementia can be challenging, but multimodal hallucinations, abrupt deterioration in behaviour or orientation and evi-dence of physical ill health should raise suspicions. Identification and effective treatment of precipitating factors (including poor functional or nutritional status, inactivity, pain, hypoxia, dehydration, infection, alcohol withdrawal, or poor metabolic control) may abolish the hallucinations.

Visual impairment due to age-related eye disease is common in demented patients. Furthermore, demented patients may have difficulties expressing their visual complaints and are at risk of mislaying or losing their visual aids and may have limited access to oph-thalmologists (Mitchell et al., 1997). It is therefore important to exclude visual impair-ment as a possible cause for hallucinations in dementia (Chapman et al., 1999).

> Mr F was troubled by figures whom he saw in the early evening in the garden and whom he interpreted as intruders. His hallucinations were abolished by drawing the curtains early, before the light faded.

Non-pharmacological treatment strategies

The treatment models covered earlier in this volume are relevant to people with halluci-nations and dementia, though they may need adapting to be suitable for people with limited recall. Simplifying approaches, repeating and writing information, and enlisting support from families and staff can all lead to effective interventions even in people with moderately severe dementia.

Environmental manipulations

The evidence supporting non-pharmacological management options is limited. Theory-driven approaches suggest that reducing risk factors for hallucinations by improving sensory function (Ishikura *et al.*, 1998, Chapman *et al.*, 1999, Terao, 2000) and improving under or over stimulation should be effective strategies (Cohen-Mansfield, 2003). In our clinical experience, such strategies may help some patients. We have had some success with managing activity levels and improving illumination, but systematic evidence is still lacking (Rongve & Aarsland, 2006).

Mr G had a diagnosis of LBD. He had experienced ill-formed hallucinations of figures for several years, but lately, he had been seeing people carrying placards outside his house saying that he was a paedophile. He was greatly upset. He was unable to benefit from a cognitive behavioural approach since he could not retain information or reason from evidence. Cholinesterase inhibitors reduced but did not abolish his hallucinations and he remained distressed. A low dose of neuroleptics reduced his distress but at the cost of some increase in his parkinsonism. After three months, his medication could be reduced without a recurrence of the distress.

Education

As with clinicians in other areas (Garrett, this volume), we routinely educate patients and carers as to the meaning of hallucinations. Our main messages are that hallucinations are common and an expected feature in some people with cognitive or visual impairments. They are not generally a sign of madness and are usually transitory, reducing and disappearing in time with no specific treatment. This information appears to be sufficient for the majority of people who have not developed an elaborated explanation of their experiences. If hallucinations are associated with delusions, particularly emotionally significant ones, it is hard for patients to accept alternative explanations. Written information, specific to the individual patient, can be very useful.

Psychological interventions analogous to those used in psychosis (this volume) may be tried, but there is, as yet, no evidence for effectiveness, and the cognitive impairments associated with dementia may reduce the potential benefit. We have rarely found that people with dementia can use formal attentional or coping strategies (Valmaggia & Morris; Farhall, both this volume). More commonly, a patient will either adopt an alternative perspective if this is supported by a professional, or resist all attempts to change their mind. Self-help material (May & Longden, this volume) can be directed at carers, even when the person with dementia cannot use it. Carer education and support can be critical in reducing carer burden and postpone carer breakdown.

Pharmacological management of hallucinations

Deciding whether to actively treat

Many hallucinations are transient. Active treatments need to balance effectiveness with side effects, particularly in LBD (Aarsland *et al.*, 2004; Boeve, 2005) in which hallucinations, motor symptoms, and confusion may have inverse relationships with improvements in one balanced by worsening in others. Effect size may be modest, and adverse events with consequent treatment dropouts are common. Though medication lends itself more easily to systematic assessment than do some of the other strategies for managing hallucinations in dementia, the evidence is generally lacking for specific effects on hallucinations. At present, there is little evidence that, within classes, one specific drug is more effective or that there are systematic variations in outcome depending upon the type of dementia or modality of hallucination.

Reduction strategies

Initial pharmacological management needs to focus on reducing the number of medication before starting new drugs (Mosimann & McKeith, 2003). Though street-drug-induced hallucinations are uncommon in elderly people with dementia, prescribed drugs, particularly those with anticholinergic effects or side effects, may contribute to hallucination onset. The list of such medication is long. The main exponents are antimuscarinic drugs for bladder control (Kay *et al.*, 2005), tricyclic antidepressants with anticholinergic side effects (Cancelli *et al.*, 2004), or anticholinergic drugs to treat tremor in Parkinson's disease. Dose reduction or stopping these drugs, where justifiable, is likely to reduce hallucination frequency or abolish them entirely.

Typical and atypical neuroleptics

Some 50 reports of trials of typical and atypical neuroleptics in dementia have now been published. In contrast to other clinical areas (Sanjuan *et al.*, this volume), recent systematic reviews (Sink & Yaffe, 2005, Schneider *et al.*, 2006a,b, Katz *et al.*, 2007) have indicated that effectiveness in general is modest in treating behavioural and psychological symptoms in people with dementia. There appears to be no specific effect on hallucinations *per se* (Rabinowitz *et al.*, 2007).

Neuroleptics are dopamine antagonists. Patients with LBD and PDD (who have the highest rates of hallucinations) have a dopaminergic deficit and are at significant risk of experiencing neuroleptic sensitivity when treated with typical and atypical neuroleptics. Aarsland and colleagues (Piggott *et al.*, 1998, Aarsland *et al.*, 2005) reported severe neuroleptic sensitivity in around 50% of patients with LBD, 40% of those with PDD, but none of those with Alzheimer's disease.

Excess morbidity is also common with somnolence, extrapyramidal symptoms, and cognitive decline frequently reported adverse events (Schneider *et al.*, 2007). For these reasons, discontinuation of medication is frequent, with up to a third of participants in treatment trials dropping out (Schneider *et al.*, 2006a,b). Furthermore, in 2005, several reports have indicated that patients with dementia are at increased risk for cerebrovascular accidents especially when treated with atypical neuroleptics. Schneider and colleagues

(Schneider *et al.*, 2006a,b) have reported a 50% increase in the risk of death (from 2.3% to 3.5%) during treatment. These concerns were major reasons for the US and UK regulatory authorities to restrict their use. This modest efficacy and side effects have changed the prescription practice for neuroleptics in patients with dementia. Economic analysis suggests that watchful waiting is often as effective as the treatment with neuroleptics (Rosenheck *et al.*, 2007) when managing behavioural and psychological symptoms of dementia. Neuroleptics are therefore not the first choice of treatment for demented patients with visual hallucinations. Despite the above, neuroleptics remain commonly, and poorly prescribed, especially in nursing home residents. Standards are low, with a quarter of prescriptions for non-indicated symptoms, a fifth above recommended doses, and less than a half compliant with guidelines (Briesacher *et al.*, 2005).

Cholinesterase inhibitors

The effectiveness of cholinesterase inhibitors (rivastigmine, donepezil, and galantamine) is similarly modest in terms of managing general non-cognitive symptoms in dementia. There is preliminary evidence of a more specific relationship between treatment response and visual hallucinations (Burn *et al.*, 2006, Edwards *et al.*, 2007, Emre *et al.*, 2007b, Rozzini *et al.*, 2007, Lemstra *et al.*, 2008). Patients with hallucinations show a better general response to cholinesterase inhibitors compared to those without.

As with neuroleptics, delayed prescribing and careful titration reduces the chance of excess morbidity. The most common adverse events are gastrointestinal (Ellis, 2005). If one cholinesterase inhibitor is ineffective, increasing the dose, or switching to another drug from the same class, may be an effective strategy (Bhanji & Gauthier, 2005; Sadowsky *et al.*, 2004). There have also been reports of effective augmentation with neuroleptics, though the evidence so far is preliminary (Drach, 2007; Rayner, 2007). There have been no head-to-head comparisons of neuroleptics and cholinesterase inhibitors for the treatment of hallucinations, and due to the risks associated with neuroleptic treatment in demented patients, it is unlikely that such trials will ever be done.

Other drugs

Antidepressants, mood stabilizers, and memantine have been tested for the treatment of behavioural and psychological symptoms (Sink *et al.*, 2005). Most reports are case studies or case series. Results of randomized controlled trials of memantine for behavioural and psychological symptoms of dementia in PDD are awaited. If hallucinations are associated with REM sleep behaviour disorder (Boeve *et al.*, 2004), clonazepam and melatonin may be effective treatment strategies.

In conclusion, a review of medication, with reducing or stopping drugs with anticholinergic side effects, and the treatment with a cholinesterase inhibitor, may be the first pharmacological consideration, with neuroleptics only the last resort in patients with distressing hallucinations and delusions or severe agitation. When prescribed, it is important to seek the consent of the patient and the nearest relative after explaining potential effects or side effects.

Future Directions

There is a need to develop valid and reliable measures of hallucinations and their consequences—emotional, behavioural, and cognitive—in modalities other than the visual,
suitable for people with dementing illnesses. These measures need to be sensitive for
change in order to be useful for treatment studies and suitable across different disorders,
including delirium, psychosis, and eye disease as well as dementia, to allow different types
of hallucinations in different disorders to be compared. Accurate measures will overcome
the underreporting of hallucinations. Better measurement of phenomenology will make
it easier to relate clinical symptoms to the pathophysiology involved in hallucination
generation, e.g., when using new neuroimaging techniques. We need an improved understanding of pathophysiology. Research to date has indicated that specific brain areas and
pathologies are associated with hallucinations, but the links are still tenuous and not
clinically applicable. Better specified models of hallucination generation are needed to
allow testable predictors of hallucinations in different patient groups.

Evidence-based treatment using pharmacological and non-pharmacological strategies
is urgently needed for patients with distressing hallucinations and patients at risk of early
nursing home placement due to their hallucinations. Current data suggests that multiple
causes contribute to the onset of hallucinations and that some of the risk factors contributing to hallucinations are likely modifiable (e.g., medication, visual acuity) but large
scale randomized trials are still some way off.

Conclusions

In the last 15 years, there has been an explosion of hallucination research in dementing
illnesses driven primarily by the recognition that hallucinations are a frequent and disabling feature of dementia, and that they are a diagnostic feature of LBD and PDD.
Recognition of the roles of co-existing visual impairment, medication with anticholinergic effects, and of physical illness contributing to delirium has lead to treatment strategies
that can improve hallucinations for some patients.

The field is now moving beyond simple recognition and classification of hallucinations
towards increasingly sophisticated measurement and model building. Specific treatment
strategies for hallucinations have lagged behind, but there are numerous promising
treatment approaches that can be tested in the near future. Adverse reactions and lack of
established efficacy currently limit pharmacological interventions. Risk and benefit are
finely balanced with treatment primarily dependent not on the presence of hallucinations
but on the distress experienced by the hallucinator. Non-pharmacological interventions
have little risk of harm, but lack systematic evidence of efficacy. Well-designed prospective studies are needed to test which is the most efficient treatment strategy. In the interim,
careful systematic assessment and treatment of known factors (poor attention, sensory
impairment, under- or over-stimulating environments, and distressing attributions) in
the context of an informing and supportive relationship can be effective for many
patients.

List of abbreviations

CAMCOG	Cambridge cognitive assessment
CDR	Clinical dementia rating
CT	Computer tomography
LBD	Lewy Body Dementia
MMSE	Mini mental state examination
MRI	Magnetic resonance imaging
NPI	Neuropsychiatric inventory
NEVHI	North East visual hallucinations interview
PAD model	Perception attention deficit model
PDD	Parkinson's disease dementia
SPECT	Single photon computer tomography

References

Aarsland, D., Mosimann, U. P., & McKeith, I. G. (2004). Role of cholinesterase inhibitors in Parkinson's disease and dementia with Lewy Bodies. *J Geriatr Psychiatry Neurol,* **17**, 164–71.

Aarsland, D., Perry, R., Larsen, J. P., *et al.* (2005). Neuroleptic sensitivity in Parkinson's disease and parkinsonian dementias. *J Clin Psychiatry,* **66**, 633–7.

Aarsland, D., Brønnick, K., Ehrt, U., *et al.* (2007). Neuropsychiatric symptoms in patients with Parkinson's disease and dementia: Frequency, profile and associated care giver stress. *J Neurology, Neurosurgery Psychiatry,* **78**, 36–42.

Aleman, A., & Larøi, F. (2008). *Hallucinations. The Science of Idiosyncratic Perception,* Washington: American Psychological Association.

Allan, L. M., Ballard, C. G., Burn, D. J., & Kenny, R. A. (2005). Prevalence and severity of gait disorders in Alzheimer's and non-Alzheimer's dementias. *J Am Geriatr Soc,* **53**, 1681–7.

Allegri, R. F., Sarasola, D., Serrano, C. M., *et al.* (2006). Neuropsychiatric symptoms as a predictor of caregiver burden in Alzheimer's disease. *Neuropsychiatric Dis Treatment,* **2**, 105–110.

APA (1994). *Diagnostic and Statistical Manual of Mental Disorders,* Washington DC, American Psychiatric Association.

Awata, S., Matsuoka, H., & Shimabukuro, J. (2005). Behavioral and psychological symptoms of dementia characteristic of mild Alzheimer patients. *Psychiatry Clin Neurosci,* **59**, 274–9.

Ballard, C. G., Saad, K., Patel, A., *et al.* (1995). The prevalence and phenomenology of psychotic symptoms in dementia sufferers. *Int J Geriatr Psychiatry,* **10**, 477–85.

Ballard, C. G., Jacoby, R., Del Ser, T., *et al.* (2004). Neuropathological substrates of psychiatric symptoms in prospectively studied patients with autopsy-confirmed dementia with Lewy bodies. *Am J Psychiatry,* **161**, 843–9.

Behrendt, R. P., & Young, C. (2004). Hallucinations in schizophrenia, sensory impairment, and brain disease: A unifying model. *Behav Brain Sci,* **27**, 771–87.

Bhanji, N. H., & Gauthier, S. (2005). Emergent complications following donepezil switchover to galantamine in three cases of dementia with Lewy bodies. *J Neuropsychiatry Clin Neurosci,* **17**, 552–55.

Boeve, B. F., Silber, M. H., & Ferman, T. J. (2004). REM sleep behavior disorder in Parkinson's disease and dementia with Lewy bodies. *J Geriatr Psychiatry Neurol,* **17**, 146–57.

Boeve, B. F. (2005). Clinical, diagnostic, genetic and management issues in dementia with Lewy bodies. *Clin Sci*, **109**, 343–54.

Bozzali, M., Falini, A., Cercignani, M., *et al.* (2005). Brain tissue damage in dementia with Lewy bodies: An in vivo diffusion tensor MRI study. *Brain*, **128**, 1595–604.

Briesacher, B. A., Limcangco, M. R., Simoni-Wastila, L., *et al.* (2005). The quality of antipsychotic drug prescribing in nursing homes. *Arch Inter Med*, **165**, 1280–5.

Brodaty, H. (2007). Meaning and measurement of caregiver outcomes. *Int Psychogeriatr*, **19**, 363–81.

Burn, D., Emre, M., McKeith, I., *et al.* (2006) Effects of rivastigmine in patients with and without visual hallucinations in dementia associated with Parkinson's disease. *Mov Disord*, **21**, 1899–907.

Cancelli, I., Marcon, G., & Balestrieri, M. (2004). Factors associated with complex visual hallucinations during antidepressant treatment. *Human Psychopharmacol: Clin Exp*, **19**, 577–584.

Capitani, E., Francescani, A., & Spinnler, H. (2007). Are hallucinations and extrapyramidal signs associated with a steeper cognitive decline in degenerative dementia patients? *Neurol Sci*, **28**, 245–50.

Chadwick, P., & Birchwood, M. (1994). The omnipotence of voices. A cognitive approach to auditory hallucinations. *Br J Psychiatry*, **164**, 190–201.

Chapman, F. M., Dickinson, J., McKeith, I., & Ballard, C. (1999). Association among visual hallucinations, visual acuity, and specific eye pathologies in Alzheimer's disease: treatment implications. *Am J Psychiatry*, **156**, 1983–5.

Cohen-Mansfield, J. (2003). Nonpharmacologic interventions for psychotic symptoms in dementia. *J Geriatr Psychiatry Neurology*, **16**, 219.

Collerton, D., & Dudley, R. (2004). A cognitive behavioural framework for the treatment of distressing visual hallucinations in older people. *Behav Cogn Psychother*, **32**, 1–13.

Collerton, D., Perry, E., & McKeith, I. (2005). Why people see things that are not there: A novel perception and attention deficit model for recurrent complex visual hallucinations. *Behav Brain Sci*, **28**, 737–57.

Court, J. A., Ballard, C. G., Piggott, M. A., *et al.* (2001). Visual hallucinations are associated with lower alpha bungarotoxin binding in dementia with Lewy bodies. *Pharmacol Biochem Behav*, **70**, 571–9.

Craig, D., Mirakhur, A., Hart, D. J., Mcilroy, S. P., & Passmore, A. P. (2005). A cross-sectional study of neuropsychiatric symptoms in 435 patients with Alzheimer's disease. *Am J Geriatr Psychiatry*, **13**, 460–468.

Cummings, J. L., Mega, M., Gray, K., Rosenberg-Thompson, S., Carusi, D. A., & Gornbein, J. (1994). The neuropsychiatric inventory: comprehensive assessment of psychopathology in dementia. *Neurology*, **44**, 2308–14.

De Vugt, M. E., Riedijk, S. R., Aalten, P., Tibben, A., Van Swieten, J. C., & Verhey, F. R. (2006). Impact of behavioural problems on spousal caregivers: A comparison between Alzheimer's disease and frontotemporal dementia. *Dement Geriatr Cogn Disord*, **22**, 35–41.

Diederich, N. J., Goetz, C. G., & Stebbins, G. T. (2004). Repeated visual hallucinations in Parkinson's disease as disturbed external/internal perceptions: Focused review and a new integrative model. *Mov Disord*, **20** (2), 130–140.

Djamgoz, M. B., Hankins, M. W., Hirano, J., & Archer, S. N. (1997). Neurobiology of retinal dopamine in relation to degenerative states of the tissue. *Vision Res*, **37**, 3509–29.

Donnemiller, E., Heilmann, J., Wenning, G. K., *et al.* (1997). Brain perfusion scintigraphy with 99mTc-HMPAO or 99mTc-ECD and 123I-beta-CIT single-photon emission tomography in dementia of the Alzheimer-type and diffuse Lewy body disease. *Eur J Nucl Med*, **24**, 320–5.

Drach, L. M. (2007). Dementia with lewy bodies—state of the art. *demenz mit lewy-ko?rperchen—State of the art, 33*, 239–43.

Dubois, B., Feldman, H. H., Jacova, C., *et al.* (2007). Research criteria for the diagnosis of Alzheimer's disease: Revising the NINCDS-ADRDA criteria. *Lancet Neurol, 6*, 734–46.

Edwards, K., Royall, D., Hershey, L., *et al.* (2007). Efficacy and safety of galantamine in patients with dementia with Lewy bodies: A 24-week open-label study. *Dementia Geriatr Cogn Disord, 23*, 401–5.

Ellis, J. M. (2005). Cholinesterase inhibitors in the treatment of dementia. *J Am Osteopathic Association, 105*, 145–58.

Emre, M. , Aarsland, D., Brown, R., *et al.* (2007a). Clinical diagnostic criteria for dementia associated with Parkinson's disease. *Mov Disord, 22*, 1689-707.

Emre, M., Cummings, J. L. & Lane, R. M. (2007b). Rivastigmine in dementia associated with Parkinson's disease and Alzheimer's disease: Similarities and differences. *J Alzheimer's Dis, 11*, 509–19.

Ferri, C. P., Prince, M., Brayne, C., *et al.* (2005). Global prevalence of dementia: A Delphi consensus study. *Lancet, 366*, 2112–7.

Firbank, M. J., Colloby, S. J., Burn, D. J., McKeith, I. G., & O'Brien, J. T. (2003). Regional cerebral blood flow in Parkinson's disease with and without dementia. *Neuroimage, 20*, 1309–19.

Flynn, W. R. (1962). Visual hallucinations in sensory deprivation. A review of the literature, a case report and a discussion of the mechanism. *Psychiatr Q, 36*, 55–65.

Folstein, M. F., Folstein, S. E., & Mchugh, P. R. (1975). 'Mini-mental state'. A practical method for grading the cognitive state of patients for the clinician. *J Psychiatr Res, 12*, 189–98.

Fujishiro, H., Umegaki, H., Suzuki, Y., *et al.* (2007). Clinical profiles of autopsy-confirmed dementia with Lewy bodies at institutionalization: Comparison with Alzheimer's disease. *Psychogeriatr, 7*, 98–103.

Gomez-ISLA, T., Growdon, W. B., Mcnamara, M., *et al.* (1999). Clinicopathologic correlates in temporal cortex in dementia with Lewy bodies. *Neurology, 53*, 2003–9.

Graham, G., Dean, J. L., Mosimann, U. P., *et al.* (In press) Specific attentional impairments and complex visual hallucinations in eye disease. *Int J Geriatr Psychiatry.*

Grand, M. G., Kaine, J., Fulling, K., *et al.* (1988). Cerebroretinal vasculopathy. A new hereditary syndrome. *Ophthalmology, 95*, 649–59.

Hamuro, A., Isono, H., Sugai, Y., *et al.* (2007). Behavioral and psychological symptoms of dementia in untreated Alzheimer's disease patients. *Psychogeriatr, 7*, 4–7.

Harding, A. J., Broe, G. A., & Halliday, G. M. (2002). Visual hallucinations in Lewy body disease relate to Lewy bodies in the temporal lobe. *Brain, 125*, 391–403.

Harnois, C., & Di Paolo, T. (1990). Decreased dopamine in the retinas of patients with Parkinson's disease. *Invest Ophthalmol Vis Sci, 31*, 2473–5.

Harris, J. P., Calvert, J. E., & Phillipson, O. T. (1992). Processing of spatial contrast in peripheral vision in Parkinson's disease. *Brain, 115* (Pt 5), 1447–57.

Heron, W., Doane, B. K., & Scott, T. H. (1956). Visual disturbances after prolonged perceptual isolation. *Can J Psychol, 10*, 13–8.

Higuchi, M., Tashiro, M., Arai, H., *et al.* (2000). Glucose hypometabolism and neuropathological correlates in brains of dementia with Lewy bodies. *Exp Neurol, 162*, 247–56.

Hikosaka, O., Takikawa, Y., & Kawagoe, R. (2000). Role of the basal ganglia in the control of purposive saccadic eye movements. *Physiol Rev, 80*, 953–78.

Holroyd, S., Currie, L., & Wooten, G. F. (2001). Prospective study of hallucinations and delusions in Parkinson's disease. *J Neurol Neurosurg Psychiatry, 70*, 734–8.

Horowitz, M. J. (1975). Hallucinations: An information-processing approach. IN Siegel, R. K. & West, L. J. (Eds.) *Hallucinations. Behav, Exp Theory.* New York: Wiley.

Howard, R., David, A., Woodruff, P., *et al.* (1997) Seeing visual hallucinations with functional magnetic resonance imaging. *Dement Geriatr Cogn Disord,* **8**, 73–7.

Imamura, T., Hirono, N., Hashimoto, M., *et al.* (1999). Clinical diagnosis of dementia with Lewy bodies in a Japanese dementia registry. *Dementia Geriatr Cogn Disord,* **10**, 210–16.

Imamura, T., Ishii, K., Hirono, N., *et al.* (2001). Occipital glucose metabolism in dementia with Lewy bodies with and without Parkinsonism: A study using positron emission tomography. *Dement Geriatr Cogn Disord,* **12**, 194–7.

Ishii, K., Imamura, T., Sasaki, M., *et al.* (1998). Regional cerebral glucose metabolism in dementia with Lewy bodies and Alzheimer's disease. *Neurology,* **51**, 125–30.

Ishikura, N., Asada, T., Kimura, M., Saitoh, H., & Uno, M. (1998). Visual hallucination in demented elderly with visual impairment. *Seishin Igaku (Clinical Psychiatry),* **40**, 1163–9.

Iuvone, P. M., Galli, C. L., Garrison-Gund, C. K., & Neff, N. H. (1978). Light stimulates tyrosine hydroxylase activity and dopamine synthesis in retinal amacrine neurons. *Science,* **202**, 901–2.

Johnson, M. R., Shafi, N., Parker, J. C., Jr., & Parker, J. R. (2005). Dementia with Lewy bodies: A commonly unrecognized cause of dementia. *J Ky Med Assoc,* **103**, 559–62.

Katz, I., De Deyn, P. P., Mintzer, J., Greenspan, A., Zhu, Y., & Brodaty, H. (2007). The efficacy and safety of risperidone in the treatment of psychosis of Alzheimer's disease and mixed dementia: A metal-analysis of 4 placebo-controlled clinical trials. *Int J Geriatr psychiatry,* **22**, 475–84.

Kay, G. G., Abou-Donia, M. B., Messer J. R., W. S., Murphy, D. G., Tsao, J. W., & Ouslander, J. G. (2005). Antimuscarinic drugs for overactive bladder and their potential effects on cognitive function in older patients. *J the Am Geriatr Soc,* **53**, 2195–201.

Kimura, F. (2000). Cholinergic modulation of cortical function: A hypothetical role in shifting the dynamics in cortical network. *Neurosci Res,* **38**, 19–26.

Kitagawa, M., Fukushima, J., & Tashiro, K. (1994). Relationship between antisaccades and the clinical symptoms in Parkinson's disease. *Neurology,* **44**, 2285–9.

Kobayashi, Y., Saito, Y., & Isa, T. (2001). Facilitation of saccade initiation by brainstem cholinergic system. *Brain Dev,* **23** Suppl 1, S24–7.

Kobayashi, Y., & Isa, T. (2002). Sensory-motor gating and cognitive control by the brainstem cholinergic system. Neural Netw, **15**, 731–41.

Lee, K. H., Williams, L. M., Breakspear, M., & Gordon, E. (2003). Synchronous gamma activity: A review and contribution to an integrative neuroscience model of schizophrenia. *Brain Res Brain Res Rev,* **41**, 57–78.

Lemstra, A. W., Kuiper, R. B., Schmand, B., & Van Gool, W. A. (2008). Identification of responders to rivastigmine: A prospective cohort study. *Dementia Geriatr Cogn Disord,* **25**, 60–6.

Liang, T. S., Duda, J. E., Trojanowski, J., Stern, M. B., & Hurtig, H. I. (2005). Visual hallucinations and a-synuclein pathology in Parkinson's disease and dementia with Lewy bodies. *Neurology,* **64**, P02–089.

Litvan, I. C. G., Mangone, C.A., Verny, M., *et al.* (1997). Which clinical features differentiate progressive supranuclear palsy (Steele-Richardson-Olszewski syndrome) from related disorders? A clinicopathological study. *Brain,* **120**, 65–74.

Lobotesis, K., Fenwick, J. D., Phipps, A., *et al.* (2001). Occipital hypoperfusion on SPECT in dementia with Lewy bodies but not AD. *Neurology,* **56**, 643–9.

Maher, B. A. (1974). Delusional thinking and perceptual disorder. *J Individ Psychol,* **30**, 98–113.

Maher, B. (2005). Delusional thinking and cognitive disorder. *Integr Physiol Behav Sci,* **40**, 136–46.

Manford, M., & Andermann, F. (1998). Complex visual hallucinations. Clinical and neurobiological insights. *Brain,* **121** (Pt 10), 1819–40.

McKeith, I. G., & Mosimann, U. P. (2004). Dementia with Lewy bodies and Parkinson's disease. *Parkinsonism Relat Disord,* **10** Suppl 1, S15–8.

McKeith, I. G., Dickson, D. W., Lowe, J., *et al.* (2005). Diagnosis and management of dementia with Lewy bodies: Third report of the DLB Consortium. *Neurology,* **65**, 1863–72.

McKhann, G., Drachman, D., Folstein, M., Katzman, R., Price, D., & Stadlan, E. M. (1984). Clinical diagnosis of Alzheimer's disease: Report of the NINCDS-ADRDA work group under the auspices of department of health and human services task force on Alzheimer's disease. *Neurology,* **34**, 939–44.

McKhann, G. M., Albert, M. S., Grossman, M., Miller, B., Dickson, D., & Trojanowski, J. Q. (2001). Clinical and pathological diagnosis of frontotemporal dementia: Report of the work group on frontotemporal dementia and Pick's disease. *Arch Neurol,* **58**, 1803–9.

Merdes, A. R., Hansen, L. A., Jeste, D. V., *et al.* (2003). Influence of Alzheimer pathology on clinical diagnostic accuracy in dementia with Lewy bodies. *Neurology,* **60**, 1586–90.

Metzler-Baddeley, C. (2007). A review of cognitive impairments in dementia with Lewy bodies relative to Alzheimer's disease and Parkinson's disease with dementia. *Cortex,* **43**, 583–600.

Minoshima, S., Foster, N. L., Sima, A. A., Frey, K. A., Albin, R. L., & Kuhl, D. E. (2001). Alzheimer's disease versus dementia with Lewy bodies: cerebral metabolic distinction with autopsy confirmation. *Ann Neurol,* **50**, 358–65.

Mitchell, P., Hayes, P., & Wang, J. J. (1997). Visual impairment in nursing home residents: The Blue Mountains Eye Study. *Med J Aust,* **166**, 73–6.

Mollenhauer, B., Bibl, M., Esselmann, H., *et al.* (2007). Tauopathies and synucleinopathies: Do cerebrospinal fluid beta-amyloid peptides reflect disease-specific pathogenesis? *J Neural Transm,* **114**(7), 919–927.

Morris, J. (1993). The clinical dementia rating (CDR): Current version and scoring rules. *Neurology,* **43**, 2412–14.

Morrison, A. (1998). A cognitive analysis of the maintenance of auditory hallucinations: Are voices to schizophrenia what bodily sensations are to panic. *Behav Cogn Psychother,* **26**, 289–302.

Mosimann, U. P., & McKeith, I. G. (2003). Dementia with Lewy bodies—diagnosis and treatment. *Swiss Med Wkly,* **133**, 131–42.

Mosimann, U. P., Rowan, E. N., Partington, C. E., *et al.* (2006). Characteristics of visual hallucinations in Parkinson disease dementia and dementia with Lewy bodies. *Am J Geriatr Psychiatry,* **14**, 153–60.

Mosimann, U. P., Collerton, D., Dudley, R., *et al.* (2008). A semi-structured interview to assess visual hallucinations in older people. *Int J Geriatr Psychiatry,* **23**, 712-8.

Neary, D., Snowden, J. S., Gustafson, L., *et al.* (1998). Frontotemporal lobar degeneration: A consensus on clinical diagnostic criteria. *Neurology,* **51**, 1546–54.

O'Brien, J. T. (2006). Vascular cognitive impairment. *Am J Geriatr Psychiatry,* **14**, 724–33.

O'Connor, D. W. (1990). The contribution of CAMDEX to the diagnosis of mild dementia in community surveys. *Psychiatr J Univ Ott,* **15**, 216–20.

Pasquier, J., Michel, B. F., Brenot-Rossi, I., Hassan-Sebbag, N., Sauvan, R., & Gastaut, J. L. (2002). Value of (99m)Tc-ECD SPET for the diagnosis of dementia with Lewy bodies. *Eur J Nucl Med Mol Imaging,* **29**, 1342–8.

Pelaez, J. R. (2000). Towards a neural network based therapy for hallucinatory disorders. *Neural Netw,* **13**, 1047–61.

Perry, E. K., Curtis, M., Dick, D. J., *et al.* (1985). Cholinergic correlates of cognitive impairment in Parkinson's disease: Comparisons with Alzheimer's disease. *J Neurol Neurosurg Psychiatry,* **48**, 413–21.

Perry, E. K., Morris, C. M., Court, J. A., *et al.* (1995). Alteration in nicotine binding sites in Parkinson's disease, Lewy body dementia and Alzheimer's disease: Possible index of early neuropathology. *Neuroscience,* **64**, 385–95.

Piggott, M. A., Perry, E. K., Marshall, E. F., *et al.* (1998). Nigrostriatal dopaminergic activities in dementia with Lewy bodies in relation to neuroleptic sensitivity: Comparisons with Parkinson's disease. *Biol Psychiatry,* **44**, 765–74.

Pliskin, N. H., Kiolbasa, T. A., Towle, V. L., *et al.* (1996). Charles Bonnet syndrome: An early marker for dementia? *J Am Geriatr Soc,* **44**, 1055–61.

Rabinowitz, J., Katz, I., de Deyn, P. P., Greenspan, A., & Brodaty, H. (2007). Treating behavioral and psychological symptoms in patients with psychosis of Alzheimer's disease using risperidone. *Int psychogeriatr/IPA,* **19**, 227–40.

Rayner, A. (2007). Managing psychotic symptoms in the older patient. *Geriatr Aging,* **10**, 241–245.

Roman, G. C., Tatemichi, T. K., Erkinjuntti, T., *et al.* (1993). Vascular dementia: Diagnostic criteria for research studies. Report of the NINDS-AIREN International Workshop. *Neurology,* **43**, 250–60.

Roman, G. C., Sachdev, P., Royall, D. R., *et al.* (2004). Vascular cognitive disorder: A new diagnostic category updating vascular cognitive impairment and vascular dementia. *J Neurol Sci,* **226**, 81–7.

Rongve, A., & Aarsland, D. (2006). Management of Parkinson's disease dementia: Practical considerations. *Drugs Aging,* **23**, 807–22.

Ropacki, S. A., & Jeste, D. V. (2005). Epidemiology of and risk factors for psychosis of Alzheimer's disease: A review of 55 studies published from 1990 to 2003. *Am J Psychiatry,* **162**, 2022–30.

Rosenheck, R. A., Leslie, D. L., Sindelar, J. L., *et al.* (2007). Cost-benefit analysis of second-generation antipsychotics and placebo in a randomized trial of the treatment of psychosis and aggression in Alzheimer disease. *Arch Gen Psychiatry,* **64**, 1259–68.

Rozzini, L., Chilovi, B. V., Bertoletti, E., *et al.* (2007). Cognitive and psychopathologic response to rivastigmine in dementia with Lewy bodies compared to Alzheimer's disease: A case control study. *Am J Alzheimer's Dis Other Dement,* **22**, 42–7.

Sadowsky, C., Edwards, K., Etemad, B., & Farlow, M. (2004). Maintaining effective treatment in dementia: A case series on patients switched to rivastigmine. *Primary Care Psychiatry,* **9**, 71–5.

Sauer, J., Ffytche, D. H., Ballard, C., Brown, R. G., & Howard, R. (2006). Differences between Alzheimer's disease and dementia with Lewy bodies: an fMRI study of task-related brain activity. *Brain,* **129**(Pt 7),1780–8.

Scarmeas, N., Brandt, J., Albert, M., *et al.* (2005). Delusions and hallucinations are associated with worse outcome in Alzheimer disease. *Arch Neurol,* **62**, 1601–8.

Schneider, L. S., Tariot, P. N., & Dagerman, K. S. (2007). Atypical antipsychotics minimally effective in Alzheimer's. *J Family Practice,* **56**, 14.

Schneider, L. S., Dagerman, K., & Insel, P. S. (2006a). Efficacy and adverse effects of atypical antipsychotics for dementia: Meta-analysis of randomized, placebo-controlled trials. *Am J Geriatr Psychiatry,* **14**, 191–210.

Schneider, L. S., Dagerman, K. S., & Insel, P. (2006b). Risk of death with atypical antipsychotic drug treatment for dementia: Meta-analysis of randomized placebo-controlled trials: Reply. *JAMA: J Am Med Assoc,* **295**, 496–7.

Sink, K.M., Holden, K. F., & Yaffe, K. (2005). Pharmacological treatment of neuropsychiatric symptoms of dementia. A review of the evidence. *J Am Med Assoc,* **293**, 596–608.

Sink, K. M., Covinsky, K. E., Barnes, D. E., Newcomer, R. J., & Yaffe, K. (2006). Caregiver characteristics are associated with neuropsychiatric symptoms of dementia. *J Am Geriatr Soc,* **54**, 796–803.

Steinberg, M., Corcoran, C., Tschanz, J. T., *et al.* (2006). Risk factors for neuropsychiatric symptoms in dementia: The Cache County Study. *Int J Geriatr Psychiatry,* **21**, 824–30.

Stevens, T., Livingston, G., Kichen, G., Manela, M., Walker, Z., & Katona, C. (2002). Islington study of dementia subtypes in the community. *Br J Psychiatry,* **180**, 270–6.

Terao, T. (2000). Visual hallucinations in Alzheimer's disease: Possible involvement of low visual acuity and dementia with Lewy bodies. *J Neuropsychiatry Clin Neurosci,* **12**, 516–17.

Tiraboschi, P., Hansen, L. A., Alford, M., *et al.* (2002). Early and widespread cholinergic losses differentiate dementia with Lewy bodies from Alzheimer disease. *Arch Gen Psychiatry,* **59**, 946–51.

Tiraboschi, P., Salmon, D. P., Hansen, L. A., *et al.* (2006). What best differentiates Lewy body from Alzheimer's disease in early-stage dementia? *Brain,* **129**, 729–35.

Wada-Isoe, K., Ohta, K., Imamura, K., *et al.* (2008). Assessment of hallucinations in Parkinson's disease using a novel scale. *Acta Neurol Scand,* **117**, 35–40.

Waldemar, G., Dubois, B., Emre, M., *et al.* (2007). Recommendations for the diagnosis and management of Alzheimer's disease and other disorders associated with dementia: EFNS guideline. *Eur J Neurol,* **14**, e1–26.

Weinberger, L. M. (1940). Visual hallucinations and their neurooptical correlates. *Arch Ophthalmol,* **23**, 166–99.

WHO (2003). *Classification of Mental and Behavioural Disorders. Clinical Descriptions and Diagnositc Guidelines,* Geneva: Churchill and Livingstone.

Williams, D. R., & Lees, A. J. (2005). Visual hallucinations in the diagnosis of idiopathic Parkinson's disease: A retrospective autopsy study. *Lancet Neurol,* **4**, 605–10.

Wink, B., & Harris, J. (2000). A model of the Parkinsonian visual system: Support for the dark adaptation hypothesis. *Vision Res,* **40**, 1937–46.

Witkovsky, P. (2004). Dopamine and retinal function. *Doc Ophthalmol,* **108**, 17–40.

Zarroug, E. T. (1975). The frequency of visual hallucinations in schizophrenic patients in Saudi Arabia. *Br J Psychiatry,* **127**, 553–5.

Chapter 18

Hallucinations in Parkinson's disease

Gilles Fénelon

Parkinson's disease (PD) is the second most common neurodegenerative disease (Alves *et al.*, 2008). Primarily, PD is a disorder of the nigrostriatal dopaminergic pathway that results in the cardinal motor symptoms of bradykinesia, tremor, and rigidity. However, other dopaminergic and non-dopaminergic transmitter systems are also affected, mediating a large spectrum of non-motor symptoms, including cognitive impairment and neuropsychiatric disturbances. Hallucinations are common in patients with PD. Originally considered as coincidental or end-stage non-specific phenomena, they were later viewed as a mere side effect of anti-parkinsonian treatment, mainly dopaminergic agents, and more recently as the product of complex interactions between treatment- and disease-related factors. Hallucinations and other psychotic symptoms lead to increased disability and poor quality of life in patients (Schrag, 2004) and to greater stress in caregivers (Aarsland *et al.*, 2007). The treatment of hallucinations is often challenging for the clinician, but has become noticeably easier since the introduction of atypical anti-psychotics, especially clozapine.

Hallucinations in Parkinson's disease: An overview

Definitions and evaluation

Hallucinations in PD are usually included in the broader entity of PD-associated psychosis. The term psychosis has been defined in various ways, none of which is universally accepted (Ravina *et al.*, 2007). Applied to PD, the term psychosis usually refers to a mental state characterized by hallucinations and/or delusions. However, the typical hallucinatory syndrome in PD encompasses other related phenomena such as a sense of presence and illusions—that is misperceptions or misinterpretations of a real external stimulus. Recently, diagnostic criteria for PD-associated psychosis have been proposed (Box 18.1). These criteria describe a constellation of clinical features that are not shared by other psychotic syndromes and that are coupled with a clear sensorium and a chronic course, thus excluding delirium.

   To identify hallucinations or psychosis and rate their severity, the examiner relies on the patient and/or caregiver to describe the relevant symptoms. As few patients (10–20%)

Box 18.1 Proposed diagnostic criteria for PD-associated psychosis

A. Characteristic symptoms

Presence of at least one of the following symptoms (specify which of the symptoms fulfill the criteria):

♦ Illusions

♦ False sense of presence

♦ Hallucinations

♦ Delusions

B. Primary diagnosis

♦ UK Brain Bank criteria for PD

C. Chronology of the onset of symptoms of psychosis

♦ The symptoms in Criterion A occur after the onset of PD

D. Duration

♦ The symptom(s) in Criterion A are recurrent or continuous for 1 month

E. Exclusion of other causes

♦ The symptoms in Criterion A are not better accounted for by another cause of parkinsonism such as Lewy Body Dementia (LBD), psychiatric disorders such as schizophrenia, schizoaffective disorder, delusional disorder, or mood disorder with psychotic features, or a general medical condition including delirium

F. Associated features (specify if associated)

♦ With/without insight

♦ With/without dementia

♦ With/without treatment for PD (specify drug, surgical, other).

Diederich, N.J., Pieri, V., & Goetz, C.G. (2003). Coping strategies for visual hallucinations in Parkinson's disease. *Movement Disorder*, **18**, 831–8. Reprinted with permission of John Wiley & Sons, Inc.

report their hallucinations spontaneously (Fénelon *et al.*, 2000; Holroyd *et al.*, 2001), the information has to be sought by use of specific questions or scales. To identify psychosis, single items from part I of the Unified Parkinson's Disease Rating Scale (thought disorder item) or from the neuropsychiatric inventory (NPI) have been used, as well as self-developed questionnaires or inventories. The latter are useful to record the variety of psychotic symptoms, but they do not allow examiners to rate the symptoms. There is no gold-standard scale for the rating of PD-associated psychosis (Miyasaki *et al.*, 2006;

Fernandez *et al.*, 2008). Scales for rating hallucinations and other psychotic symptoms of PD include scales, which have been specifically designed for PD but are generally insufficiently validated or scales from the psychiatry field (e.g., the positive and negative syndrome scale or the scale for assessment of positive symptoms) or the dementia field, such as the NPI. Although some of these scales have interesting characteristics, a Movement Disorder Society task force noted the need to develop a new scale (Fernandez *et al.*, 2008).

Phenomenology

Complex visual hallucinations are the most common type of hallucinations in patients with PD (Fénelon *et al.*, 2000; Barnes & David 2001; Holroyd *et al.*, 2001; Mosimann *et al.*, 2006). They mostly consist of people, who may or may not be known to the patient and, if known, may be alive or deceased, and less often of animals or objects. Although there may be many people in a hallucination, there is usually only one or a few. Typically, the hallucinated figures appear suddenly, in dim light, with the patient's eyes open. They are moving or static, and seem real. They usually vanish suddenly. Hallucinatory images are seen superimposed on the normal background scene. They may be relatively stereo-typed in a given patient. For instance, a patient repeatedly saw a man dressed in black walking slowly through his garden, but he experienced no other type of hallucination. In most instances, the patient is an observer rather than an actor in the hallucinated scene. Simple visual hallucinations, consisting of elementary phenomena with geometrical pat-terns, are uncommon in PD. Auditory hallucinations (Inzelberg *et al.*, 1998; Fénelon *et al.*, 2000) can be elementary (ringing, knocks, etc.) or, more often, complex (music, voices). When auditory verbal hallucinations are present, they are emotionally neutral (or some-times incomprehensible) in most cases and clearly different from the pejorative or threat-ening auditory hallucinations characteristic of schizophrenia. Auditory hallucinations can accompany visual hallucinations as a 'soundtrack'; for example, the patient may hear a conversation between the hallucinated people. Hallucinations in other sensory modali-ties have been less frequently investigated. Tactile hallucinations typically involve contact with small animals, or the feeling of being touched by someone (Fénelon *et al.*, 2002). Olfactory and gustatory hallucinations have also been reported in some series and case reports (Chou *et al.*, 2005; Fénelon *et al.*, 2010).

PD patients also frequently experience minor hallucinatory phenomena, such as visual illusions, passage hallucinations, and presence hallucinations (Fénelon *et al.*, 2000; Williams *et al.*, 2008). Visual illusions in PD almost invariably consist of the perception of an inanimate object as a living being. For example, a branch of a tree is seen as a cat, a stone, or a tree trunk as a face. Passage hallucinations consist of the brief vision of an animal, passing sideways. A sense of presence involves the vivid sensation that somebody is present nearby, when in fact there is no-one there and no-one is seen. In most cases, the patient can precisely locate the perceived presence behind or beside himself or herself. The perceived presence can be that of a person who is either identified (a living or, less frequently, a deceased relative or spouse) or unidentified.

In most cases, several types of hallucinatory phenomena appear in combination. The simultaneous occurrence of hallucinations in different modalities (for instance seeing and hearing persons in a room, or seeing and feeling a mouse on the legs) enhances the realistic, and sometimes unpleasant, nature of the phenomenon. Hallucinations can occur at any time of day or night, but are more frequent in the evening and during the night. When visual hallucinations occur at night, it can be difficult to differentiate them from dreams, nightmares or rapid-eye-movement sleep behavior disorder, especially in persons with cognitive impairment. Visual hallucinations last from seconds to minutes and, in most cases, occur at least once a week. Nearly all PD patients who are free from cognitive impairment realize the hallucinatory nature of their hallucinations. Patients with dementia commonly lose this insight. Some patients with cognitive impairment can have partial and/or fluctuating insight (Holroyd et al., 2001).

Few studies on PD-associated psychosis have been specifically devoted to the evaluation of delusions (Marsh et al., 2004). Although delusions can be present in isolation, they often accompany hallucinations. Delusions are often of a systematized paranoid type, with jealousy and persecution being frequent themes. They are usually independent of mood disorder.

Prevalence

Epidemiological studies of hallucinations and psychosis in PD (reviewed by Fénelon & Alves, 2009) are constrained by several methodological issues, including the selection of symptoms that are to be systematically assessed, the methods used to assess these symptoms, the study population, and the study period. Most studies are prospective point-prevalence studies in patients under dopaminergic treatment. Visual hallucinations are present in about one-quarter to one-third of these patients and auditory hallucinations in up to 20%. Tactile/somatic and olfactory hallucinations are usually not systematically evaluated and their frequency is probably underestimated. Minor phenomena (sense of presence, visual illusions) affect 17–72% of PD patients. Delusions are recorded in about 5% of patients. The lifetime prevalence of visual hallucinations reaches about 50%. The prevalence of hallucinations is higher in PD patients with dementia, reaching figures between 50 and 87%, which is close to the prevalence observed in LBD. The prevalence of delusions in PD patients with dementia is also increased, with up to 25–35% of patients being affected.

Clinical course and prognosis

In most patients, hallucinations occur late in the course of PD (Williams & Lees, 2005). Early hallucinations occurring in the first months of dopaminergic treatment are suggestive of other psychiatric or degenerative conditions (Goetz et al., 1998b). Once hallucinations have emerged, they tend to persist. In two independent follow-up studies, it was found that more than 80% of the patients who had hallucinations at baseline still reported hallucinations at one year (Doe et al., 2005) and at four years (Goetz et al., 2001). In the latter study, the presence of hallucinations at baseline and at any given assessment was a strong predictor of continued hallucinations being present at all subsequent assessments. Hallucinations do not only persist, but they also worsen: during a three-year follow-up, 39 (81%) of 48 PD patients with hallucinations and retained insight had progressed to more severe forms of psychosis characterized by loss of insight and/or delusions (Goetz *et al.*, 2006).

Hallucinations in PD have been found to predict nursing home placement. In a small case–control study, hallucinations were more frequent in patients admitted to nursing homes than in matched controls in the community (Goetz & Stebbins, 1993). During a 26-month prospective study of 59 patients enrolled in a trial of clozapine, the proportion of patients admitted to nursing homes increased from 12% to 42% (Factor *et al.*, 2003). However, in this study predictors of nursing home placement were older age and paranoia, but not hallucinations. Finally, in a 4-year prospective study of a community-based sample of 178 patients, Aarsland *et al.* (2000) found that 26% of patients were admitted to a nursing home, and that hallucinations were an independent predictor of this endpoint, together with old age, functional impairment, and dementia. Two longitudinal studies have shown that hallucinations in PD are also an independent risk factor for the subsequent development of dementia (Hobson & Meara, 2004; Galvin *et al.*, 2006). Finally, a higher mortality was found in PD patients with hallucinations who lived in a nursing home, compared with controls living in the community (Goetz & Stebbins, 1995). Psychosis is associated with dementia, which in turn predicts an increased mortality risk in PD (Levy *et al.*, 2002). However, hallucinations could constitute an independent risk factor for mortality (Lo *et al.*, 2009).

Associated factors

Historically, dopaminergic treatments were seen to have a central role in the development of psychosis in PD, hence terms such as 'dopaminergic' or 'dopamimetic' psychosis (Factor *et al.*, 1995b). However, other medications, including other anti-parkinsonian drugs, analgesics, psychopharmaceuticals, or non-anti-parkinsonian drugs with anticholinergic properties, can also induce psychotic symptoms. Although pharmacological agents probably do contribute to the development of psychosis, there is now a consensus that disease-related factors have a more prominent role in this context (Fénelon, 2008). Clinical factors associated with the development of psychosis in PD are summarized in Box 18.2.

Pharmacological factors

The prevalence of hallucinations in untreated PD patients is unknown. Data from the pre-levodopa era are scarce and difficult to interpret. Although the early literature contains cases of hallucinations or delusions in PD patients with severe depression, confusion, or dementia, there is no description of the typical hallucinatory syndrome encountered nowadays, which is characterized by a chronic course and a clear sensorium (Fénelon *et al.*, 2006). In a recent prospective study of untreated PD patients, visual hallucinations were present in 8 (27%) of 30 cases and in none of 31 controls (Biousse *et al.*, 2004).

Box 18.2 Clinical factors associated with chronic hallucinations in PD

Pharmacological factors

- Anti-PD drugs
- Psychoactive drugs, opioid analgesics, drugs with anticholinergic properties

Endogenous factors

- Cognitive impairment
- Older age/longer duration of PD
- Disease severity (axial motor impairment)
- Altered dream phenomena (vivid dreams, nightmares, rapid-eye-movement sleep behaviour disorder), daytime somnolence
- Dysautonomia
- Depression (?)*
- Genetic factors

* The facilitating role of depression on hallucinations is debated.

However, in a study of 175 drug naïve patients with incident PD, only 1.2% had a positive score at the hallucinations item of the NPI (Aarsland *et al.*, 2009).

Although clinical experience and early open-label studies of levodopa in PD suggest that levodopa may trigger hallucinations, no evidence-based data support this statement. By contrast, two meta-analyses demonstrated that hallucinations in patients with early PD were more frequent in those randomized to a dopamine agonist than in those randomized to placebo or levodopa (Baker *et al.*, 2008, Stowe *et al.*, 2008). This effect was due to non-ergot dopaminergic agonists (ropinirole, pramipexole) as it was not observed when only ergot derivatives studies (e.g., bromocriptine, pergolide) were taken into account (Stowe *et al.*, 2008). This difference may be due to different pharmacological properties of ergot and non-ergot dopaminergic agonists or to bias such as underreporting psychosis in ergot dopaminergic agonists studies, which were generally performed earlier than non-ergot studies, before an emphasis was put on the frequency of non-motor symptoms in PD (Fénelon & Alves, 2009). There is no simple dose–response relationship between dopaminergic treatment and the presence and/or severity of hallucinations: most cross-sectional studies on hallucinations found that hallucinators did not receive a higher mean daily levodopa or levodopa-equivalent dose than did non-hallucinators (reviewed by Fénelon & Alves, 2009), and in PD patients with hallucinations, there is no relationship between visual hallucinations and high plasma levels of levodopa or sudden changes in plasma levels (Goetz *et al.*, 1998a). The specific influence of the dose and type of dopaminergic treatment (ergot versus non-ergot derivative) has not been assessed, but it might be critical.

Disease-related factors

In clinical studies, the main disease-related factor associated with the development of hallucinations in PD is the presence of severe cognitive impairment or dementia. In community-based studies, prevalence rates of dementia range from 18% to 41% (Alves *et al.*, 2008). As stated above, the prevalence of hallucinations is significantly higher in PD patients with dementia than in those without, and severe cognitive impairment and dementia are independent risk factors for hallucinations. Several studies have investigated the association of hallucinations with specific types of cognitive dysfunction by evaluating hallucinating and non-hallucinating PD patients with various neuropsychological tests. Hallucinations were found to be associated with a wide range of cognitive defects, including visuoperceptual, executive, reality-monitoring, and memory dysfunctions. Other disease-related factors in this context include advanced age, a long disease duration, a more-severe form of PD, and the presence of sleep disorders, including altered dream phenomena (vivid dreams, nightmares, rapid-eye-movement sleep behavior disorder) and daytime somnolence. Patients with visual hallucinations are also more likely to suffer visual disorders, namely low visual acuity resulting from coincidental ocular disease or PD-related disturbances, such as reduced contrast sensitivity and color discrimination. Finally, studies of the relationships between depression and psychosis or hallucinations have yielded conflicting results (reviewed by Fénelon, 2008).

Genetic factors

In one study, hallucinations were associated with a positive family history of dementia (Paleacu *et al.*, 2005), suggesting a role for genetic factors. Several studies have investigated the association of hallucinations or psychosis with genetic polymorphisms (reviewed by Fénelon, 2008). Studies examining the distribution of allele or genotype frequencies of dopamine receptor and transporter genes in PD subjects with and without hallucinations have yielded inconsistent results. Two studies found an association of visual hallucinations with the cholecystokinin *CT/TT* genotype and with a combination of the cholecystokinin *CT/TT* and the cholecystokinin-A receptor *TC/CC* genotype, suggesting that the cholecystokinin system may influence the development of hallucinations in PD. Finally, no association was found between PD-associated visual hallucinations and polymorphisms of the serotonin 5-HT$_2$A receptor and transporter genes or HLA type.

Pathophysiology

Neuroimaging and biological studies in this field have so far been inconclusive. Neuroimaging studies in PD have yielded heterogeneous results, but have generally suggested alterations in the cortical processing of visual stimuli in patients with visual hallucinations, in particular, a decreased visual input (bottom–up processing) and a disinhibition of top–down cortical processing (review in Diederich *et al.*, 2009). In PD and LBD, pathological studies have shown an association between visual hallucinations and increased densities of Lewy bodies in the temporal lobe and the amygdala, but also in other cortical areas. The involvement of widespread dopaminergic, serotoninergic and/or cholinergic projection pathways in the genesis of hallucinations has been postulated, mainly on the basis of indirect pharmacological evidence and theoretically based considerations. The dopaminergic hypothesis essentially states that hallucinations in PD result from an overstimulation of mesocorticolimbic dopaminergic receptors. Variants of this model imply the involvement of several neurotransmitter systems through a cascade of activations and inhibitions, a serotoninergic–dopaminergic imbalance, or a monoaminergic–cholinergic imbalance.

Obviously, no simple model can account for the full diversity and heterogeneity of factors associated with hallucinations in PD. Complex visual hallucinations are probably associated with abnormal activity in the ventral extrastriate visual cortex. This has not been demonstrated in PD, but activation of the extrastriate (non primary) visual cortical areas during visual hallucinations was elegantly shown in a functional MRI study of patients with Charles Bonnet syndrome (Ffytche *et al.*, 1998). In PD, hallucinations might constitute a common endpoint of several underlying mechanisms that may act alone or in combination, including (a) dopaminergic overactivity and/or imbalance between monoaminergic (relatively preserved) and cholinergic (altered) neurotransmission, (b) alteration of brainstem sleep–wake and dream regulation, (c) dysfunction of visual pathways, which can be non-specific (i.e., coincidental ocular disease) and/or specific (i.e., PD-associated retinal dysfunction or functional disturbances in the ventral stream of visual cortical processing), (d) dysfunction of top-down mechanisms of visual information processing, such as impaired attentional focus, and (e) contributory effect of antiparkinsonian drugs and other pharmacological agents that can interfere with the previously mentioned mechanisms at many levels. In an attempt to integrate seemingly disparate pathophysiologic clues on PD associated hallucinations, Diederich *et al.* (2005) proposed an integrative model based on Allan Hobson's work on factors regulating consciousness. In this model, visual hallucinations in PD are due to dysregulation of the gating and filtering of external perceptions and/or aberrant internal image productions, both strongly influenced by various pharmacological modulations. A more general model of complex visual hallucinations involves cognitively based models of scene perception (Collerton *et al.*, 2005).

General measures and first-line treatment options

Evaluating the impact of hallucinations in PD

Careful evaluation of the impact of PD-related hallucinations is critical when determining a therapeutic strategy. Most PD-associated hallucinations are non-threatening: only about one-quarter of patients report coexisting anxiety (Fénelon *et al.*, 2000). Patients with lost or partial insight may have behavioral disturbances directly related to the hallucinations. For example, in one instance a patient tried to climb over the railing of his balcony on the fourth floor, because he wanted to join a group of hallucinated persons in a virtual garden. Others have seized a knife or a stick to defend themselves against imagined individuals of whom they were frightened. Thus, in a minority of cases, behavioral disturbances can have potentially hazardous consequences for patients or caregivers.

The impact of PD-associated hallucinations on caregivers should also be evaluated, as hallucinations are often poorly understood and accepted by those who care for the patient. In a study of PD patients with dementia who were drawn from a large clinical trial of rivastigmine, psychosis and agitation were associated with the highest caregiver distress scores (Aarsland *et al.*, 2007).

Evaluating contributory factors

As discussed, PD-associated hallucinations are associated with a number of clinical characteristics. Although in most cases no causal relationship can be demonstrated, these potential contributors should be considered when choosing an approach to the treatment of hallucinations. Medical records should be checked for current medications and recent dose increases. A search for an underlying illness, such as infection, dehydration, or metabolic disturbances, should be undertaken. The cognitive status should be evaluated using brief cognitive tests. Recommended screening tools for the diagnosis of cognitive impairment in PD are the Mini Mental Status (cutoff < 26), giving the months reversed, the lexical fluency, and the clock drawing test (Dubois *et al.*, 2007). The impact of cognitive impairment on daily living activities that cannot be attributed to motor symptoms should be assessed. If the presence of severe cognitive impairment or dementia remains uncertain or equivocal after this first level evaluation, a more detailed neuropsychological assessment is advisable (Dubois *et al.*, 2007). Patients should also be tested for depression and, if visual hallucinations are reported, ocular disease.

Non-pharmacological measures

Studying 46 PD patients with hallucinations, Diederich *et al.* (2003) identified potentially useful coping strategies that reduce the frequency and severity of visual hallucinations; about three-quarters of the patients frequently used these coping strategies without any instructions given by the neurologists. Potentially useful coping strategies are listed in Box 18.3.

Caregivers also need reassurance. It has been shown that patient nonmotor psychological symptoms have a greater impact on caregiver strain and depression than patient motor symptoms (Carter *et al.*, 2008). In a study exploring neuropsychiatric symptoms in patients with PD and dementia, psychosis and agitation was associated with high caregiver distress scores (Aarland *et al.*, 2007). Professionals should provide information to the caregiver throughout the course of Parkinson's disease to support the adjustment process. The tactics aiming at reducing the effects of hallucinations (Box 18.3) should be explained to the caregiver, as well as how to react when patients lack insight and respond to hallucinations or delusions, and when to seek additional help (Marsh, 2006; Williamson *et al.*, 2008).

Box 18.3 Coping strategies for visual hallucinations in PD

Visual techniques

- Looking in another direction or focusing on another object
- Better focusing the hallucinatory object
- Turning the lights on

Cognitive techniques

- Reassuring oneself that the hallucinations are not real and will resolve shortly
- Approaching or 'touching' the hallucinations

Interactive techniques

- Discussions with family and other caregivers:
  - to gain comfort and reassurance
  - to check for the non-reality of the hallucinations

Diederich, N.J., Pieri, V., & Goetz, C.G. (2003). Coping strategies for visual hallucinations in Parkinson's disease. *Movement Disorder*, **18**, 831–8. Reprinted with permission of John Wiley & Sons, Inc.

Pharmacological measures, excluding anti-psychotics

As soon as hallucinations become troublesome for the patient, even in the absence of anxiety or behavioral disorders, a review of current treatments is warranted. First, a small dose decrease or the withdrawal of some anti-parkinsonian medications should be considered, following a last-in, first-out strategy, or beginning with less potent drugs (i.e., anticholinergics, amantadine, and selegiline). If necessary, dopaminergic agonists should be decreased or withdrawn before decreasing levodopa doses. The challenge is to find the optimal dose that reduces the hallucinations while maintaining an acceptable motor status—a goal that is not always achieved. In the past, authors also proposed the transient withdrawal of dopaminergic treatment (drug holiday) to alleviate hallucinations (Koller *et al.*, 1981), but interest in this approach is limited because of the risk of major complications (lengthy hospitalizations, aspiration, pulmonary emboli, neuroleptic-like malignant syndrome) (Goetz *et al.*, 2009). Treatment with other potentially aggravating drugs, including opioid analgesics and psychoactive drugs, should also be reviewed. However, the role of antidepressants in this context is not clear-cut. Lauterbach (1993) reported a case of worsened psychosis when a demented patient with PD was treated with fluoxetine to exclude depressive pseudodementia, whereas antidepressants may be beneficial in PD patients with psychotic symptoms and comorbid depression (Voon & Lang, 2004).

Treatment with cholinesterase inhibitors could be of interest in the context of coexisting dementia, but, at present, evidence for their efficacy in PD-associated hallucinations is weak. A large randomized, placebo-controlled study of rivastigmine in PD patients with dementia demonstrated a moderate beneficial effect of these agents on cognitive variables (Emre *et al.*, 2004). Patients with visual hallucinations at baseline had the greatest therapeutic benefit (Burn *et al.*, 2006). However, although the total NPI score was significantly improved, a significant effect on the NPI hallucination item was not demonstrated. Similarly, two small randomized controlled trials of donepezil showed a mild improvement of cognition, but the drug had no effect on hallucinations (Aarsland *et al.*, 2002, Ravina *et al.*, 2005). The only evidence that cholinesterase inhibitors might improve hallucinations in PD patients with cognitive impairment comes from small studies with an open-label design (Reading *et al.*, 2001; Bergman & Lerner, 2002; Aarsland *et al.*, 2003). However, in the context of cognitive impairment, it seems reasonable to consider treatment with a cholinesterase inhibitor and to re-evaluate psychosis before deciding to introduce an atypical anti-psychotic agent (Box 18.4). Most adverse events associated with cholinesterase inhibitors are mild or moderate, but these drugs can aggravate parkinsonian tremors (Emre *et al.*, 2004). The usefulness of rivastigmine can be limited because of nausea and/or vomiting, but studies in patients with Alzheimer's disease suggest that the incidence of these side effects is reduced when using the transdermal patch formulation of the drug. Patients should be warned that sudden withdrawal of a cholinesterase inhibitor may produce acute cognitive decline and/or exacerbate hallucinations (Minett *et al.*, 2003).

Memantine, a drug with a complex pharmacological profile, is approved for the treatment of moderate to severe Alzheimer's disease, but not for the treatment of PD dementia. This drug may trigger psychosis in patients with PD or LBD (Seeman *et al.*, 2008) and should therefore not be used in this setting.

Second-line treatment option: Atypical anti-psychotics

When should atypical anti-psychotics be initiated?

The majority of patients do not need anti-psychotics because they respond to first-line, general measures. In a group of 26 PD patients with psychosis, the symptoms resolved sufficiently in the short term in 16 (62%) patients, precluding the need for anti-psychotic therapy (Thomsen *et al.*, 2008). There is no doubt that anti-psychotics should be prescribed when the consequences of the hallucinations are severe, especially when the hallucinations are associated with anxiety and/or behavioral disorders. Anti-psychotics should either be started after general measures and first-line treatment options have been tried with insufficient results, or they should be given concomitantly with first-line treatment options if a behavioral disorder puts the patient or caregivers in danger. The benefit of initiating anti-psychotic treatment earlier in the disease course, when the patient is not yet distressed by the hallucinations, is not clear. As mentioned above, PD-associated hallucinations tend to persist and worsen in the long term. A retrospective study has suggested that the risk of subsequent deterioration is reduced if patients with mild hallucinations are treated with anti-psychotic medication (Goetz *et al.*, 2008).

Box 18.4 Management of hallucinations in PD

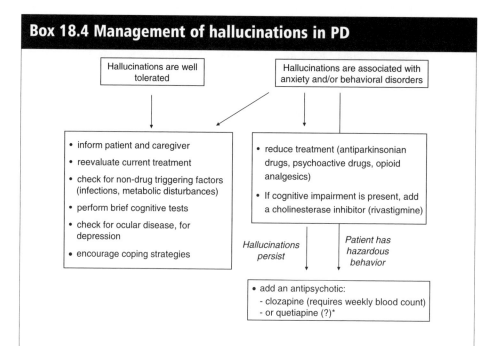

*The use of quetiapine is frequent in this setting but is not supported by controlled studies (see text)

Seeing fish on the bed

A 70-year-old woman, a widow and a former shopkeeper, had Parkinson's disease for 9 years. Her motor state was fair, with mild fluctuations and dyskinesias. The patient reported hallucinatory phenomena, including visual illusions, sense of presence of an unidentified person, feeling 'the wind of a bird's wing' on her face, feeling slaps behind her head when falling asleep, and hearing 'mice nibbling'. The patient was not anxious and remained ambiguous about the reality of the phenomena: she wondered whether her house was haunted. Her treatment consisted of levodopa (600 mg/day) + benserazide, lisuride (0.6 mg/day), bromazepam, amitriptyline, zolpidem, and analgesics (paracetamol + codeine). At this stage, psychoactive drugs were reduced or stopped, and hallucinations became less frequent but did not cease.

One year later, the hallucinations had worsened. The patient saw lizards running on her skin and felt bites in her back. She saw marks of blood on her dressing gown (she would try to wipe them off), chests of unidentified persons, and dead fish on her bed ('The other day, I wrapped one in a dishcloth; it looked like a seabream. When I wanted to show it to my son, it had gone'). The patient also reported visual illusions (e.g., a cushion on the settee was seen as the head of a dog), a sense of presence ('a crowd, or my guardian angel, far away or very near, just behind me'), and rubbing noises. She thought that 'people' would eat her sweets and turn her TV on. These phenomena occurred daily, predominately in the evening, and generated moderate to severe anxiety. The patient wondered, 'Am I dreaming, or could all this be possible?' Her motor status remained fair. The patient had no complaint about sleep. She was not depressed. On neuropsychological evaluation, the Mattis Dementia Rating Scale score was 98 (normal score: ≥ 136). At this stage, as a first step, lisuride was withdrawn, leaving levodopa as a monotherapy (550 mg/day), and rivastigmine was added, but poorly tolerated (nausea). These measures had no efficacy on the hallucinations. The second step was to introduce clozapine (12.5 mg/day, then 25 mg/day), which was well tolerated and had a clear beneficial effect on the hallucinations: these persisted, but were less dramatic, with no concomitant anxiety and better insight.

This clinical vignette illustrates several typical aspects of a chronic hallucinatory syndrome in PD: the variety of hallucinatory phenomena (multimodal hallucinations, visual illusions, sense of presence); the contributory role of pharmacological factors and the association with cognitive impairment; the progression from 'benign' to more-severe forms, with loss of insight, associated delusions, and anxiety; and finally the response to pharmacological interventions. However, the prognosis of such clinical pictures is poor because of a high risk of developing PD-associated dementia.

Whether this results from a symptomatic effect or from a modification of the disease course remains to be elucidated.

What is the rationale for using atypical anti-psychotics?

Conventional anti-psychotics are contraindicated in patients with PD as they can dramatically worsen parkinsonism. The main advantage of new-generation anti-psychotics over conventional drugs is a reduced risk of extrapyramidal side effects. Therefore, these 'atypical' anti-psychotics could theoretically be valuable for the treatment of PD-associated psychosis. However, two points need to be considered: first, a meta-analysis of controlled studies in patients with schizophrenia suggested that the risk of extrapyramidal side effects associated with atypical anti-psychotics is not reduced when these drugs are compared with low-potency conventional anti-psychotics (clozapine is an exception) (Leucht *et al.*, 2003); second, the exact characteristics that make these new anti-psychotics 'atypical' are a matter of debate, and there may be significant differences between the drugs within this class. The atypical anti-psychotic effect could, at the molecular level, be due to a fast dissociation of the drug from the D_2 receptor, rather than a high 5-HT_2 occupancy. Clozapine and quetiapine occupy less than 60% of D_2 receptors when occupancy levels are measured 12 h after administration of the drug. This level is below the threshold of 78–80%, above which extrapyramidal side effects develop. Olanzapine and risperidone exceed this threshold in a dose-dependent fashion and may thus give rise to worsening of parkinsonism (Kapur & Seeman, 2001).

Which atypical anti-psychotic should be used?

A number of atypical anti-psychotic drugs have been tested to see whether they can control psychotic symptoms in patients with PD-associated hallucinations with a low risk of worsening motor function and generating tardive dyskinesia. Although many open-label studies and case reports have claimed that certain atypical anti-psychotics could be effective in controlling hallucinations in patients with PD, controlled trials have been less numerous and less convincing. They are summarized in Table 18.1

Clozapine. Clozapine is a tricyclic dibenzodiazepine derivative. It has a complex receptor pharmacology, with antagonist activity at dopaminergic (D_1, D_2), serotoninergic (5-HT_2A, 5-HT_2C, 5-HT_3), adrenergic (alpha$_1$, alpha$_2$), histaminergic (H_1), and muscarinic (M_1) receptors. The efficacy and tolerability of clozapine in PD patients with hallucinations were suggested by a number of open-label trials that began in 1985 (Friedman and Factor 2000) and were confirmed in two randomized, placebo-controlled, double-blind trials, both of which investigated the effect of clozapine over a period of 4 weeks (Table 18.1). Importantly, the clinical trials demonstrating the efficacy of clozapine were restricted to non-demented PD patients with hallucinations. This exclusion makes its impossible to extrapolate the efficacy of clozapine directly to the large population of hallucinating PD-dementia patients.

Over 80% of PD patients respond to clozapine with a complete or partial resolution of their psychosis. Clozapine is the only atypical anti-psychotic that has been fully recommended for the treatment of PD-associated psychosis, both in a meta-analysis (Frieling et al., 2007) and in several evidence-based reviews (Goetz et al., 2002, Miyasaki et al., 2006). The required doses are generally low. The recommended initial daily dose is 6.25 mg or 12.5 mg given at night, with a slow incremental increase until symptoms are adequately controlled or adverse effects occur (Goetz et al., 2009; Poewe, 2008). In most cases, efficacy is achieved at doses of 50 mg or less, but sometimes higher doses may be required. Clozapine does not appear to worsen parkinsonism and may even improve some motor symptoms such as tremor and dyskinesias (Friedman & Factor, 2000). Hematologic monitoring for potential agranulocytosis is mandatory and should be performed weekly during the first 18 weeks of treatment and monthly thereafter. In a large study of schizophrenia, 0.80% of patients had developed agranulocytosis at one year, with the risk being highest in the six first months of treatment (Alvir et al., 1993). Agranulocytosis is idiosyncratic and not dose-related. Clozapine is also associated with a low (<0.2%) risk of potentially fatal myocarditis or cardiomyopathy (Merrill et al., 2005). However, the most common side effects are more-benign and dose-related: sedation, orthostatic hypotension, confusion, and drooling.

Quetiapine. Quetiapine is an atypical anti-psychotic with a structure and preclinical profile similar to clozapine, but with no risk of agranulocytosis (Dev & Raniwalla, 2000). The hope that this drug could have similar efficacy and better tolerability than clozapine in PD-associated hallucinations was reinforced by a number of open-label trials that provided positive results (reviewed by Friedman & Factor, 2000; Juncos, 2004). Two controlled trials failed to show that quetiapine was more effective than placebo in the treatment

Table 18.1 Randomized controlled trials of atypical anti-psychotics for PD with hallucinations or delusions (modified from Frieling et al., 2007 and Zahodne et al., 2008)

Study	Comparison	Patients (n) randomized/ completed study	Dosage (mg) range/mean	Duration	Psychosis outcome	Motor worsening
Clozapine						
Parkinson Study Group 1999	Clozapine vs. placebo (a)	60/54	6.25–50/25	4 weeks	Improvement on the CGI, the BPRS, and the SAPS	None
French Clozapine Parkinson Study Group 1999	Clozapine vs. placebo (a)	60/46	6.25–50/36	4 weeks	Improvement on the CGI and the positive subscore of the PANSS	None
Quetiapine						
Morgante et al., 2004	Clozapine vs. quetiapine (b)	45/40	12.5–50/26 25–200/91	12 weeks	Improvement on the CGI and the BPRS with no differences between groups	None. Dyskinesia decreased
Merims et al., 2006	Clozapine vs. quetiapine (b)	27/16	NA/13 NA/91	22 weeks	Improvement on the CGI with no difference between groups. No major change in hallucinations (NPI item). Decrease in delusions frequency (NPI item)	None
Ondo et al., 2005	Quetiapine vs. placebo (a)	31/26	75–200/169	12 weeks	No change on the BPRS and the Baylor PD Hallucination Questionnaire compared with placebo	None
Rabey et al., 2007	Quetiapine vs. placebo (a)	58/32	NA/119	3 months	No change on the BPRS and the CGI	None

(Continued)

Table 18.1 (continued) Randomized controlled trials of atypical anti-psychotics for PD with hallucinations or delusions (modified from Frieling et al., 2007 and Zahodne et al., 2008)

Study	Comparison	Patients (n) randomized/ completed study	Dosage (mg) range/mean	Duration	Psychosis outcome	Motor worsening
Olanzapine						
Breier et al., 2002: USA study	Olanzapine vs. placebo (a)	83/60	NA/4.2	4 weeks	Improvement on the CGI, the BPRS (total and positive symptom subscore), and the NPI (total and hallucinations item), with no differences between groups	Worsening of UPDRS total, motor, and activities of daily living scores compared with placebo
Breier et al., 2002: European study	Olanzapine vs. placebo (a)	77/61	NA/4.1			
Ondo et al., 2002	Olanzapine vs. placebo (a)	30/27	NA/4.6	9 weeks	No significant improvement on item 2 of the UPDRS part I and a structured interview for hallucinations compared with placebo	Worsening of UPDRS motor score and time tapping compared with placebo
Risperidone						
Ellis et al., 2000	Risperidone vs. clozapine (a)	10/9	1–1.5/1.2 25–100/62.5	3 months	Improvement on the BPRS psychosis cluster subscore in both groups (significant in the risperidone group) but no significant difference between groups	Not significant worsening of UPDRS motor score with risperidone and improvement with clozapine

BPRS, brief psychiatric rating scale; CGI, clinical global impression; NA, not available; NPI, neuropsychiatric inventory; PANSS, positive and negative syndrome scale; SAPS, scale for the assessment of positive symptoms; UPDRS, unified Parkinson's disease rating scale.
(a) double-blind design; (b) rater-blinded design.

of PD-related hallucinations, while two trials with a rater-blinded design that compared quetiapine with clozapine suggested that both drugs were effective (Table 18.1). Because of methodological limitations (Frieling *et al.*, 2007), these results have to be interpreted with caution and this issue needs to be clarified based on further studies. The results from the placebo-controlled trials are in conflict with the widespread utilization of quetiapine in clinical settings, the positive results from open-label studies, and personal reports of an overall favourable experience with the drug (Weintraub and Hurtig 2007, Goetz *et al.*, 2009). Goetz *et al.* (2009) have suggested that this discrepancy between clinical experience and evidence-based data could be explained by the fact that quetiapine has not only antihallucinatory properties but also sleep-promoting qualities, and that the clinical perception of improvement could simply result from improved sleep. On the basis of evidence-based reviews, quetiapine cannot be recommended for the treatment of PD-associated hallucinations, although some guidelines consider that for patients with PD and psychosis, quetiapine may be useful (Horstink *et al.*, 2006b, Miyasaki *et al.*, 2006).

Other atypical anti-psychotics. Olanzapine has been shown to worsen parkinsonism and should not be used in this setting (Table 18.1). The same holds true for risperidone, which has been used mainly in open-label trials (Factor *et al.*, 2001). No controlled trails are available for other anti-psychotic drugs. In pilot studies, remoxipride (Lang *et al.*, 1995) and zotepine (Arnold *et al.*, 1994) were shown to aggravate parkinsonism. A few case reports and small series suggested that ziprasidone could improve hallucinations in PD, but some patients had motor worsening and/or pathological laughing (Schindehütte & Trenkwalder, 2007). Some case reports and an open-label pilot study also showed that aripiprazole could improve PD-associated hallucinations, but, again, a majority of patients experienced an exacerbation of motor symptoms (Friedman *et al.*, 2006). Finally, a few open-label studies showed that the serotonin receptor 5-HT$_3$ antagonist ondansetron could attenuate PD-associated psychosis without inducing motor deterioration (Zoldan *et al.*, 1995; Friedberg *et al.*, 1998). These promising results have not been replicated in a controlled study, and the high cost of ondansetron would preclude the widespread use of this drug in the treatment of PD-associated hallucinations. However, it has been suggested that ondansetron could be used transiently in emergency situations when hallucinations are associated with acute agitation (Marsh, 2006).

What is the risk–benefit ratio of atypical anti-psychotics in PD?

As described above, atypical anti-psychotics can have potentially serious adverse effects, such as agranulocytosis in the case of clozapine. Moreover, in recent years, regulatory agencies have issued recommendations and warnings concerning the use of atypical anti-psychotic drugs in the elderly because a meta-analysis of 17 placebo-controlled trials found an increased risk of mortality of 1.6–1.7 in elderly patients with dementia who used an atypical anti-psychotic (reviewed by Friedman, 2006). Given the fact that PD patients with hallucinations are often elderly and may have cognitive impairment, these warnings need to be taken into consideration (Friedman, 2006; Goetz *et al.*, 2009). However, the recommendations were made on the basis of short-term controlled studies, and large retrospective studies do not confirm these findings (Friedman, 2006). When evaluating the risk–benefit ratio of atypical anti-psychotics, it should also be kept in mind that an improvement of hallucinations or psychosis translates into a reduced risk of nursing home placement and, possibly, reduced rates of mortality (Factor *et al.*, 2003).

For how long should treatment be prescribed?

Only a few long-term studies of patients on anti-psychotic treatment have been performed. In a longitudinal follow-up study of 59 PD patients with psychosis who had been enrolled in a trial of clozapine, 64% of the survivors had persistent psychosis and most remained on clozapine or another anti-psychotic (Factor *et al.*, 2003). In a retrospective study of 32 patients who were receiving clozapine, mostly for hallucinations, nine patients stopped taking the drug because their symptoms had improved; the symptoms did not recur after discontinuation of clozapine (Klein *et al.*, 2003). However, in a prospective longitudinal study, three-quarters of patients relapsed after clozapine withdrawal, leading the authors to conclude that 'although it can be said that a low dose of clozapine has excellent efficacy on psychotic symptoms, the effect wears off once the treatment stops' (Pollak *et al.*, 2004). In some patients, the 'rebound' psychosis after quetiapine or clozapine withdrawal is worse than the original psychotic episode, requiring higher anti-psychotic medication doses (Fernandez *et al.*, 2004). Current evidence therefore favors chronic, maintenance therapy for patients who respond to an anti-psychotic.

Other therapeutic considerations and perspectives

Primary prevention

The primary prevention of hallucinations in PD consists in screening for and addressing risk factors that predispose to psychosis on an ongoing basis, especially when cognitive impairment is present (Marsh, 2006). Moreover, when symptomatic treatment is required in older patients with early PD, the use of levodopa is recommended, as older patients are more sensitive to neuropsychiatric adverse reactions associated with the use of dopamine agonists and are less prone to developing levodopa-induced motor complications (Horstink *et al.*, 2006a).

Electroconvulsive therapy

Some PD patients with hallucinations might benefit from electroconvulsive therapy. In PD patients, this treatment may improve severe depression, especially if mood-congruent delusions are present, and has also been shown to improve parkinsonism in PD patients. It has also been successfully used to treat psychosis (Factor *et al.*, 1995a, Hurwitz *et al.*, 1988) and might be an option for the treatment of PD-associated hallucinations, especially in the context of depression. However, the level of evidence supporting this option is low, and this approach should only be considered if atypical anti-psychotics are inefficient or not tolerated (Marsh, 2006). Because of the risk of delirium after electro-convulsive therapy, this treatment approach is not suitable for patients with dementia.

Hallucinations and deep brain stimulation

In recent years, deep brain stimulation, in most cases subthalamic stimulation (STN-DBS) has been increasingly used for the treatment of PD patients with severe motor complications of levodopa therapy, i.e., motor fluctuations and abnormal involuntary movements (dyskinesias). STN-DBS carries risks, and candidates for this procedure have to be carefully selected. In patients evaluated for STN-DBS, a chronic hallucinatory syndrome is not explicitly considered to be a definite contraindication for surgery (Lang *et al.*, 2006). However, patients experiencing chronic hallucinations commonly have cognitive impairment and are therefore not eligible for STN-DBS. There are no guidelines concerning patients with chronic hallucinations who have no, or mild, cognitive impairment. Given the fact that dopaminergic drugs have a contributory role in the development of hallucinations, and that STN-DBS allows a dose reduction of dopaminergic treatment, it can be postulated that deep brain stimulation could have a beneficial effect on chronic hallucinations, or that it would at least not aggravate them. Indeed, a retrospective study of 18 patients, 13 of whom had a history of hallucinations, suggested that STN-DBS did not worsen pre-existing hallucinations (Yoshida *et al.*, 2009). In a large study comparing STN-DBS with best medical treatment in patients with advanced PD (78 patients per group), psychosis was more common (seven vs. four patients) in the group receiving best medical treatment (Witt *et al.*, 2008). On the other hand, STN-DBS has been reported to induce hallucinations in a few cases (Diederich *et al.*, 2000). It should be emphasized that patients with STN-DBS can develop dementia and/or hallucinations in the long term, as part of the natural progression of PD (Deuschl *et al.*, 2006). In those who develop dementia after STN-DBS, the pre-operative presence of hallucinations seems to be a predictor for the subsequent deterioration of cognitive function (Aybek *et al.*, 2007). Thus, the presence of hallucinations in a patient considered for STN-DBS should prompt a detailed neuropsychological assessment before deciding whether the patient should undergo surgery.

Therapeutic perspectives

There remains an unmet clinical need for drug treatments that have a proven efficacy for PD-associated psychosis, and that do not worsen motor symptoms or have potentially serious adverse effects. Recently, phase III trials of pimavanserin tartrate, a $5-HT_2A$ inverse agonist, have been initiated following encouraging results from phase II studies (Abbas & Roth, 2008). In recent years, it has been shown that low-frequency repetitive transcranial magnetic stimulation (rTMS) over the left temporoparietal cortex may improve medication-resistant auditory hallucinations in schizophrenic patients (Tranulis *et al.*, 2008). So far, no trial of rTMS in PD patients with hallucinations has been reported. The main obstacle to the application of this technique to the treatment of PD-associated hallucinations would be to specify the cortical target, as cortical areas implied in the genesis of hallucinations are unknown, and are likely to vary widely according to the patients and the types of hallucinations.

Finally, it should be kept in mind that hallucinations and other psychotic symptoms tend to occur late in the course of PD. There is great excitement surrounding the possibility that future neuroprotective therapies could slow the progression of PD or even prevent or delay its onset at a preclinical stage (Poewe, 2009). Hopefully, neuroprotective therapies will have a beneficial effect on both motor and non-motor symptoms of PD, including hallucinations.

References

Aarsland, D., Brønnick, K., Ehrt, U., *et al.* (2007). Neuropsychiatric symptoms in patients with Parkinson's disease and dementia: frequency, profile and associated care giver stress. *J Neurol Neurosurg Psychiatry*, **78**, 36–42.

Aarsland, D., Bronnick, K., Alves, G., *et al.* (2009). The spectrum of neuropsychiatric symptoms in patients with early untreated Parkinson's disease. *J Neurol Neurosurg Psychiatry*, **80**, 928–930.

Aarsland, D., Hutchinson, M., & Larsen, J.P. (2003). Cognitive, psychiatric and motor response to galantamine in Parkinson's disease with dementia. *Int J Geriatr Psychiatry*, **18**, 937–41.

Aarsland, D., Laake, K., Larsen, J.P., & Janvin, C. (2002). Donepezil for cognitive impairment in Parkinson's disease: a randomised controlled study. *J Neurol Neurosurg*, **72**, 708–12.

Aarsland, D., Larsen, J.P., Tandberg, E., & Laake, K. (2000). Predictors of nursing home placement in Parkinson's disease: a population-based, prospective study. *J Am Geriatr Soc*, **48**, 938–42.

Abbas, A., & Roth, B.L. (2008). Pimavanserin tartrate: a 5-HT2A inverse agonist with potential for treating various Neuropsychiatric disorders. *Expert Opin Pharmacother*, **9**, 3251–9.

Alves, G., Forsaa, E.B., Pedersen, K.F., Gjerstad, M.D., & Larsen, J.P. (2008). Epidemiology of Parkinson's disease. *J Neurol*, **255** (suppl 5), 18–32.

Alvir, J.M.J., Lieberman, J.A., Safferman, A.Z., Schwimmer, J.L., & Schaaf, J.A. (1993). Clozapine-induced agranulocytosis. Incidence and risk factors in the United States. *N Engl J Med*, **329**, 162–7.

Arnold, G., Trenkwalder, C., Schwarz, J., & Oertel, W.H. (1994). Zotepine reversibly induces akinesia and rigidity in Parkinson's disease patients with resting tremor or drug-induced psychosis. *Mov Disord*, **9**, 238–40.

Aybek, S., Gronchi-Perrin, A., Berney, A., *et al.* (2007). Long-term cognitive profile and incidence of dementia after STN-DBS in Parkinson's disease. *Mov Disord*, **22**, 974–81.

Baker, W.L., Silver, D., & White, C.M. (2008). Dopamine agonists in the treatment of early Parkinson's disease: a meta-analysis. *Parkinsonism Relat Disord*, **15** (4), 287–294.

Barnes, J., & David, A.S. (2001). Visual hallucinations in Parkinson's disease: a review and phenomenological survey. *J Neurol Neurosurg Psychiatry*, **70**, 727–33.

Bergman, J., & Lerner, V. (2002). Successful use of donepezil for the treatment of psychotic symptoms in patients with Parkinson's disease. *Clin Neuropharmacol*, **25**, 107–110.

Biousse, V., Skibell, B.C., Watts, R.L., *et al.* (2004). Ophthalmologic features of Parkinson's disease. *Neurology*, **62**, 177–80.

Breier, A., Sutton, V.K., Feldman, P.D., *et al.* (2002). Olanzapine in the treatment of dopamimetic-induced psychosis in patients with Parkinson's disease. *Biol Psychiatry*, **52**, 438–45.

Burn, D., Emre, M., McKeith, I., *et al.* (2006). Effects of rivastigmine in patients with and without visual hallucinations in dementia associated with Parkinson's disease. *Mov Disord*, **21**, 1899–907.

Carter, J.H., Stewart, B.J., Lyons, K.S., & Archbold, P.G. (2008). Do motor and nonmotor symptoms in PD patients predict caregiver strain and depression? *Mov Disord*, **23**, 1211–16.

Chou, K., Messing, S., Oakes, D., Feldman, P.D., Breier, A., & Friedman, J.H. (2005). Drug-induced psychosis in Parkinson disease: phenomenology and correlations among psychosis rating instruments. *Clin Neuropharmacol*, **28**, 215–9.

Collerton, D., Perry, E., & McKeith, I. (2005). Why people see things that are not there: a novel perception and attention deficit model for recurrent complex visual hallucinations. *Behav Brain Sci*, **28**, 737–57.

Dev, V., & Raniwalla, J. (2000). Quetiapine. A review of its safety in the management of schizophrenia. *Drug Safety*, **23**, 295–307.

Deuschl, G., Herzog, J., Kleiner-Fisman, G., *et al.* (2006). Deep brain stimulation: postoperative issues. *Mov Disord*, **21**(suppl 14), S219–37.

Diederich, N.J., Alesch, F., & Goetz, C.G. (2000). Visual hallucinations induced by deep brain stimulation in Parkinson's disease. *Clin Neuropharmacol*, **23**, 287–9.

Diederich, N.J., Goetz, C.G., & Stebbins, G.T. (2005). Repeated visual hallucinations in Parkinson's disease as disturbed external/internal perceptions: focused review and a new integrative model. *Mov Disord*, **20**, 130–40.

Diederich, N.J., Fénelon, G., Stebbins, G., & Goetz, C.G. (2009). Hallucinations in Parkinson's disease. *Nature Rev Neurol*, **5**, 331–342.

Diederich, N.J., Pieri, V., & Goetz, C.G. (2003). Coping strategies for visual hallucinations in Parkinson's disease. *Mov Disord*, **18**, 831–8.

Doé de Maindreville, A., Fénelon, G., & Mahieux, F. (2005). Hallucinations in Parkinson's disease: a follow-up study. *Mov Disord*, **20**, 212–7.

Dubois, B., Burn, D., Goetz, C.G., *et al.* (2007). Diagnostic procedures for Parkinson's disease dementia: recommendations from the Movement Disorder Society Task Force. *Mov Disord*, **22**, 2314–24.

Ellis, T., Cudkowicz, M.E., Sexton, P.M., & Growdon, J.H. (2000). Clozapine and risperidone treatment of psychosis in Parkinson's disease. *J Neuropsychiatry Clin Neurosci*, **12**, 364–9.

Emre, M., Aarsland, D., Albanese, A., *et al.* (2004). Rivastigmine for dementia associated with Parkinson's disease. *New Engl J Med*, **351**, 2509–18.

Factor, S.A., Feustel, P.J., Friedman, J.H., *et al.* (2003). Longitudinal outcome of Parkinson's disease patients with psychosis. *Neurology*, **60**, 1756–61.

Factor, S.A., Mohlo, E.S., & Brown, D.L. (1995a). Combined clozapine and electroconvulsive therapy for the treatment of drug-induced psychosis in Parkinson's disease. *J Neuropsychiat Clin Neurosci*, **7**, 304–7.

Factor, S.A., Mohlo, E.S., & Friedman, J.H. (2001). Risperidone and Parkinson's disease. *Mov Disord*, **17**, 221–5.

Factor, S.A., Molho, E.S., Podskalny, G.D., & Brown, D. (1995b). Parkinson's disease: drug-induced psychiatric states. *Adv Neurol*, **65**, 115–38.

Fénelon, G. (2008). Psychosis in Parkinson's disease: phenomenology, frequency, risk factors, and current understanding of pathophysiologic mechanisms. *CNS Spectr*, **13** (suppl 4), 18–25.

Fénelon, G., & Alves, G. (2009). Epidemiology of psychosis in Parkinson's disease. *J Neurol Sci* (in press)

Fénelon, G., Goetz, C.G., & Karenberg, A. (2006). Hallucinations in the prelevodopa era in Parkinson's disease. *Neurology*, **66**, 93–8.

Fénelon, G., Mahieux, F., Huon, R., & Ziégler, M. (2000). Hallucinations in Parkinson's disease. Prevalence, phenomenology and risk factors. *Brain*, **123**, 733–45.

Fénelon, G., Thobois, S., Bonnet, A.-M., Broussolle, E., & Tison, F. (2002). Tactile hallucinations in Parkinson's disease. *J Neurol*, **249**, 1699–703.

Fénelon, G., Soulas, T., Zenasni, F., & Cleret de Langavant, L. (2010). The changing face of Parkinson's disease-associated psychosis: a cross-sectional study based on the new NINDS-NIMH criteria. *Mov Disord* (in press).

Fernandez, H.H., Aarsland, D., Fénelon, G., *et al.* (2008). Scales to assess psychosis in Parkinson's disease: critique and recommendations. *Mov Disord*, **23**, 484–500.

Fernandez, H.H., Trieschmann, M.E., & Okun, M.S. (2004). Rebound psychosis: effect of discontinuation of antipsychotics in Parkinson's disease. *Mov Disord*, **20**, 104–5.

Ffytche, D.H., Howard, R.J., Brammer, M.J., David, A., Woodruff, P., & Williams, S. (1998). The anatomy of conscious vision: an fMRI study of visual hallucinations. *Nature Neurosci*, **1**, 738–42.

French Clozapine Parkinson Study Group (1999). Clozapine in drug-induced psychosis in Parkinson's disease. *Lancet*, **353**, 2041–2.

Friedberg, G., Zoldan, J., Weizman, A., & Memamed, E. (1998). Parkinson psychosis Rating Scale: a practical instrument for grading psychosis in Parkinson's disease. *Clin Neuropharmacol*, **21**, 280–4.

Friedman, J.H. (1992). The management of levodopa psychoses. *Clin Neuropharmacol*, **14**, 283–95.

Friedman, J.H. (2006). Atypical antipsychotics in the elderly with Parkinson's disease and the 'black box' warning. *Neurology*, **67**, 564–6.

Friedman, J.H., Berman, R.M., Goetz, C.G., *et al.* (2006). Open-label flexible-dose pilot study to evaluate the safety and tolerability of aripiprazole in patients with psychosis associated with Parkinson's disease. *Mov Disord*, **21**, 2078–81.

Friedman, J.H., & Factor, S.A. (2000). Atypical antipsychotics in the treatment of drug-induced psychosis in Parkinson's disease. *Mov Disord*, **15**, 201–11.

Frieling, H., Hillemacher, T., Ziegenbein, M., Neundörfer, B., & Bleich, S. (2007). Treating dopamimetic psychosis in Parkinson's disease: structured review and meta-analysis. *Eur Neuropsychopharmacol*, **17**, 165–71.

Galvin, J.E., Pollack, J., & Morris, J.C. (2006). Clinical phenotype of Parkinson disease dementia. *Neurology*, **67**, 1605–11.

Goetz, C.G., Diederich, N.J., & Fénelon, G. (2009). Psychosis in Parkinson's disease, in K.R. Chaudhuri, E. Tolosa, A. Schapira, and W. Poewe (eds). *Non-Motor Symptoms of Parkinson's Disease*. (Oxford: Oxford University Press).

Goetz, C.G., Fan, W., & Leurgans, S. (2008). Antipsychotic medication treatment for mild hallucinations in Parkinson's disease: positive impact on long-term worsening. *Mov Disord*, **23**, 1541–5.

Goetz, C.G., Fan, W., Leurgans, S., Bernard, B., & Stebbins, G.T. (2006). The malignant course of 'benign hallucinations' in Parkinson's disease. *Arch Neurol*, **63**, 713–6.

Goetz, C.G., Koller, W.C., Poewe, W. *et al.* (2002). Management of Parkinson's disease: an evidence-based review. Drugs to treat dementia and psychosis. *Mov Disord*, **17** (suppl 4), S120–7.

Goetz, C.G., Leurgans, S., Pappert, E.J., Raman, R., & Stemer, A.B. (2001). Prospective longitudinal assessment of hallucinations in Parkinson's disease. *Neurology*, **57**, 2078–82.

Goetz, C.G., Pappert, E.J., Blasucci, L.M., *et al.* (1998a). Intravenous levodopa infusions in hallucinating Parkinson's disease patients: high-dose challenge does not precipitate hallucinations. *Neurology*, **50**, 515–7.

Goetz, C.G., & Stebbins, G.T. (1993). Risk factors for nursing home placement in advanced Parkinson's disease. *Neurology*, **43**, 2227–9.

Goetz, C.G., & Stebbins, G.T. (1995). Mortality and hallucinations in nursing home patients with advanced Parkinson's disease. *Neurology*, **45**, 669–71.

Goetz, C.G., Vogel, C., Tanner, C.M., & Stebbins, G.T. (1998b). Early dopaminergic hallucinations in parkinsonian patients. *Neurology*, **51**, 811–4.

Hobson, P., & Meara, J. (2004). Risk and incidence of dementia in a cohort of older subjects with Parkinson's disease in the United Kingdom. *Mov Disord*, **19**, 1043–9.

Holroyd, S., Currie, L., & Wooten, G.F. (2001). Prospective study of hallucinations and delusions in Parkinson's disease. *J Neurol Neurosurg Psychiatry*, **70**, 734–8.

Horstink, M., Tolosa, E., Bonucelli, U., *et al.* (2006a). Review of the therapeutic management of Parkinson's disease. Report of a joint task force of the European Federation of Neurological Societies (EFNS) and the Movement Disorder Society-European Section (MDS-ES). Part I: early (uncomplicated) Parkinson's disease. *Eur J Neurol*, **13**, 1170–85.

Horstink, M., Tolosa, E., Bonucelli, U., *et al.* (2006b). Review of the therapeutic management of Parkinson's disease. Report of a joint task force of the European Federation of Neurological Societies (EFNS) and the Movement Disorder Society-European Section (MDS-ES). Part II: late (complicated) Parkinson's disease. *Eur J Neurol*, **13**, 1186–202.

Hurwitz, T.A., Calne, D.B., & Waterman, K. (1988). Treatment of dopaminomimetic psychosis in Parkinson's disease with electroconvulsive therapy. *Can J Neurol Sci*, **15**, 32–4.

Inzelberg, R., Kippervasser, S., & Korczyn, A.D. (1998). Auditory hallucinations in Parkinson's disease. *J Neurol Neurosurg Psychiatry*, **64**, 533–5.

Juncos, J.L., Roberts, V.J., Evatt M.L. *et al.* (2004). Quetiapine improves psychotic symptoms and cognition in Parkinson's disease. *Mov Disord*, **19**, 29–35.

Kapur, S., & Seeman, P. (2001). Does fast dissociation from the dopamine D2 receptor explain the action of atypical antipsychotics? A new hypothesis. *Am J Psychiatry*, **158**, 360–9.

Klein, C., Gordon, J., Pollak, L., & Rabey, J.M. (2003). Clozapine in Parkinson's disease psychosis: 5-year follow-up review. *Clin Neuropharmacol*, **26**, 8–11.

Koller, W.J., Perlik, S., Nausieda, P.A., Goetz, C.G., & Klawans, H.L. (1981). Complications of chronic levodopa therapy: long-term efficacy of drug holiday. *Neurology*, **31**, 473–6.

Lang, A.E., Houéto, J.-L., Krack, P., *et al.* (2006). Deep brain stimulation: preoperative issues. *Mov Disord*, **21** (suppl 14), S171–96.

Lang, A.E., Sandor, P., & Duff, J. (1995). Remoxipride in Parkinson's disease: differential response in patients with dyskinesias fluctuations versus psychosis. *Clin Neuropharmacol*, **18**, 39–45.

Lauterbach, E.C. (1993). Dopaminergic hallucinosis with fluoxetine in Parkinson's disease. *Am J Psychiatry*, **150**, 1750.

Leucht, S., Wahlbeck, K., Hamann, J., & Kissling, W. (2003). New generation antipsychotics versus low-potency conventional antipsychotics: a systematic review and meta-analysis. *Lancet*, **361**, 1581–9.

Levy, G., Tang, M.-X., Louis, E.D., *et al.* (2002). The association of incident dementia with mortality in PD. *Neurology*, **59**, 1708–13.

Lo, R.Y., Tanner, C.M., Albers, K.B., *et al.* (2009). Clinical features in early Parkinson disease and survival. *Arch Neurol*, **66**, 1353–58.

Marsh, L. (2006). Psychosis, in M. Menza & L. Marsh (ed) *Psychiatric Issues in Parkinson's Disease*, pp. 155–174, (London and New-York: Taylor and Francis).

Marsh, L., Williams, J.R., Rocco, M. *et al.* (2004). Psychiatric comorbidities in patients with Parkinson disease and psychosis. *Neurology*, **63**, 293–300.

Meltzer, H.Y., Mills, R., Revell, S., *et al.* (2010). Pimavanserin, a serotonin2A receptor inverse agonist, for the treatment of Parkinson's disease psychosis. *Neuropsychopharmacol*, **35**, 881–892.

Merims, D., Balas, M., Peretz, C., Shabtai, H., & Giladi, N. (2006). Rater-blinded, prospective comparison: quetiapine versus clozapine for Parkinson's disease psychosis. *Clin Neuropharmacol*, **29**, 331–7.

Merrill, D.B., William, G., & Goff, D.C. (2005). Adverse cardiac effects associated with clozapine. *J Clin Psychopharmacol*, **25**, 32–41.

Minett, T.S., Thomas, A., Wilkinson, L.M., *et al.* (2003). What happens when donepezil is suddenly withdrawn? An open label trial in dementia with Lewy bodies and Parkinson's disease with dementia. *Int J Geriatr Psychiatry*, **18**, 988–93.

Miyasaki, J.M., Shannon, K., Voon, V., *et al.* (2006). Practice parameter: Evaluation and treatment of depression, psychosis, and dementia in Parkinson disease (an evidence-based review). *Neurology*, **66**, 996–1002.

Morgante, L., Epifanio, A., Spina, E., *et al.* (2004). Quetiapine and clozapine in parkinsonian patients with dopaminergic psychosis. *Clin Pharmacol*, **27**, 153–6.

Mosimann, U.P., Rowan, E.N., Partington, C.E., *et al.* (2006). Characteristics of visual hallucinations in Parkinson disease dementia and dementia with Lewy bodies. *Am J Geriatr Psychiatry*, **14**, 153–60.

Ondo, W.G., Levy, J.K., Vuong, K.D., Hunter, C., & Jankovic, J. (2002). Olanzapine treatment for dopaminergic-induced hallucinations. *Mov Disord*, **17**, 1031–5.

Ondo, W.G., Tintner, R., Dat Voung, K., Lai, D., & Ringholz, G. (2005). Double-blind, placebo-controlled, unforced titration parallel trial of quetiapine for dopaminergic-induced hallucinations in Parkinson's disease. *Mov Disord*, **20**, 958–63.

Paleacu, D., Schechtman, E., & Inzelberg, R. (2005). Association between family history of dementia and hallucinations in Parkinson disease. *Neurology*, **64**, 1712–15.

Parkinson Study Group (1999). Low-dose clozapine for the treatment of drug-induced psychosis in Parkinson's disease. *New Engl J Med*, **340**, 757–63.

Poewe, W. (2008). When a Parkinson's disease patient starts to hallucinate. *Pract Neurol*, **8**, 238–41.

Poewe, W. (2009). Treatments for Parkinson disease—past achievements and current clinical needs. *Neurology*, **72 (suppl 2)**, S65–73.

Pollak, P., Tison, F., Rascol, O., *et al.* (2004). Clozapine in drug induced psychosis in Parkinson's disease: a randomised, placebo-controlled study with open follow-up. *J Neurol Neurosurg Psychiatry*, **75**, 689–95.

Rabey, J.M., Prokhorov, T., Miniovitz, A., Dobronevsky, E., & Klein, C. (2007). Effect of quetiapine in psychotic Parkinson's disease patients: a double-blind labeled study of 3 months duration. *Mov Disord*, **22**, 313–8.

Ravina, B., Marder, K., Fernandez, H.H., *et al.* (2007). Diagnostic Criteria for Psychosis in Parkinson's disease: Report of an NINDS/NIMH Work Group. *Mov Disord*, **22**, 1061–8.

Ravina, B., Putt, M., Siderow, A. *et al.* (2005). Donepezil for dementia in Parkinson's disease: a randomised, double blind, placebo-controlled, crossover study. *J Neurol Neurosurg Psychiatry*, **76**, 934–9.

Reading, P.J., Luce, A.K., & McKeith, I.G. (2001). Rivastigmine in the treatment of parkinsonian psychosis and cognitive impairment: preliminary finfings from an open trial. *Mov Disord*, **16**, 1171–95.

Schindehütte, J., & Trenkwalder, C. (2007). Treatment of drug-induced psychosis in Parkinson's disease with ziprasidone can induce severe dose-dependent off-periods and pathological laughing. *Clin Neurol Neurosurg*, **109**, 188–91.

Schrag, A. (2004). Psychiatric aspects of Parkinson's disease—an update. *J Neurol*, **251**, 795–804

Seeman, P., Caruso, C., & Lasaga, M. (2008). Memantine agonist action at dopamine D2High receptors. *Synapse*, **62**, 149–53.

Stowe, R.L., Ives, N.J., Clarke, C., *et al.* (2008). Dopamine agonist therapy in early Parkinson's disease. *Cochrane Database Syst Rev*, **15** (4), 287–294.

Thomsen, T.R., Panisset, M., Suchowersky, O., Goodridge, A., Mendis, T., & Lang, A.E. (2008). Impact of standard of care of psychosis in Parkinson disease. *J Neurol Neurosurg Psychiatry*, **79**, 1413–5.

Tranulis, C., Sepehry, A.A., Galinowski, A., & Stip, E. (2008). Should we treat auditory hallucinations with repetitive transcranial magnetic stimulation? A metaanalysis. *Can J Psychiatry*, **53**, 577–86.

Voon, V., & Lang, A.E. (2004). Antidepressants in the treatment of psychosis with comorbid depression in Parkinson disease. *Clin Neuropharmacol*, **27**, 90–2.

Weintraub, D., & Hurtig, H.I. (2007). Presentation and management of psychosis in Parkinson's disease and dementia with Lewy bodies. *Am J Psychiatry*, **164**, 1491–8.

Williams, D.R., & Lees, A.J. (2005). Visual hallucinations in the diagnosis of idiopathic Parkinson's disease: a retrospective autopsy study. *Lancet Neurol*, **4**, 605–10.

Williams, D.R., Warren, J.D., & Lees, A.J. (2008). Using the presence of visual hallucinations to differentiate Parkinson's disease from atypical parkinsonism. *J Neurol Neurosurg Psychiatry*, **79**, 652–5.

Williamson C, Simpson, J., & Murray, C.D. (2008). Caregivers' experiences of caring for a husband with Parkinson's disease and psychotic symptoms. *Social Sci Med*, **67**, 583–9.

Witt, K., Daniels, C., Reiff, J., *et al.* (2008). Neuropsychological and psychiatric changes after deep brain stimulation for Parkinson's disease: a randomised; multicentre study. *Lancet Neurol*, **7**, 605–14.

Yoshida, F., Miyagi, Y., Kishimoto, J., *et al.* (2009). Subthalamic nucleus stimulation does not cause deterioration of preexisting hallucinations in Parkinson's disease patients. *Stereotact Funct Neurosurg*, **87**, 45–9.

Zahodne, L.B., & Fernandez, H.H. (2008). Course, prognosis, and management of psychosis in Parkinson's disease: are current treatment really effective? *CNS Spectrums*, **13** (suppl 4), 26–33.

Zoldan, J., Friedberg, G., Livneh, M., & Melamed, E. (1995). Psychosis in advanced Parkinson's disease: treatment with ondansetron, a 5-HT3 receptor antagonist. *Neurology*, **45**, 1305–8.

Chapter 19

Assessment of hallucinations

Vaughan Bell, Andrea Raballo, and Frank Larøi

Introduction

Although the classification of a hallucination as a 'sensory perception in the absence of sensory stimulation' (Sims, 1995) is, perhaps, one of the clearest definitions in psychiatry, it is also remarkably limited in its ability to capture fully the meaning and experience of the many perceptual distortions to which we are susceptible. To most clinicians, the distinction between hallucinations occurring in different senses, and with or without 'insight', will be familiar. This belies the fact that the experience of hallucination can entail a change to multiple realms of personal and environmental experience that are described in light of each person's personal, social, and cultural influences (Al-Issa, 1995; Thomas *et al.*, 2007). These layers pervade not only the experience as described to the clinician, but also the development and emergence of perceptual change from the point where they may not even be describable or noticeable as perceptual anomalies to the point where they are no longer just aberrant perceptions, but part of a fundamental change in the way in which the sensory world is perceived and understood (see Jaspers, 1963; Ey, 1973; Stanghellini, 2004).

One of the challenges of clinical psychology and psychiatry is to understand the lived experience of another person, which, as years of struggling with the problem of consciousness has told us, is still not even within our conceptual reach. Those wishing to understand the hallucinatory experience of another person are additionally challenged by the fact the person may be experiencing the world in a way that we cannot clearly conceive of, perhaps, by virtue of the fact that the experiences are beyond what the person has ever encountered before or what is considered to be within the possibilities of normal human experience.

Indeed, anomalous perceptions are anomalous not so much due to the fact that they occur in the absence of sensory stimulation (in this sense, we are all hallucinating to some degree owing to the constructive nature of visual perception itself) but by the fact that the perception is accompanied by other feelings, such as urgency, certainty, and vividness. Jaspers (1963, p. 66) illustrated this point when discussing hallucinations in psychosis by noting that 'hallucinations…spring up on their own as something quite new and occur simultaneously with and alongside real perceptions'. Here, he alludes to the fact that hallucinations can affect the experience of immersion in the world at such a deep level as to share the same primitive immediacy of sensory experience but there are, of course, many ways in which a hallucinatory experience can be subjectively experienced. However, Jaspers' example illustrates why understanding the phenomenology of the experience, both in the mundane sense of 'symptoms' and the broader meaning of 'subjective experience', is critical in both clinical assessment and therapy.

This understanding will necessarily be incomplete but can be enriched by both clinical interview, grounded in the empathic quality of interpersonal rapport and focusing on narratives to 'situate particular experiences in the broader life context' (Stanghellini, 2004), and by the use of standardized assessments which attempt to quantify different aspects of the experience. A full exploration of the subtleties of the clinical interview in exploring atypical mental states is beyond the scope of this chapter, but we will focus on some of the better researched aspects of hallucinatory phenomena and indicate where standardized instruments exist to capture different facets of the experience. Thankfully, there are now a wide range of psychometrically validated assessments for this purpose, thanks both to the growing interest in a single-symptom approach to psychopathology (cf., Persons, 1986; Costello, 1992; Bentall, 2003) and to a resurgence of research activity examining hallucinations (cf., Aleman & Larøi, 2008).

It is important to note that not only should assessment include a detailed evaluation of the hallucinations themselves, as well as the contexts in which they appear, but also on the consequences for the person and their entourage (e.g., carers, family members, friends, etc.). The assessment of medical and psychiatric problems and the presence of adverse life events are also essential. See Goëb and Jardri (this volume) for a detailed presentation of recommended complementary examinations to be carried out in children and adolescents. Also, see Read *et al.* (2006, 2005) for discussions concerning the assessment of adverse life events (trauma) in psychotic patients.

Where appropriate, assessment of hallucinations should include instruments with documented adequate psychometric properties, including, for example, construct validity (i.e., whether a scale measures or correlates with the theorized psychological construct), internal consistency (whether items of a same scale correlate with each other), inter-rater reliability, and test-retest reliability. It is preferable that all hallucination modalities (e.g., verbal-auditory, visual, tactical, olfactory, and gustative) are assessed. It is also recommended that the following hallucination characteristics be evaluated: Frequency, severity, duration, physical characteristics (e.g., localization, volume, clarity), hallucination triggers, coping strategies, role of medication, beliefs concerning the origin of the hallucination, and degree of controllability of hallucinations (ability to make them appear and disappear). Also emotional aspects should be included in assessments including emotional reactions (e.g., distress, depression, anxiety, worry) that hallucinations may elicit in individuals experiencing them and in those in contact with the person, emotional content of hallucinations (negative and positive or an absence of emotional content), and emotional states preceding hallucinations (e.g., distress, depression, anxiety, worry). This chapter will not provide an exhaustive list of available instruments (for a more complete list, see Aleman & Larøi, 2008), but we hope to highlight how an understanding of the phenomenology of hallucinations can translate into practical strategies for assessment.

Clinical considerations

There are significant clinical implications of taking the multitude of hallucination characteristics into account, as can be done with some of the aforementioned assessment strategies (also see Larøi, 2006; Aleman & Larøi, 2008). For instance, it may provide patients with important information regarding their own experiences. Patients who are assessed with a (comprehensive) assessment instrument may gain new insight regarding their anxieties and fears, and perhaps even offer them new or different coping strategies for dealing with them. On the contrary, not taking these experiences into account might have disastrous effects. In many patients, for example, these experiences have been going on for a number of years and have become a part of their identity. Therefore, allowing the patient to talk about these experiences may have important positive clinical implications, whereas not being able to talk about them could have serious negative consequences.

The therapeutic alliance may also be improved if one takes into account the phenomenological diversity of hallucinations. Indeed, this may convey to the patient some understanding of the hallucinatory experience, which may ease communication with patients, in turn increasing empathy with patients. Taking into account the phenomenological diversity of hallucinations may help individualize treatment and management. For instance, treatment would be fundamentally different for a patient with primarily disturbing hallucinations versus patients with pleasurable hallucinations. In the latter case, the patient might not be very motivated to change because he or she does not perceive the hallucinations as negative or problematic. Also, in such patients, noncompliance with treatment might be related to this.

Research shows that it is the phenomenological characteristics of hallucinations (and not simply, for instance, the presence of hallucinations) that are improved after effective treatment or that are associated with important risk factors (e.g., Miller, 1996). Indeed, change is often not simply an on–off switch phenomenon but in most cases involves a qualitative change with, for example, changes in intensity, frequency, control, duration, or emotional impact.

Finally, taking into account the phenomenological diversity of hallucinations may also help provide important information concerning changes in the patient's condition. Research shows that localizations of hallucinations may change over time (e.g., Larkin, 1979; Romme *et al.*, 1992). For example, voices that were initially heard as coming from outside via the ears may eventually be perceived as being located within the hearer's own head or body. Furthermore, these changes may occur according to the hearer's mental and emotional state (e.g., when a person is stressed or upset, their voices may be loud and they may experience them as coming from outside). Also, patients sometimes observe that the voices are at one time 'telling jokes,' whereas at another point in time they 'become mean.' It is therefore plausible that these variations in the phenomenology reflect important changes in the patient's emotional state.

Dimensions and categories

For the purposes of fulfilling criteria in diagnostic categories, hallucinations have often been assessed as being 'present' or 'absent' in clinical practice (Sims, 2002). Over the last two decades, the application of a psychometric approach to measuring psychosis-like experience in the general population has reconceptualized perceptual distortions as occurring on a continuum throughout the population, and to differing degrees within each individual (Tien, 1991; Ohayon, 2000; Johns & van Os, 2001). Measures that have been taken from the traditional approach tend to be designed specifically for clinical settings, involve structured interviews, and require the assessor to make a judgement whether hallucinations are present or absent before rating their characteristics.

Along these lines, the Mental Health Research Institute Unusual Perception Schedule (MUPS; Carter *et al.*, 1995) and the Psychotic Symptom Rating Scales (PSYRATS; Haddock *et al.*, 1999) are semi-structured interviews that require an *a priori* clinical judgment as to whether the patient is hallucinating or not before they can be used. The MUPS is probably the most complete scale in terms of its ability to take into account the greatest number of phenomenological characteristics, although the PSYRATS is considerably shorter and better suited for repeated clinical monitoring. The specific aspects of the experience that they assess will be discussed in the section on auditory hallucinations.

Although not specifically designed as assessments solely for hallucinations, it is worth briefly mentioning how hallucinations are assessed in two of the most widely used assessment strategies for schizophrenic and psychotic patients: the Positive and Negative Syndrome Scale (PANSS; Kay *et al.*, 1987) and the Scale for the Assessment of Positive Symptoms (SAPS; Andreasen, 1984) both of which allow quasi-dimensional ratings from structured clinical interviews. In the PANSS, there is only one hallucinations dimension, in which hallucinations are assessed along a 7-point severity scale (absent, minimal, slight, average, moderately severe, severe, and extreme). However, different hallucination modalities are not assessed, and neither are hallucination characteristics (e.g., frequency, control, triggers, emotional aspects, localization, and physical qualities). In the SAPS, auditory (general, voices commenting, voices conversing), somatic or tactile, olfactory, and visual hallucinations are assessed individually along a 6-point severity scale (none, questionable, mild, moderate, marked, severe). However, here too, hallucination characteristics (e.g., frequency, control, triggers, emotional aspects, localization, and physical qualities) are not assessed.

Measures that focus on a dimensional approach to hallucinations are typically designed as self-report questionnaires that ask about both non-clinical sensory distortions (e.g., vivid daydreams and changes in sensory intensity) as well as frank hallucinatory experiences (e.g., hearing voices in the absence of any environmental source). These encompass both the traditional psychiatric definitions of a hallucination proper, and an illusion, or a distortion in genuine sensory experience. Although designed to cover both the non-clinical spectrum they are widely used in clinical settings and are typically validated on both healthy participants and psychotic in-patients samples. One of the most widely studied is the Launay-Slade Hallucinations Scale (LSHS; Launay & Slade, 1981), a self-report questionnaire for measuring hallucinatory experiences in both the clinical and nonclinical populations. Although the LSHS may be used in a clinical context, its particular strength is its usefulness in research contexts, especially in studies including both clinical and nonclinical subjects. Originally a 12-item scale designed to assess hallucinatory experiences in a prison population, a number of changes have since been made to the LSHS, including changing the negative response items to positive ones and substituting the true-and-false format with a 5-point scale (Bentall & Slade, 1985); incorporating additional items measuring predisposition to visual hallucinations, predisposition to auditory hallucinations, vividness of imagery, and daydreaming (Morrison *et al.*, 2002); and adding items assessing other subtypes of hallucinations, including visual, olfactory, haptic, gustatory, hypnagogic, and hypnopompic hallucinations (Larøi *et al.*, 2004; Larøi & Van der Linden, 2005). The internal structure of the LSHS has been examined on numerous occasions (Levitan *et al.*, 1996; Morrison *et al.*, 2000; Aleman *et al.*, 2001; Waters *et al.*, 2003; Larøi *et al.*, 2004; Larøi & Van der Linden, 2005; Serper *et al.*, 2005; Paulik *et al.*, 2006). Larøi and Van der Linden (2005) performed principal-components analysis on a revised version of the LSHS and found evidence of five factors that were characterized as representing items related to (a) sleep-related hallucinatory items, (b) vivid daydreams, (c) intrusive or vivid thoughts, (d) auditory hallucinations, and (e) visual hallucinations.

Notably, the LSHS focuses on a conception of hallucinations and sensory distortion drawn from clinical psychiatry, where visual and auditory distortions are given specific importance. The Cardiff Anomalous Perceptions Scale (CAPS; Bell *et al.*, 2006) is a 32-item scale designed to include distortions of proprioception, time perception, somatosensory, sensory flooding, and changes in intensity as well as frank hallucinations in the five main sensory modalities. It also includes additional ratings for distress, intrusiveness and frequency, and attempts to account for differences in insight. Despite being in an interview format, the Structured Interview for Assessing Perceptual Anomalies (SIAPA) does provide fully dimensional ratings although only measures changes in sensory intensity, lack of perceptual focus, and feelings of perceptual 'flooding' (Bunney *et al.*, 1999).

Insight

One important aspect in the experience of hallucinations is the extent to which the person considers them to be true or veridical perceptions, captured somewhat clumsily by the clinical concept of insight. The traditional 3-point psychiatric concept of insight (does the patient realize the experience is abnormal? Attribute it to a mental illness? Accept treatment?) is focused on the clinical needs of a diagnostic system (David, 1990), whereas the question of to what extent someone believes a perception to be an accurate reflection of the world is complex and multi-faceted. As Sackheim (1998, p. 9) noted 'since virtually all waking perceptual experiences are veridical, a long personal history of validated perception would dictate accepting hallucinations as veridical.' Many psychometric scales rely on variations of the question 'Do you ever experience things that aren't really there or seem strange?' and rely on the fact that a patient will know which perceptions are genuine and which are not, something which is clearly problematic. Instead, Bell *et al.* (2006) approached the problem from three angles, using questions that attempt to assess the likelihood of hallucinations regardless of the patient's understand of their experience. These include asking about whether a perceptual experience is not shared by others (e.g., 'Do you ever see things that other people cannot?'), whether the experience seems strange or unusual (e.g., 'Do you ever think that everyday things look abnormal to you?') and whether the perception arises form an unexplained source (e.g., 'Do you ever hear noises or sounds when there is nothing about to explain them?'). It is also clear that insight may fluctuate for some patients (Berrios & Brook, 1984) and that there can be a difference between 'spontaneous' and 'assisted' insight. Although not well researched, clinical experience suggests that hallucinatory perceptions accepted as veridical by a patient can be subsequently accepted as illusory after discussion with another person (assisted insight) or derived from the behaviour of others as they fail to react to something that seems to occur in shared space (spontaneous insight).

Auditory hallucinations

Perhaps the most striking form of hallucinations are Auditory Verbal Hallucinations (AVHs) that classically take the form of one or more 'voices' that talk to or about the patient. While the most clinically important, owing to their intrusive nature and association with psychosis, they are not the only form of auditory hallucinations that may also take the form of noises, sounds, or quite often, music.

However, AVHs are a common symptom of schizophrenia and other florid psychotic conditions and, hence, have been a particular focus of assessment research. Audible thoughts and imperative voices, for example, have been almost consistently considered of important clinical value since Kraepelin and Bleuler and are explicitly indicated as symptoms of primary diagnostic importance (so-called First-Rank Symptoms, FRS) by Kurt Schneider. Such primacy is still maintained in DSM-IV-TR, where FRS are recoded as bizarre delusions and hallucinations consisting of 'hearing one voice participating in a running commentary of the patient's actions or of hearing two or more voices conversing with each other'.

Despite having been given such diagnostic weight, AVHs can be difficult to fully assess in the clinical context. First, they are not fully captured by operational criteria, as the experience of 'hearing voices' varies greatly between individuals and may involve numerous disturbances of agency, autonomy, and the 'stream of consciousness'. Second, they are associated with profound transformations of self-awareness that may be difficult to describe, which can lead to feelings of estrangement from common human experience and communication (Straus, 1966; Stanghellini, 2004; Dalle Luche, 2006; Cermolacce, 2007). Finally, most patients note how even the most common description of AVH as 'voices' is a rather poor metaphor, which does not fully capture the richness of their experience.

As can be seen from the quotes below, one common difficulty is that AVHs are not clearly distinguished from other environmental sounds or from other aspects of the 'stream of consciousness'.

> At these times my ear took some part in hearing the voices. This was not so before when I responded to the voices without any auditory sensation. Now even though I distinguished them readily from real voices, I could say I actually heard them resounding in my room. And then I kept seeing everything in a confusion of terrible unreality: each object cut off, under a cold and blinding light. (Sechehaye, 1951)
>
> The voices and so on were not that important. I think that the enduring and pervasive feeling of being unreal is the disease itself. When I realized this condition of looking at myself as in a movie was permanent, I understood it would eventually destroy the core of my life. (Møller & Husby, 2000)

Needless to say, it is easy to impose our own ideas about what the experience of 'hearing voices' might be like, typically focusing on the vocal, perceptual-like features of AVHs, but we would be in danger of missing many of the equally as significant aspects of the total change in experience brought about by the psychotic experience.

The emergence of auditory verbal hallucinations

Detailed phenomenological analyses of hallucinations reveal that a broad metamorphosis of psychotic consciousness precedes the appearance of florid hallucinations. Specifically, transitional sequences from more subtle, not-yet psychotic disturbances of subjectivity have been empirically identified and documented (Klosterkötter, 1988, 1992). In particular, disturbances of the stream of consciousness, such as thought pressure, thought interference, thought block, obsessive-like perseveration, and failure to discriminate between thought and perception, seem to precede the emergence of AVHs (Klosterkötter, 1988, 1992). As the prodromal state progresses, there can be an increasing gap between the sense of self and the flow of consciousness: inner speech becomes more and more objectified, spatially localized and externally perceived even before well-established auditory hallucinations emerge (Sass & Parnas, 2003). Qualitative changes in the immediacy and familiarity of the thought stream can be some of the first manifestations of a later psychotic episode.

Notably, both contemporary psychiatry and the cognitive neurosciences almost exclusively investigate hallucinations in their frank form, neglecting the changes in consciousness and experience that lead to these psychopathological end-points. This has some clear implications with respect to both research and clinical practice. Needless to say, an exclusive focus on florid symptoms, such as overt AVHs, does not allow an in-depth examination of etiological mechanisms (e.g., like investigating heart attacks in order to understand hypertension) and is not always informative for the purpose of early diagnosis and timely preventative intervention.

However, several phenomenologically inspired scales have been developed, which attempt to capture some of these processes. These include the Bonn Scale for the Assessment of Basic Symptoms (Gross *et al.*, 1987), the Schizophrenia Proneness Instrument (Schultze-Lutter *et al.*, 2007), and the Examination of Anomalous

Self-Experience (Parnas *et al.*, 2005), all which address subtle and 'not-yet-psychotic' changes in subjective experience. The Bonn scale for the Assessment of Basic Symptoms (BSABS) is a semi structured interview, originally published in German (Gross *et al.*, 1987) but currently available in an English translation (Gross *et al.*, 2008), which addresses subtle, subjectively experienced disturbances termed 'basic symptoms' in the domains of perception, cognition, language, motor function, will, initiative and level of energy, and stress tolerance. These disturbances are closely linked to the hypothetical core vulnerability of schizophrenia and are presumed to be the first experiential correlate of the underlying neurobiological disorder. The scale consists of five subsets of the basic symptoms: (a) dynamic deficits, (b) cognitive disturbances, (c) coenesthetic experiences, (d) central vegetative disturbances, and (e) self-protective behaviour/coping. Each basic symptom is rated as present or absent and some of them-particularly those inhering disturbances of cognition, speech, and perception-reveal a highly predictive value for the subsequent development of schizophrenia (Klosterkötter *et al.*, 2001). The Schizophrenia Proneness Instrument (SPI-A) was developed by Schultze-Lutter *et al.* (2007; 2010) with a specific focus on early detection of prodromal patients. It is based on a selection of BSABS items drawn from cluster and facet analyses, performed on data from the Cologne early recognition study (Klosterkötter *et al.*, 2001). The SPI-A consists of six subscales: (a) affective-dynamic disturbances, (b) cognitive-attentional impediments, (c) cognitive disturbances, (d) disturbances in experiencing the self and surroundings, (e) body perception disturbances, and (f) perception disturbances. The Examination of Anomalous Self-Experience (EASE) is a symptom checklist to assist the semi-structured exploration of disorders of subjectivity which was developed by Parnas and colleagues (Parnas, 1999; Parnas & Handest, 2003; Parnas *et al.*, 2005). The EASE addresses phenomena that are regarded as important phenomenological aspects in the pre-onset phase and as core features of schizophrenia spectrum disorders. The interview consists of five subscales: (a) cognition and stream of consciousness, (b) disorders of self-awareness and presence, (c) bodily experience, (d) transitivism/demarcation, and (e) existential reorientation/solipsism.

Perceptual properties of auditory verbal hallucinations

While there are clearly changes in meaning and subjective experience of the mind itself that accompany the experience of AVHs, it is most common for assessments to focus on the perceptual properties of the voices. These can include factors such as how many voices are present, whether the voice appears to originate from inside or outside the head, whether they are male or female, seem loud or soft, clear or indistinct, or coherent or nonsensical (Wykes, 2004). Other typical targets for assessment might be the frequency and durations of voices and their intrusiveness.

The MUPS (Carter *et al.*, 1995) is a semi-structured interview for auditory hallucinations and has items assessing various aspects of hallucinations, such as physical characteristics (e.g., frequency, when during the day, localization, volume, clarity), personal characteristics (e.g., sex of the voice; number of voices; known voice or not; whether in first, second, or third person), relations and emotion (e.g., relation with the voice, emotional state during the experience, associated emotions), form and contents (e.g., linguistic complexity, repeated contents, commands), cognitive processes (e.g., delusional activity, language or accent), perception of the experience (e.g., imaginary vs. real, hallucinations in other modalities), and psychosocial aspects (e.g., triggers, strategies used, role of medication).

Although less detailed compared to the MUPS, the PSYRATS (Haddock *et al.*, 1999) consists of 11 items assessing dimensions (based on a 5-point scale) of frequency, duration, location, loudness, beliefs concerning the origin of voices (varying from the belief that they are solely internally generated to solely from external causes), amount of negative content of voices, degree of negative content, amount of distress, intensity of distress, disruption of life caused by voices, and controllability of voices. Finally, the number of voices (over the past week) and the form of the voices (first person, second person, third person; single words, or phrases without pronouns) are assessed. The scales have been found to have excellent inter-rater reliability (Haddock *et al.*, 1999).

Similar hallucination characteristics are included in the Auditory Vocal Hallucination Rating Scale (AVHRS; Jenner *et al.*, 2002), and also included in this instrument are items on hypnagogic and hypnopompic voices, the degree to which voices interfere with thinking, and a question verifying whether voices are talking one by one or simultaneously. Results from Bartels-Velthuis *et al.* (submitted) revealed that the AVHRS has good internal consistency and inter-rater reliability.

Emotional and social aspects of auditory verbal hallucinations

The impact of auditory hallucinations is usually one of the most clinically significant aspects of the experience and is affected by the person's attributions for the experience, their perception of control over the voices, their emotional state, culture, prior social experience, and ability to resist commands or requests. Indeed, AVHs in schizophrenia can be part of a wide array of 'passivity experiences', characterized by a disturbance of the sense of agency and autonomy. Rather than the perceptual qualities of the hallucinated voice, it is the clients' understanding and beliefs about the experience, which typically drives distress and disability and is typically the target of psychological treatment.

Emotional factors may play a significant role in the experience of AVHs. This is particularly the case for psychiatric hallucinations and somewhat less so for neurological and pharmacologically-induced hallucinations. Three aspects can be distinguished: emotional antecedents, emotional content, and emotional consequences. Certain affective states have been associated with the onset of psychotic symptoms. For instance, a stage of heightened awareness and emotionality combined with a sense of anxiety and impasse has consistently been described as preceding psychosis. AVHs often have a negative, maladaptive quality. Indeed, voices may insult and criticize the patient, tell the patient to do something unacceptable (e.g., to commit suicide or to harm someone), or threaten the patient. However, AVHs are not exclusively perceived as negative by patients—some AVHs may not have a particular emotional content (i.e., are more or less neutral) and some patients may even state that their voices serve an adaptive function (help feel privileged or protected, they relieve boredom, provide an outlet for hostility, help raise self-esteem, provide comfort, etc.). Finally, for a large majority of patients, their AVHs elicit negative emotional responses such as fear, distress, anxiety, and depression.

The MUPS provides a relatively sophisticated assessment of affective aspects of AVHs. In particular, the tone of the voice (e.g., as harsh, angry, gentle, bossy, menacing, loving, etc.) is assessed, in addition to whether the tone has changed over time. Similarly, content of voices (e.g., as persecutory, abusive, obscene, derogatory, guiding, affirming, inspiring, threatening, etc.), and if the content has changed over time, is evaluated. Finally, feelings associated with AVHs (e.g. feeling terrified, irritated, sad, helpless, angry, anxious, comforted, assured, depressed, excited, frightened, confused, inspired, happy, intruded upon, etc.) is also assessed. Another instrument, the Positive and Useful Voices Inventory (PUVI; Jenner *et al.*, 2008), provides an assessment of positive (e.g., 'Want to protect me', 'Make me confident') and useful (e.g., 'Give me advice, 'Help me to make decisions') AVHs and emotional attribution.

Using the MUPS, Copolov *et al.* (2004) examined the affective impact of AVHs in detail in a group of 199 patients (the majority with schizophrenia and affective psychosis). Patients' responses to auditory hallucinations were combined into two (uncorrelated) indexes: one assessing total affective impact (i.e., the strength of affective response) and the other, assessing the affective direction (i.e., the degree of positivity or negativity). The authors argued that this suggests that (at least) two dimensions are required to characterize subjects' positive and negative experiences of and responses to auditory hallucinations. That is, even subjects who assess the tone, content, and feeling of their auditory hallucinations as extremely negative may also rate part of their experience in positive terms. Also, in this study, various differential associations (too many to detail here) were found based on this more sophisticated dimensional assessment of affective impact. For instance, it was found that frequent, long, and loud auditory hallucinations were more often perceived as negative. The auditory hallucinations of patients with grandiose delusions were found to be more pleasant than those of patients without such delusions. Also, auditory hallucinations addressing the patient in the second person were found to be significantly more unpleasant than those that did not address the patient in the second person.

Another striking and persuasive feature of AVHs can be the omnipotence and seeming omnipresence of the voices. They have been described as 'atmospheric, they behave like the elements—the wind, the rain, the fire—and yet they speak, deride, and threaten.' (Straus, 1966, p. 287). Hearing voices can seem like being 'at the centre of a *network of disembodied voices*' (Stanghellini, 2004, p. 161), which undoubtedly plays a part in a perception of their power over the individual, as noted by Chadwick and Birchwood (1994):

> without exception, voices were seen as omnipotent…For many patients this […] was supported by an experience of control […] and by the patient having no influence over the voice. Also, all voices were seen as omniscient, again emphasizing their superhuman quality.

These aspects of the experience can have a profound impact on the voice hearer but can be neglected in many assessments that focus on perceptual qualities.

In light of this, the Beliefs About Voices Questionnaire (BAVQ; Chadwick & Birchwood, 1995) does not elicit detailed and wide-ranging information concerning phenomeno-logical characteristics of hallucinations—its unique contribution is that it provides the clinician and researcher with related and crucial information concerning how subjects react in the face of hallucinatory experiences. The BAVQ is a 30-item self-report instrument that measures how people perceive and respond to their verbal auditory hallucinations. It includes five subscales: (a) Malevolence (e.g., 'My voice is evil'), (b) benevolence (e.g., 'My voice wants to help me'), (c) omnipotence (e.g., 'My voice is very powerful'), (d) resistance (e.g., 'When I hear my voice, I usually think of preventing it from talking'), and (e) engagement (e.g., 'When I hear my voice, I usually seek its advice'). Among these five subscales, three relate to beliefs about voices (malevolence, benevolence, and omnip-otence) and two measure emotional and behavioural reactions to the voices (resistance and engagement). All responses are rated by checking 'yes' or 'no.' Individuals who hear more than one voice are asked to complete the questionnaire for their predominant voice. The BAVQ shows acceptable levels of reliability, validity, and stability on test-retest over 1 week (Chadwick & Birchwood, 1995). A revised version of the BAVQ has also been developed (the Beliefs About Voices Questionnaire-Revised; BAVQ-R; Chadwick et al., 2000) to address two weaknesses in the original BAVQ: Participants answered 'yes' or 'no' to each of the items, and there was only one item concerning omnipotence. The revised version contains 35 items (which includes 5 new items pertaining to omnipotence), and responses are rated on a 4-point scale (disagree, unsure, agree slightly, and agree strongly). Results from Chadwick et al. (2000) revealed that the BAVQ-R was more reliable and sensitive to individual differences than the BAVQ and that the BAVQ-R reliably measures omnipotence.

Another pertinent scale to mention that assesses other aspects related to hallucinations, namely, how individuals cope with these experiences, is the Maastricht Assessment of Coping Strategies (MACS; Bak et al., 2001). The MACS is a semi-structured interview that asks patients about the presence of a list of 24 symptoms related to psychosis. Both audi-tory hallucinations and nonverbal hallucinatory experiences (visual, olfactory, gustatory, or tactile hallucinations) are included in this list. If a symptom is present, subjects are asked whether it has been present in the last week or month and to indicate (on a 7-point scale) the degree of distress associated with the symptom (varying from no distress to very distressing). In terms of coping strategies, patients are asked to name all the strategies used to alleviate the distress caused by the symptom. These coping strategies are catego-rized by the interviewer on the basis of a list of 14 different coping strategies. Factor analysis has identified five coping domains: active problem solving (distraction, problem solving, help seeking), passive illness behaviour (prescribed medication, non-prescribed substances, physical change), active problem avoiding (shifted attention, socialization, task performance, indulgence), passive problem avoiding (isolation, nonspecific activities, suppression), and symptomatic behaviour. Results from Bak et al. (2001) indicate that the

MACS has good inter-rater and test-retest reliability. Also see Farhall (this volume) for a guide to how to assess coping strategies in individuals experiencing hallucinations.

Culture has a certain influence on hallucination prevalence and expression (cf. Aleman & Larøi, 2008). Al-Issa (1995) suggests that contrasting (metaphysical) attitudes between cultures, such as between Western and non-Western cultures, varying, for example, in the degree to which a given experience is considered real or imaginary, could explain these cultural variations. There is, for example, evidence of cultural variation in the frequency of different kinds of hallucinations between cultures—where auditory hallucinations are more frequently reported by patients in the West compared to visual hallucinations being more frequently reported in African and Asian countries. (see Aleman & Larøi, 2008 for a review). Studies reveal that it is common for people to see, hear, or feel the presence of the deceased person during bereavement, and that there are cultural differences in terms of the rates of hallucinatory experiences in the context of bereavement (Grimby, 1993, 1998; Yamamoto et al., 1969). Kent and Wahass (1996) observe that a religious and superstitious content was more likely to be reported by patients from Saudi Arabia, whereas instruction and running commentary were more commonly reported by patients from the UK. Also, Wahass and Kent (1997a) found that patients from the United Kingdom were more likely to use biological and psychological approaches to explain the apparition of their hallucinations, whereas patients from Saudi Arabia were more likely to evoke religious and superstitious causes. Finally, patients in Saudi Arabia tend to use coping strategies for their hallucinations that are associated with their religion, whereas patients in the United Kingdom are more likely to use distraction or physiologically based approaches (Wahass & Kent, 1997b).

Evidence of cultural variations has clinical implications. Simply put, the clinician, in addition to providing a detailed account of the hallucinations, must also take into account a person's cultural background when assessing and treating hallucinations. Thus, the treatment strategies that clinicians propose should attempt to take into account the etiological beliefs of their patients. As Bentall (2003) pointed out, failure to appreciate the cultural context may prevent clinicians from responding appropriately to the distress experienced by their patients. On the other hand, where hallucinatory experiences are culturally accepted reactions to various life events (and therefore might be quite common), the clinician may consider not intervening at all. Thus, awareness of people's attitudes toward hallucinations may help the clinician distinguish between pathological and culturally sanctioned hallucinations (Al-Issa, 1995).

Some assessment tools have been developed for use (but not exclusively) in the context of specific types of auditory hallucinations, such as command hallucinations. The Voice Compliance Scale (Beck-Sander et al., 1997) is an observer-rated scale to measure the frequency of command hallucinations and the level of compliance or resistance with each identified command. The Voice Power Differential Scale (Birchwood et al., 2000) measures the perceived relative power differential between voice and voice hearer with regard to the components of power, including strength, confidence, respect, ability to inflict harm, superiority, and knowledge. There are seven items, and each is rated on a 5-point scale and yields a total power score.

Musical hallucinations

Musical hallucinations most typically present in older people and females and are most associated with hearing loss, psychiatric disorder, focal brain lesions, epilepsy, and intoxication, although, unlike auditory verbal hallucinations, are not most commonly associated with psychotic mental illness (Evers & Ellger, 2004). Indeed, for an estimated 40% of patients, they present as the only symptom (Berrios, 1991). The music can be varied and can include both singing and instrumental arrangements, popular tunes, religious music, traditional music, and even unfamiliar and unknown melodies. Although musical hallucinations are often considered benign, it is worth noting that in their analysis of 73 cases, Evers and Ellger (2004) reported that 41% of patients found the experience frightening, although it is not clear how much this is to do with the perceptual qualities of the music or the fact that the experiences sparks distressing concerns about 'going mad'. As with Charles Bonnet syndrome, it is likely that these experiences are under-reported for this reason.

Visual Hallucinations

Visual perceptual distortions can occur in a wide range of pathological and non-pathological conditions with phenomena ranging from flashes of light, alterations in sensory acuity and stability of objects in the visual field, to fully formed complex scenes of a fantastical nature.

Curiously, impairments to the earliest stage of the visual system, the retina, can lead to some of the most spectacular hallucinations. The following description is from a case of Charles Bonnet syndrome owing to macular degeneration (Jacob *et al.*, 2004):

> Neighbours brought an 87-year-old white widower—who lived alone in a flat—to the medical assessment unit of a district general hospital. They were concerned that he was becoming demented. Apparently, he had reported seeing people and animals in his house—including bears and Highland cattle. He verified these statements and said he had been seeing them for the previous six weeks. He had also often seen swarms of flies and blue fish darting across the room. He knew that these visions were not real and they didn't bother him much, but he thought he might be losing his mind. The visions lasted for minutes to hours, and the cattle used to stare at him while quietly munching away at the grass. The visions tended to occur more in the evenings before he switched on the lights.

These hallucinations tend to appear in the area of visual field loss have a number of typical features (Plummer *et al.*, 2006): they are exacerbated by dim lighting, drowsiness, and isolation and are typically experienced with good insight with the patient feeling as if they are an 'onlooker' rather than an active participant. Despite their high prevalence in older adults, clinicians should be aware that patients may be reluctant to report the experiences for fear of appearing 'mad', even though they are rarely associated with psychiatric illness (Teunisse *et al.*, 1995).

Various forms of 'hallucinosis' are also commonly reported in the neurological literature. Hallucinosis refers to complex auditory or visual hallucinations with preserved insight (sometimes called 'pseudo hallucinations' for this reason), without delusion or concurrent disturbances to consciousness, although, in practice, the term is used some-what vaguely and can be used to refer generally to hallucinations as a consequence of organic brain disease. Most commonly discussed in the literature are alcoholic hallucino-sis, triggered by acute alcohol withdrawal and more likely to involve auditory hallucina-tions and paranoid ideation (Glass, 1989), and peduncular hallucinosis, triggered by lesions in the midbrain and pons and having a significant overlap with Charles Bonnet syndrome (Mocellin *et al.*, 2006).

Geometric patterns, grids and lines, often described as 'form constants' (Kluver, 1966) are another form of hallucinatory experience in which the subject typically retains good insight. These are associated with migraine, occipital lobe epilepsy, certain hallucinogenic drugs, and the visual flicker in the 8–13 Hz range (Panayiotopoulos, 1999; Ter Meulen *et al.*, 2009) and are thought to arise from unstable activity and desynchronized commu-nication in the early visual system (Ffytche, 2008).

Visual hallucinations that seem to have particular reference to the person experiencing them are more likely to occur in psychoses such as schizophrenia or bipolar disorder or in the context of psychoses after gross neuropathology and are less likely to be perceived as unreal and may form part of a larger delusional system (Cutting, 1987).

Sadly, there are few scales that attempt to specifically tackle visual hallucinations, although they are covered as part of more comprehensive assessments (e.g., in the LHSH, Larøi & Van der Linden, 2005; and CAPS, Bell *et al.*, 2006). One that does target the area, however, is the Institute of Psychiatry Visual Hallucinations Interview (Santhouse *et al.*, 2000) that was developed from a previous unstructured survey (Ffytche & Howard, 1999). Participants are questioned about various phenomenological categories of patho-logical visual experience, such as temporal aspects (e.g., duration of individual hallucina-tions, length of time subjects have been hallucinating, frequency), emotional content (pleasant, unpleasant, neutral), localization (e.g., in front of the subject, out of the corner of the eye, in their blind area), detail and physical characteristics (e.g., more detail than real objects, whole scenes or individual objects or figures, can you see through them, flashes, lines, colours, zigzags, regular or irregular patterns, face without a body, words, letters, musical notes, numbers), and triggers (e.g., if they appear when the participant's eyes are closed, if they disappear when the participant blinks or move his or her head). In addition, there are exclusion questions (e.g., visions associated with sound or talking, diz-ziness, or strange smells; occurrence only in bed or on waking from sleep; history of psychiatric and/or neurological disorders; frightening visions of small animals, snakes, maggots).

More recently, Mosimann *et al.* (2008) developed the North-East Visual Hallucinations Interview (NEVHI), a semi-structured interview for identifying and assessing visual hal-lucinations in older people with eye disease and/or cognitive impairment. Section 1 includes screening questions for visual hallucinations and a detailed assessment of the phenomenology, section 2 assesses the temporal aspects of hallucinations (i.e., when they first started, and duration and frequency of hallucinations), section 3 evaluates emotions, cognitions, and behaviours associated with recurrent visual hallucinations. Results from

Mosimann *et al.* (2008) revealed that the NEVHI possesses good psychometric properties including good face and content validities, internal consistency, and inter-rater reliability.

Hallucinations in other modalities

Somatic hallucinations

Although much less commonly discussed, somatic hallucinations are a remarkably diverse form of perceptual distortion that appear in numerous conditions. Although auditory verbal hallucinations are considered to be one of the main symptoms of schizophrenia, the experience of 'influences playing on the body' are also listed among Schneider's (1959) 'first rank symptoms'. In schizophrenia, they are usually linked to thematically related delusional beliefs and may include specific tactile sensations, for example, touches, stab sensations, sexual feelings, or alterations to the body image or proprioception, such as the stretching or distortion of the body (e.g., Lewandowski *et al.*, 2009). Additionally, hallucinations may occur as sensations seeming to arise in internal bodily organs, including internal movements, changes to how a part of the body 'feels' (such as the perception that a hand has 'turned to jelly'), and internal spatial distortions. These are not well studied but have been historically described as 'cenesthetic hallucinations' (Jenkins & Röhricht, 2007). 'Phantom' sensations are where patients have sensations from amputated body parts and are a normal consequence of surgery. Although typically described as a 'phantom limb', the experience can follow after removing almost any body parts including the eyes, teeth, tongue, breasts, rectum, or bladder and occur in 50% to 78% of post-amputation patients (Schley *et al.*, 2008). The sensation of 'bugs' crawling over or just under the skin is commonly associated with stimulant drugs that affect the dopamine system, such as cocaine, amphetamine, and L-DOPA treatment in Parkinson's disease and in its delusional form may present as delusional parasitosis where the patient believes they are infested with a parasite (Koo & Lee, 2001).

Olfactory and gustatory hallucinations

Hallucinations of touch and taste are among the most common reported perceptual distortions in the general population (Tien, 1991; Ohayon, 2000) but receive far less clinical attention. However, they can present in multiple conditions and in their non-delusional form are most linked to epileptic aura or simple-partial seizures (Elliot *et al.*, 2009) and in their delusional form can be associated with schizophrenia or 'olfactory reference syndrome' where the patient believes they emit an offensive odour despite evidence to the contrary (Bizamcer *et al.*, 2008).

Time and space

Changes in time perception are particularly common in patients with neurodegenerative disorders that affect the basal ganglia such as Parkinson's and Huntingdon's disease (Wild-Wall *et al.*, 2008). Specific alterations to the perception of relative size of the body or external world without other visual disturbances is usually associated with 'Alice in Wonderland' syndrome, micro- or macrosomatognosia, which is relatively more common in children and usually linked to migraine or epilepsy (Todd, 1955; Evans & Rolak, 2004).

Conclusion

Despite their seemingly simple definition, hallucinations constitute a challenging target for clinical assessment. Hallucinatory experiences, usually classified according to their sensory qualities, also entail complex cognitive and emotional aspects that need to be addressed not only for research and diagnostic purposes, but also for and adequate identification of treatment needs that will guide the therapeutic approach. Such assessment needs to be context-dependent and informed by a preliminary recognition of the layers of personal, social, and cultural influences that might affect the patient's modes of experiencing and, hence, communicating his or her own subjective experience.

Notably, besides their phenomenological heterogeneity, hallucinations are dynamic and can change in time. In this respect, assessment instruments offer a valuable support for longitudinal monitoring. Moreover, addressing the very moment of their emergence constitutes a useful entry point for a more person-tailored evaluation and a deeper understanding of their existential and psychological impact. The assessment instruments discussed in this chapter are meant to constitute strategic tools to enrich and supplement the clinical investigation of hallucinations, specifically providing reproducible quantitative frameworks. Their use provides both the patient and the clinician with a shared medium to reframe experiences. Besides the obvious implications in terms of informational gathering and consolidation of the therapeutic alliance, this can be an important part of overcoming stigma and difficulties with the verbalization of the experiences often associated with hallucinations. This is clearly an important step towards tailored treatment and can support both an understanding of the exacerbating or maintaining factors (e.g., intense emotional valences in auditory verbal hallucinations) and the strengthening of basic coping strategies.

References

Al-Issa, I. (1995). The illusion of reality or the reality of illusion. Hallucinations and culture. *Br J Psychiatry*, **166**, 368–373.

Aleman, A., Nieuwenstein, M.R., Böcker, K.B.E., & de Haan, E.H.F. (2001). Multi-dimensionality of hallucinatory predisposition: Factor structure of the Launay-Slade Hallucination Scale in a normal sample. *Personality and Individual Differences*, **30**, 287–292.

Aleman, A., & Larøi, F. (2008). *Hallucinations: The science of idiosyncratic perception*. Washington D.C.: American Psychological Association.

Andreasen, N.C. (1984). *The scale for the assessment of positive symptoms (SAPS)*. Iowa City: The University of Iowa.

Bak, M., van der Spil, F., Gunther, N., Radstake, S., Delespaul, P., & van Os, J. (2001). Maastricht assessment of coping strategies (MACS-I): A brief instrument to assess coping with psychotic symptoms. *Acta Psychiatr Scand*, **103**, 453–459.

Bartels-Velthuis, A.A., van de Willige, G., Jenner, J.A., & Wiersma, D. (submitted). The Psychometric Evaluation of the Auditory Vocal Hallucination Rating Scale (AVHRS).

Beck-Sander, A., Birchwood, M., & Chadwick, P. (1997). Acting on command hallucinations: a cognitive approach. *Br J Clin Psychol*, **36**, 139–148.

Bell, V., Halligan, P.W., & Ellis, H.D. (2006). The Cardiff anomalous perceptions scale (CAPS): A new validated measure of anomalous perceptual experience. *Schizophr Bull*, **32**, 366–377.

Bentall, R.P., & Slade, P.D. (1985). Reliability of a scale measuring disposition towards hallucination: a brief report. *Personality and Individual Differences*, **6**, 527–529.

Bentall, R.P. (2003). *Madness explained: psychosis and human nature*. London: Penguin.

Berrios, G.E., & Brook, P. (1984). Visual hallucinations and sensory delusions in the elderly. *Br J Psychiatry*, 144, 662–664.

Berrios, G.E. (1991). Musical hallucinations: a statistical analysis of 46 cases. *Psychopathology*, **24**, 356–360.

Birchwood, M., Meaden, A., Trower, P., Gilbert, P., & Plaistow, J. (2000). The power and omnipotence of voices: subordnation and entrapment by voices and significant others. *Psychol Med*, **30**, 337–344.

Bizamcer, A.N., Dubin, W.R., & Hayburn, B. (2008). Olfactory reference syndrome. *Psychosomatics*, **49**, 77–81.

Bunney, W.E. Jr, Hetrick, W.P., Bunney, B.G., *et al.* (1999). Structured interview for assessing perceptual anomalies (SIAPA). *Schizophr Bull*, **25**, 577–592.

Carter, D.M., Mackinnon, A., Howard, S., Zeegers, T., & Copolov, D.L. (1995). The development and reliability of the mental health research institute perceptions schedule (MUPS): an instrument to record auditory hallucinatory experience. *Schizophrenia Research*, **16**, 157–165.

Cermolacce, M., Naudin, J., & Parnas, J. (2007). The 'minimal self' in psychopathology: Re-examining the self-disorders in the schizophrenia spectrum. *Conscious Cogn*, **16**, 703–714.

Chadwick, P., & Birchwood, M. (1994). The omnipotence of voices: Part I. *Br J Psychiatry*, **164**, 190–201.

Chadwick, P., & Birchwood, M. (1995). The omnipotence of voices II: The beliefs about voices questionnaire (BVAQ). *Br J Psychiatry*, **166**, 773–776.

Chadwick, P., Lees, S., & Birchwood, M. (2000). The revised beliefs about voices questionnaire (BAVQ-R). *Br J Psychiatry*, **177**, 229–232.

Copolov, D.L., Mackinnon, A., & Trauer, T. (2004). Correlates of the affective impact of auditory hallucinations in psychotic disorders. *Schizophr Bull*, **30**, 163–171.

Costello, C.G. (1992). Research on symptoms versus research on syndromes: arguments in favour of allocating more research time to the study of symptoms. *Br J Psychiatry*, **160**, 304–308.

Cutting, J. (1987). The phenomenology of acute organic psychosis. Comparison with acute schizophrenia. *Br J Psychiatry*, **151**, 324–332.

Dalle Luche, R. (2006). Una ricognizione fenomenologica delle allucinazioni acustiche verbali. *Rivista Sperimentale di Freniatria*, **130**, 65–86.

David, A.S. (1990). Insight and psychosis. *Br J Psychiatry*, **156**, 798–808.

Elliott, B., Joyce, E., & Shorvon, S. (2009). Delusions, illusions and hallucinations in epilepsy: 1. Elementary phenomena. *Epilepsy Research*, **85**, 162–171.

Evans, R.W., & Rolak, L.A. (2004). The Alice in wonderland syndrome. *Headache*, **44**, 624–625.

Evers, S., & Ellger, T. (2004). The clinical spectrum of musical hallucinations. *J Neurol Sci*, **227**, 55–65.

Ey, H. (1973). *Traité des hallucinations* (2 volumes). Paris: Masson et Cie.

Ffytche, D.H., & Howard, R.J. (1999). The perceptual consequences of visual loss: 'positive' pathologies of vision. *Brain*, **122**, 1247–1260.

Ffytche, D.H. (2008). The hodology of hallucinations. *Cortex*, **44**, 1067–1083.

Glass, I.B. (1989). Alcoholic hallucinosis: a psychiatric enigma. 1. The development of an idea. *Br J Addict*, **84**, 29–41.

Grimby, A. (1993). Bereavement among elderly people: Grief reactions, post-bereavement hallucinations and quality of life. *Acta Psychiatr Scand,* **87**, 72–80.

Grimby, A. (1998). Hallucinations following the loss of a spouse: Common and normal events among the elderly. *Journal of Clinical Gerontology,* **4**, 65–74.

Gross, G., Huber, G., Klosterkoetter, J., & Linz, M. (1987). *Bonner Skala fur die Beurteilung von Basissymptomen.* Berlin: Springer.

Gross, G., Huber, G., Klosterkotter, J., & Linz, M (2008). *Bonn scale for the assessment of basic symptoms: 1st complete english edition.* Germany: Shaker Verlag GmbH.

Gruhle, H. W. (1952). Schizophrenia. *Die Medizinische,* **20**, 1585–1588.

Haddock, G., McCarron, J., Tarrier, N., & Faragher, E.B. (1999). Scales to measure dimensions of hallucinations and delusions: The psychotic symptoms rating scale (PSYRATS). *Psychol Med,* **29**, 879–889.

Jacob, A., Prasad, S., Boggild, M., & Chandratre, S. (2004). Charles Bonnet syndrome—elderly people and visual hallucinations. *Br Med J,* **328**, 1552–1554.

Jaspers, K. (1963). *General Psychopathology.* J. Hoenig & M. W. Hamilton (Trs). Chicago: The University of Chicago Press.

Jenkins, G., & Röhricht, F. (2007). From cenesthesias to cenesthopathic schizophrenia: a historical and phenomenological review. *Psychopathology,* **40**, 361–368.

Jenner J.A., & Van de Willige, G. (2002) The auditory vocal hallucination rating scale (AVHRS). Groningen: University Medical Center Groningen, University Center for Psychiatry, University of Groningen.

Jenner, J.A., Rutten, S., Beuckens, J., Boonstra, N., & Sytema, S. (2008). Positive and useful auditory vocal hallucinations: prevalence, characteristics, attributions, and implications for treatment. *Acta Psychiatr Scand,* **118**, 238–245.

Johns, L.C., & van Os, J. (2001). The continuity of psychotic experiences in the general population. *Clin Psychol Rev,* **21**, 1125–1141.

Kay, S.R., Fiszbein, A., & Opler, L.A. (1987). The positive and negative syndrome scale (PANSS) for Schizophrenia. *Schizophr Bull,* **13**, 261–276.

Kent, G., & Wahass, S. (1996). The content and characteristics of auditory hallucinations in Saudi Arabia and the UK: A cross-cultural comparison. *Acta Psychiatr Scand,* **94**, 433–437.

Klosterkötter, J. (1988). *Basissymptome und Endphänomeneder Schizophrenie. Eine empirische Untersuchung der psychopathologischen Übergangsreihen zwischen defizitären und produktiven Schizophreniesymptomen.* Berlin: Springer.

Klosterkötter, J. (1992). The meaning of basic symptoms for the genesis of schizophrenic nuclear syndrome. *Jpn J Psychiatry Neurol,* 46, 609–630.

Klosterkötter, J., Hellmich, M., Steinmeyer, E.M., & Schultze-Lutter, F. (2001). Diagnosing schizophrenia in the initial prodromal phase. *Arch Gen Psychiatry,* **58**, 158–164.

Kluver, H. (1966). *Mescal and the Mechanisms of Hallucination.* Chicago: University of Chicago Press.

Koo, J., & Lee, C.S. (2001). Delusions of parasitosis: A dermatologists guide to diagnosis and treatment. *Am J Clin Dermatol,* **2**, 285–290.

Kot, T., & Serper, M. (2002). Increased susceptibility to auditory conditioning in hallucinating schizophrenic patients. *J Nerv Ment Dis,* **190**, 282–288.

Larkin, A.R. (1979). The form and content of schizophrenic hallucinations. *Am J Psychiatry,* **136**, 940–943.

Larøi, F., Marczewski, P., & Van der Linden, M. (2004). The multi-dimensionality of hallucinatory predisposition: Factor structure of a modified version of the Launay-Slade hallucinations scale in a normal sample. *Eur Psychiatry,* **19**, 15–20.

Larøi, F., & Van der Linden, M. (2005). Normal subjects' reports of hallucinatory experiences. *Can J Behav Sci*, **37**, 33–43.

Larøi, F. (2006). The phenomenological diversity of hallucinations: Some theoretical and clinical implications. *Psychol Belg*, **46**, 163–183.

Launay, G., & Slade, P. (1981). The measurement of hallucinatory predisposition in male and female prisoners. *Personality and Individual Differences*, **2**, 221–234.

Levitan, C., Ward, P.B., Catts, S.V., & Hemsley, D.R. (1996). Predisposition toward auditory hallucinations: the utility of the Launay-Slade hallucination scale in psychiatric patients. *Personality and Individual Differences*, **21**, 287–289.

Lewandowski, K.E., DePaola, J., Camsari, G.B., Cohen, B.M., & Ongür, D. (2009). Tactile, olfactory, and gustatory hallucinations in psychotic disorders: a descriptive study. *Annals Academy of Medicine Singapore*, **38**, 383–385.

Miller, L.J. (1996). Qualitative changes in hallucinations. *Am J Psychiatry*, **153**, 265–267.

Mocellin, R., Walterfang, M., & Velakoulis, D. (2006). Neuropsychiatry of complex visual hallucinations. *Aust N Z J Psychiatry*, **40**, 742–751.

Moreau de Tours, J.J. (1845). *Du hachisch et de l'aliénation mentale: Études psychologiques*. Paris: Masson et Cie.

Morrison, A.P., Wells, A., & Nothard, S. (2000). Cognitive factors in predisposition to auditory and visual hallucinations. *Br J Clin Psychol*, **39**, 67–78.

Morrison, A.P., Wells, A., & Nothard, S. (2002). Cognitive and emotional predictors of predisposition to hallucinations in non-patients. *Br J Clin Psychol*, **41**, 259–270.

Mosimann, U.P., Rowan, E.N., Partington, C.E., *et al.* (2006). Characteristics of visual hallucinations in Parkinson disease dementia and dementia with Lewy Bodies. *Am J Geriatr Psychiatry*, **14**, 153–160.

Mosimann, U.P., Collerton, D., Dudley, R., *et al.* (2008). A semi-structured interview to assess visual hallucinations in older people. *Int J Geriatr Psychiatry*, **23**, 712–718.

Møller, P., & Husby, R. (2000). The initial prodrome in schizophrenia: searching for naturalistic core dimensions of experience and behaviour. *Schizophr Bull*, **26**, 217–232.

Ohayon, M.M. (2000). Prevalence of hallucinations and their pathological associations in the general population. *Psychiatry Res*, **97**, 153–164.

Panayiotopoulos, C.P. (1999). Elementary visual hallucinations, blindness, and headache in idiopathic occipital epilepsy: differentiation from migraine. *Journal of Neurology, Neurosurgery and Psychiatry*, **66**, 536–540.

Parnas, J. (1999). From predisposition to psychosis: progression of symptoms in schizophrenia. *Acta Psychiatr Scand*, s**395**, 20–29.

Parnas, J., & Handest, P. (2003). Phenomenology of anomalous self-experience in early schizophrenia. *Compr Psychiatry*, **44**, 121–134.

Parnas, J., Handest, P., Jansson, L., & Sæbye, D. (2005). Anomalies of subjective experience in first-admitted schizophrenia spectrum patients: empirical investigation. *Psychopathology*, **38**, 259–267.

Parnas, J., Møller, P., Kircher, T., *et al.* (2005). EASE: Examination of anomalous self-experience. *Psychopathology*, **38**, 236–258.

Paulik, G., Badcock, J.C., & Maybery, M.T. (2006). The multifactorial structure of the predisposition to hallucinate and associations with anxiety, depression and stress. *Personality and Individual Differences*, **41**, 1067–1076.

Persons, J.B. (1986). The advantages of studying psychological phenomena rather than psychiatric diagnoses. *Am Psychol*, **41**, 1252–1260.

Plummer, C., Kleinitz, A., Vroomen, P., & Watts, R. (2006). Of Roman chariots and goats in overcoats: the syndrome of Charles Bonnet. *J Clin Neurosci*, **14**, 709–714.

Read, J., van Os, J., Morrison, A. P., & Ross, C. A. (2005). Childhood trauma, psychosis and schizophrenia: a literature review with theoretical and clinical implications. *Acta Psychiatr Scand,* **112**, 330–350.

Read, J., McGregor, K., Coggan, C., & Thomas, D.R. (2006). Mental health services and sexual abuse: the need for staff training. *Journal of Trauma and Dissociation,* **7**, 33–50.

Romme, M.A., Honig, A., Noorthoorn, E., & Escher, A. (1992). Coping with hearing voices: An emancipatory approach. *Br J Psychiatry,* **161**, 99–103.

Sackheim, H.A. (1998). The meaning of insight. In: Amador, X.F., & David, A.S. (eds.), *Insight and psychosis* (pp. 1–12). 1st ed. Oxford: Oxford University Press.

Santhouse, A.M., Howard, R.J., & Fytche, D.H. (2000). Visual hallucinatory syndromes and the anatomy of the brain. *Brain,* **123**, 2055–2064.

Sass, L.A., & Parnas, J. (2003). Schizophrenia, consciousness and the self. *Schizophr Bull,* **29**, 427–444.

Schley, M.T., Wilms, P., Toepfner, S., *et al.* (2008). Painful and nonpainful phantom and stump sensations in acute traumatic amputees. *Journal of Trauma,* **65**, 858–864.

Schneider, K. (1959). *Clinical psychopathology.* New York: Grune and Stratton.

Schultze-Lutter, F., Addington, J., Ruhrmann, S., & Klosterkötter, J. (2007). *The schizophrenia proneness instrument (SPI–A).* Rome: Giovanni Fioriti.

Schultze-Lutter, F., Ruhrmann, S., Berning, J., Maier, W., & Klosterkötter, J. (2010). Basic symptoms and ultrahigh risk criteria: symptom development in the initial prodromal state. *Schizophr Bull,* **36**, 182–191.

Sechehaye, M. (1951). *Autobiography of a schizophrenic girl.* New York: Grune & Stratton.

Serper, M., Dill, C.A., Chang, N., Kot, T., & Elliot, J. (2005). Factorial structure of the hallucinatory experience: continuity of experience in psychotic and normal individuals. *J Nerv Ment Dis,* **193**, 265–272.

Sims, A. (2002). *Symptoms in the mind: an introduction to descriptive psychopathology.* Philadelphia: W. B. Saunders.

Stanghellini, G. (2004). *Disembodied spirits and deanimated bodies. The psychopathology of common sense.* Oxford: Oxford University Press.

Straus, E. W. (1966). *Phenomenology of hallucinations.* In: E.W. Straus (ed.), *Phenomenological psychology* (pp. 277–287). New York: Basic Books.

Ter Meulen, B.C., Tavy, D., & Jacobs, B.C. (2009). From stroboscope to dream machine: a history of flicker-induced hallucinations. *Eur Neurol,* **62**, 316–320.

Teunisse, R.J., Cruysberg, J.R.M., Verbeek, A., & Zitman, F.G. (1995). The Charles Bonnet syndrome: a large prospective study in The Netherlands. *Br J Psychiatry,* **166**, 254–257.

Thomas, P., Mathur, P., Gottesman, I.I., Nagpal, R., Nimgaonkar, V.L., & Deshpande, S.N. (2007). Correlates of hallucinations in schizophrenia: a cross-cultural evaluation. *Schizophr Res,* **92**, 41–49.

Tien, A.Y. (1991). Distributions of hallucinations in the population. *Soc Psychiatry Psychiatr Epidemiol,* **26**, 287–292.

Todd, J. (1955). The syndrome of Alice in Wonderland. *Can Med Assoc J,* **73**, 701–704.

Wahass, S., & Kent, G. (1997a). A comparison of public attitudes in Britain and Saudi Arabia towards auditory hallucinations. *Int J Soc Psychiatry,* **43**, 175–183.

Wahass, S., & Kent, G. (1997b). Coping with auditory hallucinations: a cross-cultural comparison between Western (British) and non-Western (Saudi Arabian) patients. *J Nerv Ment Dis,* **185**, 664–668.

Waters, F.A.V., Badcock, J.C., & Mayberry, M.T. (2003). Revision of the factor structure of the Launay-Slade hallucination scale (LSHS-R). *Personality and Individual Differences,* **35**, 1351–1357.

Wild-Wall, N., Willemssen, R., Falkenstein, M., & Beste, C. (2008). Time estimation in healthy ageing and neurodegenerative basal ganglia disorders. *Neurosci Lett*, **442**, 34–38.

Wykes, T. (2004). Psychological treatment for voices in psychosis. *Cog Neuropsychiatry*, **9**, 25–41.

Yamamoto, J., Okonogi, K., Iwasaki, T., & Yosimura, S. (1969). Mourning in Japan. *Am J Psychiatry*, **125**, 1660–1665.

Index